Psychoanalytic Perspectives on the Shadow of the Parent

Psychoanalytic Perspectives on the Shadow of the Parent explores the psychological challenges faced by the offspring of either famous or notorious parents.

Beginning with parental legacies found in mythology and the Bible, the book presents a series of case studies drawn from a range of narrative contexts, selecting personalities drawn from history, politics, psychoanalysis and literature, all viewed from an analytic perspective. The concluding section focuses on the manifestation of this parental shadow within the field of fine art, as written by artists themselves.

This is a lively and varied collection from a fascinating range of contributors. It provides readers with a new understanding of family history, trauma and reckoning screened through a psychoanalytic perspective, and will appeal to psychoanalysts, psychotherapists, counsellors and anyone interested in the dynamics of the family.

Jonathan Burke is a psychoanalytic psychotherapist working in private practice in the UK. He previously edited *The Topic of Cancer: New Perspectives on the Emotional Experience of Cancer* (Karnac, 2013).

Psychoanalytic Perspectives on the Shadow of the Parent

Mythology, History, Politics and Art

Edited by Jonathan Burke

Routledge
Taylor & Francis Group
LONDON AND NEW YORK

First published 2019
by Routledge
2 Park Square, Milton Park, Abingdon, Oxon OX14 4RN

and by Routledge
52 Vanderbilt Avenue, New York, NY 10017

Routledge is an imprint of the Taylor & Francis Group, an informa business

British Library Cataloguing-in-Publication Data
A catalogue record for this book is available from the British Library

Library of Congress Cataloging-in-Publication Data
A catalog record for this book has been requested

ISBN: 978-1-138-32295-0 (hbk)
ISBN: 978-1-78220-547-0 (pbk)
ISBN: 978-0-429-45170-6 (ebk)

Typeset in Times New Roman
by Apex CoVantage, LLC

To my parents, Jack and Marie Burke

Contents

About the editor and contributors x
Foreword xv
MARGOT WADDELL
Preface: a hard act to follow xviii
JONATHAN BURKE

Introduction 1
JONATHAN BURKE

PART I
Perspectives 5

In the Bible 7

1 **In the shadow of violence: Isaac and Abraham** 9
STEPHEN FROSH

In Greek mythology and opera 21

2 **Hard acts hard to follow: Sophocles, Hofmannsthal, Strauss and *Elektra*** 23
CHRISTOPHER WINTLE

In Shakespeare 41

3 **Under the shadow of silence: on speechless love in *King Lear*** 43
STEVEN GROARKE

4 **"Madness, yet there's method in it": the shadow of the doctor in Hamlet's mirror** 58
PAUL HERITAGE

PART II
'I'-witness accounts 71

In psychoanalysis 73

5 'Derealization': in the shadow of *the son* 75
FAYE CAREY

6 Her mother's footsteps 93
MARION BOWER

7 A tragic inheritance: the irresolvable conflict for children of perpetrators 105
COLINE COVINGTON

8 Making my way out of the shadow into the sun: a painful confrontation with my past 127
MARTIN MILLER

In socio-political life 143

9 Closed doors 145
SYLVIA PASKIN – WITH CODA BY SARA COLLINS

10 Kafka: 'parental superiority' as the act that feels hard to follow 161
STEVEN MENDOZA

In philosophy 177

11 Attachment and doubt in the work of Stanley Cavell 179
ROBBIE DUSCHINSKY AND SERENA MESSINA

In religion and family life 193

12 The eye begins to see: personal reflections on a fragmented father–son relationship, and other related matters 195
HOWARD COOPER

Reflections in fine art 209

13 Shadow, colour, glass: the family I knew and the family I never knew 211
ARDYN HALTER

14 Paddle your own canoe: negotiating the shadows **223**
JANE MCADAM FREUD

Index 243

About the editor and contributors

Jonathan Burke is an adult psychoanalytic psychotherapist who first trained in social work and health care and later became a health planning consultant to UK hospitals and ministries of health abroad. After managing the Cancer *LIFE* Project at Enfield Disability Action, he trained as a psychoanalytic psychotherapist. A member of the British Psychotherapy Foundation, he continues today to see a wide range of patients in his private psychotherapy practice. He has served as editor on *The Topic of Cancer: New Perspectives on the Emotional Experience of Cancer* and on *Psychoanalytic Perspectives on the Shadow of the Parent: Mythology, History, Politics and Art.*

Marion Bower is an adult psychotherapist. She was previously a consultant social worker at the Tavistock Clinic. The books she has edited or co-edited include *The Emotional Needs of Young Children and Their Families; Thinking under Fire; Addictive States of Mind*; and *What Social Workers Need to Know*. She is currently writing a biography of Joan Riviere and preparing an edited book on sexual exploitation.

Faye Carey is a psychoanalytic psychotherapist with a background in the visual arts. Her MA in Art Theory Goldsmiths ('Comic Relief') applies Freud's theories of jokes to the development of humour in sculpture, and her doctoral thesis in psychoanalytic studies at the University of Essex ('Seeing Hearing') concerns the clinical value of the therapist's capacity for visualisation (due to be published by Routledge in 2018). In 1994, Faye qualified as a psychoanalytic psychotherapist with the London Centre for Psychotherapy (LCP), today part of the British Psychotherapy Foundation (BPF). She remains Chair of Training for the LCP, and is Chair of Curriculum for the Psychoanalytic Psychotherapy Association (PPA) of the BPF. She was appointed a Fellow of the BPF in 2014, and teaches and writes on her chosen subjects.

Sara Collins is a training and supervising psychoanalyst with the British Psychoanalytic Association and the British Psychotherapy Foundation. She is the current Director of Training at the BPA, and a member of its Board. She has taught widely on psychoanalytic and psychotherapy courses. Her published papers, relating primarily to the analytic relationship, include 'The Voice behind the Couch: Whatever Happened to the Blank Screen?' in *Interpretive Voices – Responding to Patients* (Karnac, 2015) and 'Why Reconstruct? Perspectives on Reconstruction within the Transference' in *Transference and Countertransference: A Unifying Focus of Psychoanalysis* (Karnac 2011). Her paper 'On Authenticity: The Question of Truth in Construction and Autobiography' was published in the *International Journal of Psychoanalysis* (IJPA) in 2011. Sara was the keynote speaker at the first BPA international conference in 2017 on psychic change, on the topic 'Occasion for Change: Is There Such a Thing as a Mutative Enactment?' Her other interests include opera and psychoanalysis, on which she has published papers in *New Associations* and on the IPA World website. She works in private practice.

Howard Cooper is a rabbinic graduate of the Leo Baeck College and has a master's degree with distinction in creative writing and critical theory. He works as a psychoanalytic psychotherapist and supervisor in private practice and is the Director of Spiritual Development at Finchley Reform Synagogue, London. A workshop leader, lecturer and writer exploring religious, Judaic, spiritual and psychological themes, he is the editor of *Soul Searching: Essays in Judaism and Psychotherapy* (SCM Press, 1988) and author of, amongst other works, *The Alphabet of Paradise: An A–Z of Spirituality for Everyday Life* (Skylight Paths, 2002).

Coline Covington is a Jungian analyst with a background in political science and criminology. She is a Fellow of International Dialogue Initiative (IDI), a think tank formed by Prof. Vamik Volkan, Lord Alderdice, and Dr Robi Friedman to apply psychoanalytic concepts to understanding political conflict. Coline's publications include *Terrorism and War: Unconscious Dynamics of Political Violence* (Karnac, 2002), *Shrinking the News: Headline Stories on the Couch* (Karnac, 2014), *Sabina Spielrein: Forgotten Pioneer of Psychoanalysis*, 2nd ed. (Routledge, 2015), and *Everyday Evils: A Psychoanalytic View of Evil and Morality* (Routledge, 2016). Coline works in private practice in London.

Robbie Duschinsky is Head of the Applied Social Science Group in the Primary Care Unit, Cambridge University. He is also Director of Studies in Sociology at Sidney Sussex College. He is the co-author of *Sustaining Social Work: Between Power and Powerlessness,* and presently holds a New Investigator Award from the Wellcome Trust for a study of debates in attachment research.

Jane McAdam Freud was born in London and built her career as Jane McAdam without reference to her renowned portrait painter father, Lucian Freud, and her great-grandfather, the father of psychoanalysis, Sigmund Freud. Working in various mediums, McAdam Freud's main focus is sculpture and relief, which she has exhibited globally. Her work continues to be acquired by several major public collections including the Victoria and Albert Museum, the British Museum and Guildhall. Solo shows in the UK include the Ashmolean Museum in Oxford, Fitzwilliam Museum in Cambridge, Hunterian Museum in Glasgow and Freud Museum in London. International solo shows include the Contemporary Art Museum in Missouri, Museum Novojiínska in the Czech Republic and the Sundaram Tagore Gallery in Los Angeles.

Stephen Frosh is Professor in the Department of Psychosocial Studies at Birkbeck, University of London. He has a background in academic and clinical psychology and was Consultant Clinical Psychologist at the Tavistock Clinic, London, throughout the 1990s. He is the author of many books and papers on psychosocial studies and on psychoanalysis, most recently *Hauntings: Psychoanalysis and Ghostly Transmissions* (Palgrave Macmillan, 2013) and *Simply Freud* (New York: Simply Charly, 2017). He is a Fellow of the Academy of Social Sciences, an Academic Associate of the British Psychoanalytical Society, a Founding Member of the Association of Psychosocial Studies and an Honorary Member of the Institute of Group Analysis.

Steven Groarke is Professor of Social Thought at the University of Roehampton and a member of the British Psycho-analytical Society and the International Psychoanalytical Association. He teaches at the Institute of Psychoanalysis in London and is a member of the editorial board of the *International Journal of Psychoanalysis*. He is the author, most recently, of *Managed Lives: Psychoanalysis, Inner Security and the Social Order*. He currently works in private practice in London.

Ardyn Halter is an artist born in London and based in Israel. His oil paintings and his prints have been exhibited in museums in Europe and Israel and his work is in museum and national library collections in the United States, Europe and Israel, including the Victoria and Albert Museum; the British Library; the Open Museum, Israel; the New York Public Library; and the National Library of Ireland. His major stained glass projects include Yad LaYeled (with Roman Halter); the National Genocide Memorial, Rwanda; and numerous stained glass windows in London, one of which, *The Tree of Life* (St Johns Wood Synagogue), is celebrated in the book *The Hundred Best Stained Glass Sites of London*.

Paul Heritage is Professor of Drama and Performance and Director of People's Palace Projects, a School of English and Drama research centre. Since 1991, he has been creating arts and cultural projects between the UK and Brazil, including 15 years of performance-based human rights projects in the Brazilian prison system from São Paulo through to the Amazon region. As Associate Producer at the Barbican Centre for three years, he created a partnership with Grupo Cultural AfroReggae that included productions of *From the Favela to the World* and *Favelization* as well as community-based projects in the East End of London. His current research includes practice-based projects on cultural value, Shakespeare, Brazilian indigenous cultures, arts and homelessness. In 2004, he was made a Knight of the Order of the Rio Branco by the Brazilian government.

Steven Mendoza is a psychoanalytic psychotherapist, trainer, supervisor and teacher of psychoanalytic trainees. His secondary education was in the sciences and his professional experience in the film industry, social work and market research. Some of his writing can be read in the *British Journal of Psychotherapy*. He is a Buddhist and an amateur painter and photographer. He loves walking in Scotland and hates gardening and beach holidays.

Serena Messina is a Licensed Psychologist working at the Austin Child Guidance Center in Austin, Texas. She is also Visiting Scholar and Lecturer at the University of Texas at Austin, in the departments of Human Development and Family Science and Educational Psychology. Dr Messina's research interests focus on attachment and factors affecting children's emotional development.

Martin Miller is a member of the Swiss Federation of Psychologists, and graduate of the University in Zurich. He was also educated by Dr Jan Bastiaans in Holland and in Psychosomatics with Dr Christel Schöttler in Germany. He received further psychotherapeutic training in London along with training in organisational psychotherapy. He is author of *The True "Drama of the Gifted Child": The Tragedy of Alice Miller – How Repressed War Trauma Impact Families* (currently available only in German: *Das wahre Drama des begabten Kindes. Die Tragödie Alice Millers – wie verdrängte Kriegstraumata in der Familie wirken*, Kreuz, Verlag, 2013).

Sylvia Paskin has edited and co-edited various books of poetry, short fiction and Yiddish film. In addition she has written the scripts for two short films: *L'Esprit de L'Escalier* and *Dream Life of Debris*, both of which are set in and around Istanbul. Sylvia is a Tutor at JW3 (Jewish Community Centre, London) where she teaches creative writing. Currently she is compiling a collection of her poetry for publication and is working on a play titled *A True Friend of England*, set in Berlin and London and based on an intriguing aspect of her family history. When that is completed, then "the complex family drama of Trotsky and his household on Buyukada beckons".

Margot Waddell is a Fellow of the British Psychoanalytical Society and Visiting Lecturer at the Tavistock Clinic. She works in private clinical practice and previously worked for many years in the British National Health Service (NHS), as a Child and Adolescent Psychotherapist in the Tavistock Clinic's Adolescent Department. In addition to publishing many papers and books, she has taught extensively in the UK and around the world. For the last 20 years, she has also edited, and latterly co-edited, the Tavistock Clinic Series (recently acquired by Routledge). As Series Editor she has worked on all 50 Tavistock publications to date, a collection that represents a rich diversity of psychoanalytic and psychotherapeutic subjects springing from the Clinic's range of NHS practices.

Christopher Wintle has taught music in the University of London since 1979 and is the founding director of Plumbago Books and Arts (2000). He reviewed opera for the *Times Literary Supplement* for 20 years and has written extensively for leading opera houses in the UK. His interest in opera has been matched by an unaffiliated fascination with psychoanalysis – his monograph *What Opera Means* (2018) includes a section on psychology. He is also the literary executor of the music critic Hans Keller (1919–1985), in the 1940s a leading Freudian. His editions of Keller include *Music and Psychology* (2003) and *Britten* (2013).

Foreword

It is fitting that a book with so commanding and suggestive a title should turn out to have gathered such a fine collection of reflections, ones ranging from the intensely personal to the deeply erudite. The contributing authors offer varying interpretations of the subject, whether based in myth, in history, in literature, in biblical stories, on the stage or in intimate examinations of self and other within the family framework.

For the title draws in anyone, and everyone, who has an interest in the internal and external worlds and in the relationship between the two; between, at once, their own felt version of who their parent or parents are, or were, and also the seen version of how the world regarded them. Here, we find ourselves engrossed in chapters by the offspring of many historically significant families. Yet the pages also invite, even compel, a reader to engage with their own parent or parents' and families' legacies, of what they meant to others and to themselves. These meanings are irrespective of whether those lives were special in any external and recognised way, or how consciously they stayed part of the stories that a child carries within, as internal stories of those life experiences. Here the emphasis tends to be on the shadow cast, yet not entirely so, for in some chapters it is clear that having a parent who is felt to be 'a hard act to follow' is very much a function of a whole tangle of historical, transgenerational and personal factors that have to be taken into consideration.

In keeping with the character of the book, I shall try to draw these different registers together by recounting some of my own memories. I was first reading Jonathan Burke's fascinating collection as I travelled north to teach in Scotland. I was to give papers about 'the unhoused mind', issues of familial surrender and succession, in relation to King Lear in particular, and also about Melanie Klein and her theories of the impact on the personality of very early experiences, whether of nurture or neglect. My much-delayed Virgin train was likely to take six hours to reach Edinburgh. I found myself dwelling on the thrilling verbal accounts, from my childhood (possibly embellished) of my great-grandfather driving the *Flying Scotsman* steam train from London to Edinburgh non-stop in four hours. I had not thought about this remarkable feat for some years but, because of the book in my hands, my own story internally ran on. My great-grandfather's son, my beloved grandpa, fought in the trenches during the First World War. His son, James, my own father, was an impoverished Edinburgh scholarship boy. He earned his own way through higher education, came south, worked, enlisted and landed on D-Day on the Normandy beaches, an unsung hero, as he was to be in his subsequent life in government service. Here, too, but for the obituaries, he remained largely unknown.

I would probably not have reflected in any such terms but for the invitation to contribute to this compelling book, one that is sometimes disturbing and, at once, deeply thoughtful and moving. Here there is some joy but also much sorrow; both celebration and gratitude and also loss, misunderstanding, bitterness, pain and regret.

The title draws any reader in to some kind of reverie about what has contributed to, and what has impeded, their own growth as human beings, and with what may have enabled them to develop and to nurture something of worth in others.

For me, such reflections contributed nothing of the legacy of some of the well-known families featured in this book, but something much more modest, though certainly no less important. These pages, in inviting, as they do, personal reflection on one's forebears, can have a bearing on a possible reframing of the picture, true for me as, surely, for many readers.

That my great-grandfather drove that famous steam train; that his son fought in the trenches; that *his* son landed on D-Day did not command any place in the history books. But internally, to me, these experiences and the whole culture and politics of two world wars proffered the basis for everything that I have ever found important in life: to unsung work; the individual unnamed commitment to doing one's very best for the family, for the community, for the country and for those who were dedicated to serving it in so many ways: unknown ways – and much else – unnamed, unsung.

These qualities certainly constitute hard acts to follow, and this impressive collection of papers will surely inspire the reader not only to reflect on those who feel that their forebears cast a shadow of sorts, but also that they cast a light – perhaps one that cannot immediately be seen; perhaps one that we are too blind to see. Some may feel diminished by their inherited family legacy; others may be encouraged to re-think the legacy of their own unique make-up and experience.

Travelling to Scotland always stirs in me a powerful identification with the Waddell family history, the name stemming (as 'history' has it) from the west coast wreck of part of the Spanish Armada, the remnants of which fetched up, as I learnt from my 'Gran', and was confirmed many years later in London, by my Holloway Road electrician, in the Woedell – the place of woe.

The other half of the family story, my mother's, is totally different: ruled by my sadistic, mad and terrifying grandmother, not infrequently sectioned in the then notorious 'snake pit' mental hospital, St Bernard's, Grandma had married into the British Officer Class during the Raj. My mother's life was shadowed, from the first, by parental mental illness and bereavement, yet it led to her passionate commitment not to re-visit the horrors of her childhood and her depressed self on her own children. Isolated and largely uneducated, she did her very best. She devoured the great poets, playwrights and novelists; she danced, sang and played the piano beautifully, but suffered the well-known deprivations of a middle-class housewife in the post-war years.

These two utterly different people married during the Battle of Britain. Their two children were also utterly different, in every way. As my tutor at the Tavistock Clinic, Martha Harris, rightly put it: "No two siblings have the same parents". This simple statement, so obviously true, is, in the context of this book, also deeply important. For some, a parent's fame, status, genius even, is felt to be excluding, neglectful, crushing. For others, it carries the seeds of a different kind of self-hood – not so diminished by parental eminence, as simply part of the extraordinarily complex picture of how the human personality is formed and inwardly survives, and how it is, over time, that it develops in whatever way that it does.

This is a matter that psychoanalysis has always sought to explain and Freud's comment, well over a century ago, that we are still only in the foothills when it comes to the question of understanding human nature, is as true now as it ever was. This book casts much light on the often surprising inside stories and outcomes stirred by that question, and, most importantly, requires the reader to think anew about the manifold factors that contribute to the various disguises that others believe to be 'you'.

Margot Waddell
Child and Adult Psychoanalyst

Preface

A hard act to follow

What do we mean when we say of others, of family members and particularly of our elders that they are 'a hard act to follow'? Are we speaking of their achievements, their personalities, their talents or perhaps their overall bearing? In other words, what are these 'acts' that are so powerfully experienced by us as being hard to follow? What or who has made them appear so difficult to emulate?

In the chapters that follow we focus on personalities in the field of psychoanalysis including Freud, Melanie Klein and her daughter, Melitta Schmideberg; Alice Miller and her son, Martin. Other chapters centre on selected personalities in the Bible, Shakespeare, opera, politics and literature, religion and family life, philosophy and art, all viewed primarily, albeit not exclusively, from an analytic perspective.

As psychoanalytic enquiries traditionally begin with Freud, our preface will follow suit by referring to Freud, not Sigmund Freud this time, but for our purposes rather, his eldest son, Martin. Reporting on a long-term study of children of famous and infamous parents,[1] Dr Danielle Knafo, begins with the following statement by Martin Freud:

> The son of a genius remains the son of a genius, and his chances of winning human approval of anything he may do hardly exist if he attempts to make any claim to fame detached from that of his father.[2]

Yet the work and reputation of Anna Freud, Martin's younger sister, may already call this assertion into question. Guardian and exponent of her father's science and his legacy, at 41 she authored *The Ego and the Mechanisms of Defence*, first published in 1936 – an 80th birthday gift to her father who, on reading it, wrote:

> She has become an independent person who has been granted the gift of recognising that which only confuses others.[3]

Were these simply the words of a proud father, a man able to recognise genius in another, or shall we see them as an expression of something more aspirational, even urgent – perhaps an unconscious desire in Freud whose upper jaw and palate were by then ravaged by cancer, to see his pioneering work live on in his offspring?

In some cases the working demands of the 'genius' may be so all-consuming, or at least be experienced as such, Knafo reflects, that often little time whatsoever is left for their children and their emotional growth, thus leaving the offspring of some with feelings of neglect and abandonment – a palpable sense of not being loved.

Drafting the outlines of this book, with music in the background, my mind drifts to figures in the world of music and the accolades they are accorded. I hear the playing of the enigmatic Glenn Gould – "one of the best-known and most celebrated classical pianists of the 20th century" – reclusive and eccentric (infamous for cancelling performances!), playful and mesmerising in equal measure. Though never having fathered children of his own, he was felt to be kind, avuncular and undoubtedly playful with the children of the woman with whom he had had a love affair and planned to marry. Yet it seems the children, whose loyalties were divided between their father and their mother's lover, "bore the brunt of the emotional hit and were left with unresolved feelings after Mr Gould's untimely death at the age of 50".[4]

As I keep writing, the strings of the violinist Yehudi Menuhin are now beginning to play in the background. By this point, however, as beautiful as the music sounds, I cannot help but stop and wonder about the man himself: a hard act to follow? A day in the life of Menuhin's son, the pianist Jeremy Menuhin, as told to the journalist Judith Woods, provides us with the following snapshot of life in the Menuhin household:

> To the outside world, he [Jeremy] and his three elder siblings, including two from Yehudi's first marriage, wanted for nothing. They would be photographed for newspapers and magazines, relaxing together with their parents in the Alps, like a latter-day von Trapp family. The reality was very different.
>
> The emotional life of our family was grotesque. We barely saw our parents, and when we did, the atmosphere was dour and artificial.

Of growing up in the shadow of his father, Jeremy Menuhin put it simply:

> My father regarded me as an adjunct to his career, like some empty vessel, to be filled by him.[5]

I have thus far remarked briefly on Sigmund Freud and two of his offspring, then speculated about personalities in music – classical music in the Western world and, at that, of only two famous figures. But could a 'hard act to follow' be a theme more common than we might first imagine?

I would argue that the issues presented here are in some ways familiar to us all. We might well look up to our immediate forebears as great sources of pride – we shine in their light. Or we may experience ourselves as overshadowed by them, as if in a daily struggle to match, outdo or perhaps escape the overpowering spectre their light projects.

And so, on a more personal note, the following vignette is cautiously offered:

> "Justin Trudeau – a real Liberal!", declares my son with innocent admiration of Canada's new Prime Minister. Instinctively I respond, *"Justin Trudeau? You should have seen his father, Pierre Elliot Trudeau!"; and* in that impulsive retort I hear with startling clarity my own father's voice – joining me, teaching me but, I fear, somewhere one-upping me, as if to say, 'Yes, but I've seen better.' In bringing my father back, I know immediately why I've *subtitled* this preface "A Hard Act to Follow" – abbreviated in early communications with our authors as simply 'HAF'.

On the surface, of course, my response to my son addressed a simple desire to acquaint him with something of myself and my past. Painfully close to the surface, however, the very manner of my reply betrayed perhaps something more sinister – a proud identification with a loved and loving father and esteemed teacher, yet at the same time a desire to liberate myself from the mantle of being the son of a charming scholar too often referred to, I feared, *ad lauditum*. Without further personal analysis, how long would I assume the role of 'half' – the diffident beneficiary of the 'HAF-Master'?

I am not alone, of course. The league that I have joined, consciously or not, of proud and exasperated offspring, is in fact quite common. *'Aren't you the son of . . . ?'* What a proud legacy I was given, you might say, and what could possibly be wrong with legacy? Nothing or perhaps everything – depending on what kind of legacy we're dealing with, who the donor is and who the heir – or could it be perhaps the manner in which the transmission itself is experienced? In our book we will examine the nature of legacy and attempt to grapple with the challenges that different legacies can present.

Jonathan Burke

Notes

1 Knafo, D. (1991). What's in a Name? Psychoanalytic Considerations on Children of Famous Parents. *Psychoanalytic Psychology* 8:263–281.
2 Freud, M. (1983). *Sigmund Freud: Man and Father*. New York: Aronson.
3 Freud, E. L., ed. (1987). *The Letters of Sigmund Freud and Arnold Zweig*. New York: New York University Press.
4 Hampson, S. (2009). Christopher Foss Grew Up with Glenn Gould, but Never Got to Say Goodbye. *Globe and Mail*, 29 November and last updated 23 August 2012. See also "Genius Within: The Inner Life of Glenn Gould", 2009 film directed by Michele Hozer and Peter Raymont.
5 Woods, J. (2005). I Only Felt Loved When I Played Well. *The Telegraph* 21 February.

Introduction

Jonathan Burke

I must admit, and those closest to me would readily attest, *A Hard Act to Follow: The Shadow of the Parent* – the title with which our book was originally framed – is a theme close to my heart. The issue – at times the dilemma – inherent in the 'act' that is hard to follow is, I would suggest, familiar to us all. We may be conscious of it in our everyday lives. We might indeed have gained an appreciation of the role it has played in our development over the years. For some it may even dictate their thoughts about their past and their visions or beliefs as to what the future has in store for them.

As discussed in Part I of our book, living in the shadow of the parent is an experience tackled in biblical narrative (Chapter 1), explored in Greek mythology and dramatised with psychological intensity in opera (Chapter 2). We know it as a theme played out in myriad ways on the Shakespearean stage (Chapters 3 and 4). Indeed whilst recently watching the British actor and author Oliver Ford Davies on the stage, I was immediately transported to the theme of our book today. When later I wrote to him about *A Hard Act to Follow . . .*, he immediately cited Hamlet, who after all

> finds himself dominated by a perhaps inflated veneration of his recently dead father, "where every god did seem to set his seal to give the world assurance of a man", while his imagined revulsion at his mother's sex-life with his uncle leads him to denounce women as "breeders of sinners".

It is, of course, not only Shakespearean figures who invoke ancestral shadows, but actors themselves who may well experience themselves in the same position. Oliver Ford Davies recalls that in 1989 at the National Theatre,

> Daniel Day-Lewis was said to have felt so in thrall to his famous poet father who had died when he was fifteen, that he had visions of him on the battlements, and that this finally drove him from the stage in mid-performance.[1]

A hard act to follow so deeply experienced?

Part II, titled "'I'-Witness Accounts", begins with a range of analytic perspectives on our theme both past and present (Chapters 5–8). In Chapter 5 we examine how the theme relates to the life of Sigmund Freud and his experience of his own parents – a sensual connection to his mother and the boundary that his father signified for him. Thinking about Freud in the context of this chapter, I wondered about the extent to which he could allow himself to grapple with the parthenogenic *phallacy* of the so-called self-made man, and might even have wished, consciously or not, to defend himself against such notions.

In Chapter 6 we follow events in the lives of Melanie Klein and her daughter Melitta Schmideberg under the curious chapter title "Her Mother's Footsteps" – 'curious', as on reading the chapter the central question *What went wrong?* beckons us; moreover, *why?*

The two chapters that follow are, in a sense, two sides of the same coin as we examine the darkness of the shadow cast on offspring by parents involved in past atrocities: "the irresolvable conflict for children of perpetrators", as Jungian analyst Coline Covington, author of Chapter 7, puts it. How apt that she should begin her chapter by citing the Book of Deuteronomy (5:9) on visiting the iniquity of the fathers onto the children for generations to come. Whilst pondering the psychological conflicts posed by this 'tragic inheritance', it is hard to imagine this quote ever possessing greater meaning and power.

The next chapter continues with the 'other side of the coin' – the complex and deeply troubling account of the son of a Nazi and a well-known Jewish psychologist and psychoanalyst, and the trauma of war coupled with his parents' marriage that had beset him. Indeed in Chapter 8 the son in question, the Swiss psychologist Martin Miller, relates his own personal struggle "to make his way out of the shadow and into the sun".

In Chapters 9–12 reflections on our theme are offered from a variety of additional perspectives including, broadly speaking, socio-political and philosophical. In Chapter 9 the writer and poet Sylvia Paskin ponders the father and daughter dyad of Lev Davidovich Bronstein – the political revolutionary best known to us as Leon Trotsky, and the daughter who worshipped him yet barely got to know him. Sylvia's enquiry into this unusual relationship, if that is indeed what it can be called, is followed by an appraisal, admittedly speculative, in the form of a coda by the psychoanalyst Sara Collins.

Chapter 10 continues our theme with the story of a father who appeared unable to recognise and appreciate his son's remarkable development, his overall interests, not to mention his prodigious literary achievements – in this case, the son being the social, political and satirical author, Franz Kafka.

Might we not find ourselves on similar, albeit hardly identical grounds today? In Chapter 11 we take account of the life of the emeritus Harvard philosopher, Stanley Cavell, and the shadow curiously cast over his work by his father.

Similarly Chapter 12 offers us personal reflections on a father–son relationship: loving yet fragmented with, above all, an abiding sense of *absence* – there never having been enough time 'to mend'. The author – both psychotherapist and rabbi – also takes the wider view as he examines *life in the shadow* as experienced by the son of a Church of England minister.

Reflections in fine art

In the concluding Chapters 13 and 14, two artists offer us their unique experiences of life as the offspring of figures in creative art and expression well-known by their names, by their life stories or both.

There is much to cover in the chapters ahead, and whilst reference is made to some of the more salient points before each chapter begins, I offer these with a degree of trepidation as each of our authors are, in their own rights, for one reason or another, 'hard acts to follow'. Still, with this consideration in mind, I invite you to join me in following our authors on their own unique explorations in *the shadow of the parent.*

Note

1 In an interview with *Time* magazine Day-Lewis indicated that he had been speaking of this experience in a metaphorical rather than literal sense, adding "to some extent I probably saw my father's ghost every night, because of course if you're working in a play like Hamlet, you explore everything through your own experience".

Reflecting further on performing Shakespeare, Oliver Ford Davies writes: "*Laurence Olivier's 1944 Richard III set such a benchmark that actors felt daunted for the next forty years, perhaps until Anthony Sher created something startlingly different in 1984. Hard acts can be supplanted*".

As for his own experience, Ford Davies writes: "*When I myself played King Lear at the Almeida in 2002 I based my performance partly on my great-uncle, who in his last years suffered from ungovernable (and unwarranted) anger towards his family*".

Part I

Perspectives

In the Bible

Chapter 1

In the shadow of violence

Isaac and Abraham

Stephen Frosh

Where to start if not the beginning – with Genesis, but for our purposes with an early and certainly disturbing story which confronts us in the Bible. How are we to make sense of Abraham and Isaac – a story of a father–son relationship that could hardly possess more traumatic features? In the pivotal story of their relationship, whose 'act' could we possibly follow? Stephen Frosh reflects on the identifications made with a story that so powerfully challenges, yet whose meaning, by tradition, has also been used to inspire.

"In this chapter", he writes, "I explore the legacy of the Akedah or Binding of Isaac, a story in which Isaac is nearly killed by his father, and address the issue of recovery from paternal violence. Isaac's later blindness and his general passivity is analysed as a way of 'doing masculinity' that has been an important model for Jews. Indeed the theme of love and loss is central to Isaac's story, just as it is central to Jewish history".

Identifying with the past

There are communities that live in the shadow of their ancestors, whether or not these ancestors actually existed. The traces of these ancestral myths, if we can call them that, can be found in the lived experiences of all the later generations that are also struggling with the usual mix of ambivalence, distance and intimacy that is implicated in any 'real' relationship between a child and her or his parents. The ancestral myths, perhaps better understood as *prototypes*, feed into the ways in which identities are formed in the here-and-now. This might always be the case, but it is particularly true of communities that refer back to the prototypes constantly, as part of their heritage, in order to make conscious as well as unconscious sense of themselves. Perhaps this is a routine element in 'diasporic' identities, or perhaps it is specific to people who use traditional, reiterated texts to understand their lives. In either case, as Stuart Hall (1990) points out, the process of identity formation is a dynamic one, constantly reproducing itself differently; and to the degree that these past ancestral traces contribute to this, they remain alive.

> Cultural identities come from somewhere, have histories. But, like everything which is historical, they undergo constant transformation. Far from being eternally fixed in some essentialised past, they are subject to the continuous "play" of history, culture and power. Far from being grounded in a mere "recovery" of the past, which is waiting to be found, and which, when found, will secure our sense of ourselves into eternity, identities are the names we give to the different ways we are positioned by, and position ourselves within, the narratives of the past.
>
> (Hall, 1990, p. 225)

We keep on telling stories about our ancestors – where we came from, what we had, what was stolen from us and what passed on, what *defines* us as living in a certain cultural identity. This is an active process and it often has very powerful effects, as evidenced by the reproduction of past hurts in contemporary conflicts as well as by the gentler modes of belonging that come from nostalgia or celebration of what might in many instances be a mythologised history (Anderson, 2006). We look at the prototypical lives of these ancestors, and measure ourselves against them, using them as a way of making sense of our current situation. This mechanism of identification is perhaps especially strongly applied when the culture is genuinely diasporic; that is, when it has a history (and present/future) of needing to sustain itself through recovery and reinvention of its 'ancestors' in order to ensure its continuing vibrancy in the face of geographical and cultural challenges. Under those circumstances, the 'characters' of these past figures, as represented in the stories about them, can become ways of bonding a people together, a shared past story which also conveys strong messages about how one's life might be lived. In this way, these mythological figures also have an *ethical* role: they inhabit the imagination of a people and influence their notions of proper and improper behaviour, and of right and wrong ways of belonging.

I have described elsewhere (Frosh, 2005, 2010) how the argument for the power of religious and cultural texts in diasporic communities applies particularly strongly to classical (biblical and Talmudic) Jewish texts, which are constantly recycled through weekly synagogue readings and teaching in day schools and in religious schools. This seems even to be the case for many secular Jews, including of course Sigmund Freud, whose fascination with the Bible and avowed identification with one of its figures (Joseph) and less avowed with another (Moses) was very prominent in his writing (Freud, 1900, 1939). Showing awareness of how these stories could impact upon the mind in ways that might have powerfully material effects, Freud notes that his interest in dreams produces – and perhaps, it might be speculated, derives in part from – his identifications. "It will be noted", he writes (1900, p. 484),

> that the name Josef plays a great part in my dreams. . . . My own ego finds it very easy to hide itself behind people of that name, since Joseph was the name of a man famous in the Bible as an interpreter of dreams.

The larger point is that these texts, and particularly the figures whose stories they tell, act as a resource for collective and personal identity formation. Both deliberately and as a matter of unconscious 'transmission', 'identifying' Jews at least are affected by the material that comes at them from afar, mediated by their teachers and daily practices. Those biblical figures whose features are reasonably finely drawn – Abraham, Joseph, Moses; David, Solomon, Samson; Esther and Ruth – are material beings out of which models of cultural and ethical belonging are forged.

It is probably the figures that appear in the book of Genesis that have the most prominence and lasting impact in the pantheon of biblical identificatory models. Genesis begins cataclysmically, with the creation of the world, but rapidly focuses down on a few individuals who are all dispensed with quickly (Adam, Eve, Cain, Abel, Noah) before settling for the rest of its duration on one single family, traced over four generations – Abraham and Sarah, Isaac and Rebecca, Jacob and his wives Leah and Rachel, and Rachel's son Joseph, who becomes the leading political figure in Egypt. Each of these figures leads a life of considerable drama, but the high point – at least as measured by the subsequent literature and the hold it has had over later generations of Jews and others – comes early on, in the story of Abraham and his son Isaac. This is the moment of the 'Akedah', the binding of Isaac (Genesis 22), in which Abraham is told by God to sacrifice his son, only to have the command rescinded at the very last moment. I have written extensively about this elsewhere (Frosh, 2013), concentrating on the issue of paternal violence and also on how the Akedah becomes a template for understanding and lamenting later Jewish suffering, as if every moment of violence and loss is a reiteration of God's 'testing' of the forefathers. The consequence of this is that there is a living cultural memory of the Akedah, which has functioned as a framework for comprehending the otherwise inconceivable experiences of displacement and loss that have dogged Jewish life over the centuries, at times resulting in the actual slaying of children by their fathers to prevent them becoming victims of murderous mobs (Spiegel, 1967).

Isaac's blindness

In this brief chapter, I want to take up a different element of the Abraham–Isaac story, which I referenced but did not develop in the previous account. This concerns the question of what the figure of Isaac might be modelling in relation to feelings towards a father who is, to say the least, ambivalent in his behaviour towards him. We need to trace briefly what we 'know' about this relationship. Abraham has lived to be 100 and his only son, Ishmael, has been born from his wife's maid, Hagar; he and Sarah have long given up the idea of having a child of their own. But following a visit from three angels (Genesis 18), who amongst other things warn him of the coming destruction of Sodom (so Isaac and violence are linked from the start), a child is promised to Sarah and is duly born a year later to this 90-year-old postmenopausal woman. It hardly needs to be said that the child provokes laughter (the name Isaac is derived from the Hebrew for this) or that he is much wanted and loved, especially by his mother. But this also leads to an envious attack by Sarah on Hagar and Ishmael, who are eventually expelled from the camp – much against Abraham's wishes, it seems, perhaps on ethical grounds, perhaps out of love ("And the thing was very grievous in Abraham's sight on account of his son" – Genesis 21:11). Shortly after this – "after these things", a phrase that suggests a link between the expulsion of Ishmael and the test in relation to Isaac – Abraham receives a call from God to take Isaac on a three-day journey and sacrifice him. He gets up early in the morning to fulfil God's demand. Why early? Some say, in his eagerness to do God's will, but others think it is so that he can still the voice of objection and regret in himself; still others suggest that it is in order to take Isaac away before Sarah realises something is happening and intervenes to protect him. This later explanation is particularly relevant to my argument here: the Akedah is played out purely in the father–son domain, excluding Sarah, who is left at home and who then dies before her husband and son can return, or so it seems. Indeed, the standard explanation of why the Akedah is followed immediately by the announcement of the death of Sarah (Genesis 23:2) is that she died as a *consequence* of it. She heard what had happened, and realised that her husband had in him the capability to kill their much-loved son. The key classical commentator Rashi[1] writes in this respect: "Sarah's death is related closely after the incident of Isaac's sacrifice because it was caused by it. The shock of learning that he had nearly been sacrificed killed her". Such a discovery would be enough, one would think, to lay any mother low.

In any event, there is plenty of evidence that the story, which is told mainly with Abraham as its subject, suffers from a lack of kindness. Even the resolution of the sacrifice scene, in which Abraham holds back his knife from killing his son, is bloody. First, according to the Rabbinic story ('Midrash'[2]) drawn on by Rashi, explaining why his name has to be called twice by the angel telling him to desist ('Abraham, Abraham!' – Genesis 22: 11), Abraham asks if, having come all this way, he can at least draw some blood from his son; and second, a ram is slaughtered in Isaac's place. Although this is presented in Judaism as a radical move forward out of the mire of child sacrifice that was prevalent at the time, one has to wonder if the ram would have agreed. After this, God promises Abraham that he will keep His covenant with him and that his children will multiply and possess the land that has been promised them – another hostage to fortune, as it turns out thousands of years later. This seems like approval of Abraham's devotion to God, which clearly it is; but it should also be noted that not only does Sarah then die, but God is not recorded as having spoken to Abraham again, and nor is Isaac. Silence creeps between them; violence has put paid to intimate connection.

Isaac is a very different figure from his father. Abraham is the one who sets out on a journey ("Get away from your country, and from your kindred, and from your father's house", says God to him earlier in the story [Genesis 12:1]); dialogues with God, challenging Him; and demonstrates both generous hospitality to others, a key issue in establishing the moral standing of a figure in this kind of literature, and a capacity for ruthlessness and violence shown not only by the Akedah but also by the description of Abraham's battles with the 'kings' who abduct his nephew Lot (Genesis 14). Isaac has no such attributes. He does not seek a wife for himself, unlike his own son Jacob; instead, Abraham sends his servant to fetch one. Coming back successfully from this mission, the servant and Rebecca encounter Isaac, who has been "meditating in the field" (Genesis 24:63), suggesting a quality of otherworldliness that comes through as his strongest characteristic. Indeed, the most memorable passage in the story of Isaac, save the Akedah itself, is the record of his drastic mistake when blessing his twin sons, Esau and Jacob (Genesis 27). Isaac has gone blind; he believes it is time to bless his sons in a kind of deathbed way, though why he should do this is not clear, as he lives on for a considerable time afterwards (Genesis 35:29 records that Jacob and Esau bury him together after Jacob has returned from Aran, decades later). The main blessing is meant to go to Esau, as the firstborn of the twins, but before giving it to him, Isaac asks for some venison. At this point Rebecca takes a hand in things, dressing Jacob up in his brother's clothes and inciting him to mislead his blind father so that the blessing is given to him instead. Everything that then happens does so as a consequence of this mistake or trick. We should note that the befuddled Isaac is deeply distressed and that he shows his love and preference for Esau over Jacob; indeed, we are told expressly (Genesis 25:28), "Now Isaac loved Esau, because he did eat of his venison; and Rebecca loved Jacob". Isaac does not seem very bright here, and he certainly does not manage to pick a winner. Rebecca is too smart for him, and so is Jacob, but Isaac loves his food, and that seems to be enough.

What are we to make of this theme of blindness and stupidity – are we perhaps in the realm of the original sense of 'stupid' as 'amazed' or 'confounded', or maybe 'blinded by grief'? Isaac is regarded in Jewish literature as exceptionally pure, but also as passive and lifeless, one who spends his time meditating. His experience at the Akedah has scarred him forever; some Midrashim[3] suggest that he may even have died (Spiegel, 1967). Certainly, something died in him, at least registering the loss of his mother, but maybe something more too, some energy for life. What is most striking about Isaac is his blindness towards the things that are going on around him: the trick that is played on him; the actual nature of Esau, his impulsive, violent son; and Jacob, his wily yet deeper one. This otherworldliness, this blindness, is radically different from Abraham's impassioned connection with God. Indeed, immediately after the Akedah and then Sarah's death, Abraham is shown skilfully negotiating the business of buying her a burial place. Isaac, however, is nowhere to be found and is not mentioned in relation to the funeral; the Midrashic take on this is that he was in paradise, recovering from his wounds. Spiegel (1967, pp. 6–7) quotes the following Midrash to explain what happened: "And the angels bore him to Paradise, where he tarried three years, to be healed from the wound inflicted upon him by Abraham on the occasion of the Akedah". "Support for this legend", continues Spiegel, "was found in the Song of Songs, as Joshua ibn Shuaib, a Spanish rabbi of that generation" (ca. 1280–ca. 1340), testifies:

> In the opinion of the Midrash, Isaac was not in that city [Hebron] at the time [of his mother's funeral], because he was in Paradise to recover from the effects on his neck of what his father did to him during the Akedah, which left a mark in the shape of a bead. And that is why it is written, "With one bead of thy necklace".

This all suggests a traumatised consciousness – blindness in the form of stupidity as a response to an immense and unsymbolisable shock, namely the shock of discovering that your father is willing to sacrifice you for an idea of God.

But there is more to it than that. What we discover is that in living in the shadow of this particular kind of father, one who is relentless in his pursuit of an idea and willing to sacrifice everything for it, however much it pains him, Isaac has to forge a very different kind of way of being a man and a father – one that is easier to code as 'feminine', if we are careful about what this means. The suggestion I want to explore here is that the particular 'shadow' Isaac lives under is that of a classically violent father, and that his response to it has percolated down through Jewish history as an alternative mode of masculinity, one akin to what Daniel Boyarin (1997) ironically codes as 'unheroic masculinity'. This is a soft mode of masculinity, in which a man can love deeply and be blinded by this love.

Love and loss

In my previous work on this (Frosh, 2013, pp. 66–70), I was taken with the way Isaac is shown as having a capacity for love, and I want to go over this material again here and expand it a little. This love literally brings light into Isaac's life, whilst the loss of the loved object makes things darken. First, a small point relating to the question of why Isaac chooses the moment he does to bless his sons, when he actually has many more years to live. Rashi (on Genesis 27:2) provides an explanation, stating that Isaac was 123 years old at the time, "about five years younger than his mother at the time of her death; and when a man reaches within five years of his parent's age, he must begin thinking of his own death". This seems reasonable, and is an indication of the extent to which Isaac's mother was on his mind all the time; even 86 years later, it is her death, not Abraham's, that counts for him, psychologically speaking at least. More strongly, in the aftermath of Sarah's death, the text emphasises how Isaac's grief was intense and lasted until he learnt to love Rebecca; that is, his mourning for his mother was prolonged for three years. "And Isaac brought her into his mother Sarah's tent, and took Rebecca, and she became his wife, and he loved her. And Isaac was comforted for his mother" (Genesis 24:67). Rashi's interpretation of this is that he was only comforted when he could see that Rebecca would take Sarah's place, and it was then that he came to love her (*first* she was his wife; *then* he loved her). The discovery that Isaac makes is specifically linked to the recovery of light and sustenance. "As long as Sarah lived", Rashi continues in his comments on this verse,

> a lamp burned from the eve of the Sabbath to the eve of the following Sabbath, the dough was blessed and a divine cloud hung over the tent. When she died, it all ceased; but on Rebecca's arrival it was resumed.

And more normatively: "It is natural that whilst a man's mother is living he is wrapped up in her, but when she dies he finds comfort in his wife". Natural or not, the theme here is of love, comforting and light: the lamp that burns is the one that overcomes trauma through human closeness. It is a specifically *feminine* light that attaches itself to the mother and the wife. It is a kind of feminine *principle*, in which mother and wife are one and the same as bringers of light. Rashi adds this to his interpretation of the verse: "he brought her into the tent and behold she was his mother Sarah!" He could not tell the difference between his mother and his wife – a common joke, especially amongst Jews, but here transformed into a statement of love and also a contrast with the hyper-masculinity of the sacrifice scene. Even this early in the story, Isaac cannot see clearly without help. There is too little light in the tent; he needs his new wife, replacing his lost mother, to help him. Gradually, he becomes more and more dependent on her, until she makes all the decisions (about blessing Jacob, and about sending him away to find a wife) and he dissolves into the dimming of his eyes, immersed in his emotional world.

There is a great deal of play of light and dark in Isaac's life, with the strongest link being to blindness. Why does he go blind, and what does it signify? Whilst the loss of his mother, who we should recall is the one who is insistent on his primacy (it is she who determines that Ishmael should be expelled, against Abraham's inclinations), is the immediate source of the darkness that enters into Isaac's life "from the eve of the Sabbath to the eve of the following Sabbath", this is not the underlying cause of his blindness. Nor is it simply due to old age, as might be inferred from the plain meaning of the text (Genesis 27:1): "And it came to pass, that when Isaac was old, and his eyes were too dim to see". For the Rabbis, the loss of his sight is instead linked to the Akedah and hence to what must be constituted as the 'betrayal' of Isaac by his father, however motivated it might have been by religious fervour. Rashi comments on the verse above:

> When Isaac was bound upon the altar and his father was about to slay him, at that very moment the heavens opened, the ministering angels saw it and wept, and their tears flowed and fell upon Isaac's eyes which thus became dim.

The father's hand is lifted, the knife glints, and the sacrificial offering sees the heavens open and feels the tears of angels in his eyes. It would be enough to blind anyone; after such an experience, how could one ever see ordinary things again? Following the tradition mentioned above, that Isaac was in paradise for three years, being healed from his wounds, Isaac becomes one who has actually been sacrificed, in the sense that he is no longer fully in this world (however much he might 'sport' with his wife – Genesis 26:8) but is set apart, blind to what is going on around him. Perhaps this is not so surprising, for not only does Isaac lose his mother at this point, he also loses his father: there is no record of them speaking after the Akedah, and it takes the Rabbis' ingenuity in suggesting that Isaac is the one responsible for bringing Hagar back to re-marry Abraham (she is identified with the 'Keturah' mentioned in Genesis 25:1, with whom he has several children in his final years) to suggest an attempt at reconciliation on Isaac's part. The more general and convincing point is that Isaac, bereft in reality of his protective mother and separated from his father by the violence of Abraham's religious zealotry, finds his life obscured by melancholic darkness. In this, he really becomes divided: he is both on another plane, the one that has been in paradise, and locked into the world so that only tasty food makes any impact on him.

A compassionate masculinity

The suggestion that Isaac's response to the shadow of his father is to turn to a more 'feminine' mode of masculinity should be understood as a statement about how the Bible might be read to encompass a range of identificatory possibilities. As noted earlier, the Bible functions as a living text for the diasporic community of Jews, and whilst its primary function was as a book of law, or rather a book from which laws were derived, its strongest emotional appeal continues to be through the characters it draws and the 'lessons' that can be read out from them. In this regard, it is not far-fetched to explore the characterological issues presented by the 'patriarchs and matriarchs' of Genesis, who for generations were – and in some instances continue to be – related to as if they were real people, indeed almost as if they were the immediate ancestors and role models of the Jews of any particular time. This is what justifies the occasional psychoanalytic readings that still appear amongst biblical commentators, for example Avivah Zornberg (1995), who treat biblical material as if it is 'historical', that is as if the reference is to 'real' people and the stories of actual lives. For in many respects this is exactly how these figures function: as the most real elements of history, more real sometimes than one's actual parents, able to speak to communities struggling to make sense of the successes and struggles of their own times, and of their own lives.

This is the perspective one might also bring to bear on a contemporary reading of Isaac that stresses his 'femininity', that by Bracha Ettinger (2006). Ettinger's focus on the maternal through her notion of the 'matrixial' intimacy of the relationship between infant and mother in the womb has had some influence on theories of gender and mothering, and also more broadly on ideas on how the capacity for relating is born. Drawing on the resonance of supposedly 'telepathic' awareness – the nonverbal, automatic linking of subject and other that comes from deep intimacy – she fills out this notion with a paean to mutuality and other-absorption: "Primary compassion and empathy", she asserts (p. 119),

> are interconnected to "hypnotic" and "telepathic" transfer of waves and frequencies, and to trans-inscription and cross-inscription of psychic-mental traces – all matrixial supports for the more articulated and more conscious attitudes of respect, admiration, sorrow, awe, forgiveness, trust and gratitude, and finally the more mature compassion and full empathy, and all contributing to the creative process and to art as *transcryptum*.

Whilst the endpoint of this quotation is on art, its conjuring of the idea of compassion and empathy as arising from the prenatal absorption of one with the other both builds on and subverts the traditional gendered idea that relationality is a 'feminine' attribute. Compassion, which Ettinger sometimes rewrites as 'com-passion' to draw attention to its harmonic of 'passionate being-with' the other, is linked to the maternal and develops from this into an ability to demonstrate responsibility and care. Hence, when Ettinger asks (p. 100), "Can you imagine Isaac's compassion for his father?", she is also suggesting that the Bible is portraying Isaac's ability to relate to his father as arising from his own alertness to the link with his *mother*. We should recollect once again that Isaac's conception and gestation is a mystery. Sarah is radically postmenopausal, something emphasised in the text ("it had ceased to be with Sarah after the manner of women" [Genesis 18:11]); to say that Isaac is a desired, miracle child is not to move beyond the text at all, so we might assume that the intensity of concern and connection over him in the womb is as special as is the place he is given in Sarah's life after he is born. The link with his mother is intense (he is genuinely 'wrapped up in her', as Rashi says) and from her he gathers something into his own personality: the ability to love deeply and to feel what the other needs.

> We have to imagine Isaac's compassion for his father, Abraham. This compassion is primary; it starts before, and always also beyond, any possibility of empathy that entails understanding, before any economy of exchange, before any cognition or recognition, before any reactive forgiveness or integrative reparation. It is woven within primordial trans-sensitivity and co-re-naissance.
> (Ettinger, 2006, p. 100)

In stressing Isaac's feeling for his father, Ettinger is perhaps thinking of the way the text works with the idea of *togetherness* when describing Abraham and Isaac's journey towards the Akedah: "and they went both of them together" (Genesis 22:6) and again, "So they went both of them together" (Genesis 22:8). This is traditionally seen as a meaningful claim, showing that Isaac was not a reluctant sacrifice but shared in his father's commitment to their understanding of the will of God. For Ettinger, however, the importance of renaming it as a matrixial capacity is that it draws attention to the unspokenness of belonging together: it is only in the last stages of the ascent up the mountain that Isaac asks his father what is going on ("Behold the fire and wood; but where is the lamb for a burnt-offering?") and he then silently accepts his father's patently inadequate reply ("God will provide" [Genesis 22:7–8]). Isaac must know something is awry, but it does not matter; he sees that his father needs his complicity, and he gives it to him, whether gladly or not we do not know, but at least uncomplainingly. For Ettinger, this is all maternally induced. "Isaac's compassion toward his father", she writes (pp. 109–110), "what for Freud could have been standing for a direct identificatory love link, is based upon the infant's primary compassion toward the m/Other. . . . *In that sense Isaac is every-infant in innocent youth in passive vulnerability*". Ettinger's concentration here on passivity and vulnerability, and also on the mother's "compassionate hospitality towards her infant" – making space for the infant in the most material of ways – details how Isaac's acceptance of his father is also linked to ambivalence over the kind of masculinity this father embodies: active, passionate and conflicted, but also zealous and violent. Isaac reaches out to his father and sees the knife; he looks up and the tears of angels sear his vision; he returns to earth and finds his mother dead. When he comes across his new bride, Rebecca, she is so shocked to see him that she falls off her camel (Genesis 24:64). Why is this? Because, say the Rabbis, "what she perceived was Isaac coming down from Paradise, and he walked the way the dead walk, head down and feet up" (Spiegel, 1967, p. 6). His world turned upside down, father and mother lost; yet his compassion has been real. It also passes to his attitude to his own children. Esau sold his birthright as firstborn to Jacob (Genesis 25:33), and in so doing showed a disregard for the importance of the heritage of his father and grandfather, a disregard that is the object of radical criticism by the Rabbis. Yet Isaac loves this aberrant son Esau, and his tenderness and preference towards him demonstrates that despite his blindness, he recognises the outsider, the one who through his own stupidity and impulsivity will lose everything he has. Isaac too has lost, just as he has loved; as ever, the two go together. We get less sense of this capacity for feeling from Abraham, even though there is a reference to him 'weeping' for Sarah when she dies (Genesis 23:2). After the Akedah, he is simply the just man who passionately follows his convictions. Later on, Jacob will show a capacity for deep romantic love in his attitude to Rachel, and for misogynistic callousness in his treatment of Leah; and when Rachel dies, there is a powerful sense of tragedy. But Isaac's love is a confused blur. Having been compassionate to (complicit with, passionate alongside) his potentially murderous father, his maternal lifeline is severed and he is left adrift. After this, he never quite escapes the state of melancholy – the 'ashes' of Isaac is a trope of Jewish liturgy. He is no longer an actor; his fathering is foolish and fond. The power of the father is visited on the next generation as melancholic loss.

Amongst Jews, the story of Isaac is often overlooked between the grand deeds of Abraham and the vivid familial politics of Jacob. His is the quiet moment in-between, victim of Abraham, befuddled sire of Jacob. The textuality here is moving and confusing at once. What makes Isaac formative of Jewish identity and consciousness, if his part in the story is so passive and vague? Maybe it is precisely this shapelessness that in an odd way draws him into focus. For one thing, in Jewish liturgy his experience is drawn on as evidence for the resurrection of the dead – the hope of recovery from absolute loss, and faith in the possibility that this will be delivered at some point, in some way. Isaac survives, despite his father's violence. Perhaps we could also say that he offers another kind of possibility of recovery. We cannot all be Abrahams, striking out on our own, ready to face dislocation and uncertainty in pursuit of a grand idea, travelling without knowing when and where we will find a home. Isaac may meditate 'in the field', but he also knows where his mother's tent is, and how to fill it with love; and he knows how to reproduce this love, even if he does so blindly and in some ways foolishly. There is room for this as well – room, that is, for the one who is marked by sorrow and loss to find a way to love and be loved, and to embody this for generations to come who also do not quite know what to do with a passionate inheritance, who best to pass it on to, and how to find themselves within it.

Notes

1 The mediaeval French rabbi Shlomo Yitzchaki or Solomon ben Isaac, 1040–1105, Rashi being his generally known acronym based on the Hebrew initials of his name.
2 Midrash is a form of rabbinic literature. There are two types of Midrash: Midrash Aggadah and Midrash Halakhah. Midrash Aggadah can best be described as a form of storytelling that explores ethics and values in biblical texts. ('Aggadah' literally means 'story' or 'telling' in Hebrew.) Whilst Midrash Aggadah focuses on biblical characters as they pertain to values and ideas, Midrash Halakhah focuses on Jewish law and practice.
3 Hebrew plural of 'Midrash'.

References

Anderson, B. (2006) *Imagined Communities: Reflections on the Origin and Spread of Nationalism* (Revised Edition). London: Verso.

Boyarin, D. (1997) *Unheroic Conduct: The Rise of Heterosexuality and the Invention of the Jewish Man*. Berkeley: University of California Press.

Ettinger, B. (2006) From Proto-Ethical Compassion to Responsibility. *Athena*, *2*, 100–154.

Freud, S. (1900) The Interpretation of Dreams. In *The Standard Edition of the Complete Psychological Works of Sigmund Freud, Volume IV (1900): The Interpretation of Dreams (First Part)*, ix–627.

Freud, S. (1939) Moses and Monotheism. In *The Standard Edition of the Complete Psychological Works of Sigmund Freud, Volume XXIII (1937–1939): Moses and Monotheism, an Outline of Psycho-Analysis and Other Works*, 1–138.

Frosh, S. (2005) Fragments of Jewish Identity. *American Imago*, *62*, 179–192.

Frosh, S. (2010) Psychosocial Textuality: Religious Identities and Textual Constructions. *Subjectivity*, *3*, 426–441.

Frosh, S. (2013) *Hauntings: Psychoanalysis and Ghostly Transmissions*. London: Palgrave.

Hall, S. (1990) Cultural Identity and Diaspora. In J. Rutherford (ed.) *Identity: Community, Culture, Difference*. London: Lawrence and Wisehart.

Spiegel, S. (1967) *The Last Trial*. Woodstock: Jewish Lights, 1993.

Zornberg, A. (1995) *The Beginning of Desire: Reflections on Genesis*. New York: Doubleday.

In Greek mythology and opera

Chapter 2

Hard acts hard to follow

Sophocles, Hofmannsthal, Strauss and *Elektra*

Christopher Wintle

"I'm going to be a bit mischievous here!" This is how our next author responded to my request for an example of A Hard Act to Follow *in music – specifically opera. He knew that I was not in search of a composer and offspring couple, though J. S. Bach and some of his 20 children 'alone' would have been wonderful to explore. Instead I was looking for an opera itself, and Christopher Wintle eagerly came back to me with the following: "A hard act to follow? An act hard to follow? A hard act hard to follow? As you see I enjoy splitting hairs." Indeed he does as he opens his new reading of* Elektra *(1909), the one-act opera by Hugo von Hofmannsthal and Richard Strauss that has consistently excited psychoanalytic attention. But his hair-splitting goes further as he reminds us that whenever Freud investigated situations in literature, he was as mindful of the author and medium as he was of the circumstance depicted. To the basic question, why in the opera does Elektra die when in Sophocles (its source), she lives?, Wintle offers two answers, one derived from the situation of Hofmannsthal (and before him of the Greeks in general), the other from the psycho-dynamics of the drama. By reconstructing Hofmannsthal's stance – and the acts he and Strauss had to follow – from contemporary documentation, and by close reading of the libretto and music, he arrives at two contradictory interpretations. On the one hand, Elektra epitomizes the heroic self-sacrifice of one who fights for justice. On the other, she falls prey to the 'shadow of the object': her murdered father Agamemnon. The rhetorical power of the work, Wintle concludes, lies in this very impasse.**

From vaudeville to Freud

It is right and proper to pursue the phrase 'a hard act to follow' into the theatre – as I do here – since that is its place of origin. In her entertaining book of clichés, *The Cat's Pyjamas*, Julia Cresswell writes:

> from vaudeville [comes] a *hard* or *tough act to follow*. It developed in the USA about the beginning of the twentieth century, but did not become a

> cliché in the UK until the middle of the twentieth century. A very successful or popular act would literally be a difficult one to follow, as the audience would inevitably compare you unfavourably.[1]

From this we learn three things. First, that it is the *following* that is hard or tough, and not the act, though the act may also be hard or tough. Second, that the act, in order to be "very successful or popular", must fire and persuade the collective imagination – which, in metapoetical terms, it will do by exerting some kind of magic.[2] And third, for those obliged to do the following, failure to match or surpass a benchmark will not just arouse some degree of disappointment (or contempt) in the audience but also induce an equivalent degree of disappointment (or self-contempt) in the 'act-or'. The corresponding US injunction 'Beat that, buster!' may sound jocular, but its challenge – its aggression – isn't: there is psychic danger ahoy! What Cresswell does not specify, however, is the character of the acts – of the one that leads or the one that follows. In vaudeville these are likely to be disparate. As *The New Oxford Dictionary of English* puts it:

> *Vaudeville* [is] a type of entertainment popular chiefly in the US in the early 20th century, featuring a mixture of speciality acts such as burlesque comedy and song and dance.[3]

That is to say, its audience will not necessarily, if at all, compare like with like (one song, say, with another), but will compare the capacity of each act to cast its spell over mind, body and spirit. This is regardless of whether the act involves words, music, dance or some other form of stagecraft, be it juggling, acrobatics, mime or whatever.

When we move from vaudeville to straight theatre, we can likewise describe a 'very successful or popular drama' as 'hard to follow', whether for other authors or even for the same author. And even if an author is oblivious of following another's act, or has a suppressed memory of it, or is determined to reinvent the medium in which the act has been presented in order to bypass comparison, experienced members of an audience will know their own mind: a new work ineluctably invokes comparison with whatever work or works it follows. Authors should thus be *au fait* with the theatrical acts of their predecessors. Nor must they let lightning strike twice in the same place: to re-boot success is to court failure.

The matter becomes more complex when the drama is no longer simple but compound. Such is the case here with opera. For opera is an irreducible amalgam of dramatised music and musicalised drama put at the service of a transfiguring power more intense than that of drama or music taken singly. Opera makes manifest the 'music' that is only latent in drama, and the 'drama' that is only latent in music, and can invest the everyday with the numinous. Whereas 'music' includes singing, playing and dancing, 'drama' includes words and stagecraft; and because of its transfiguring power, musicalised stagecraft best serves the uncanny. Each element in the compound will have precedents, and some will respond to earlier acts that are 'hard to follow'. In this case study of a one-act opera, *Elektra* (1909), we need to ask how the librettist Hugo von Hofmannsthal (1874–1929) 'followed' his primary source – Sophocles' *Elektra* (an egregiously successful act) – as well as what acts the composer, Richard Strauss (1864–1949), had to follow. Only then may we analyse how 'the work itself' achieves its unprecedented rhetorical power. For within the story, the Freudian 'shadow of the object', the murdered Agamemnon, falls upon Agamemnon's daughter Elektra in a double sense: the murder is itself 'tough', and following it even tougher.

To ask questions of the 'medium' before turning to the 'message' is to affirm that "in Art . . . the delights of the Muse come before the cares of Man", and that "just as much as transmuting Life, Art transmutes Art".[4] But it is also to follow another 'act'. For the acknowledged parent of psychoanalysis, Sigmund Freud, consistently takes into account the 'medium' when addressing an artwork's 'message'. He does not treat events in drama just as if they occurred in life. This is clear from his analysis of the opening soliloquy in Shakespeare's *Richard III* (1592–1593) as it appears in "Some Character-types Drawn from Psychoanalytic Work" (1916).[5] The speaker, Richard, who is not yet king, presents himself as a social exception. It is a claim, Freud observes, "closely bound up with and . . . motivated by the circumstance of disadvantage":

> Deform'd, unfinish'd, sent before my time.
> Into this breathing world, scarce half made up.

His physiological disadvantage being irredeemable, Richard renounces love in favour of villainy (just as Alberich does at the start of Wagner's *Ring* [1876]). But, Freud argues persuasively, Richard does not forfeit our sympathy, but rather secures it: for we in the audience identify with him, as "we all demand reparation for early wounds to our narcissism, our self love", not having been granted "the lofty brow of genius or the noble profile of aristocracy". That we can do so is down to the author's skill:

> It is . . . a subtle economy of art in the poet that he does not permit his hero to give open and complete expression to all his secret motives. By this means he obliges us to supplement them; he engages our intellectual activity, diverts it from critical reflection and keeps us firmly identified with his hero.[6]

That is to say, the analysis of character is entwined with that of the relation of author to audience. Freud does not speculate as to why Shakespeare adopted this ploy – what 'hard' acts he had to follow. But, as we shall see, the clue he does give – that the bard wanted to withhold 'open and complete expression' – holds the key to our own reaction to *Elektra*.

The background in the Greeks

It was at the age of 30 that Hofmannsthal turned to Greek drama for the subjects of three plays: *Elektra* (1904), *Oedipus and the Sphinx* (1906) and *Oedipus the King* (1907). The aim, it seems, was to review the themes of Sophocles in light of unconscious motivation. To this end he looked to reinvent his diction by reining in his earlier lyric extravagance.[7] That is to say, by reviewing ancient subjects in the light of modern psychology, he was able to take on the towering themes of Greek drama (surely the acts hardest to follow), and, to an extent, express them in a new way. But what is this 'unconscious motivation'? He gives us two clues. First, referring to pairs of characters in various works, Hofmannsthal writes to Strauss in 1912:

> The similarity between Elektra and Hamlet is far greater [than with the other pairs], for in that case all the underlying motifs are identical – yet who would ever think of *Hamlet* when seeing *Elektra*?[8]

Not only does Hofmannsthal connect Sophocles with Shakespeare – both deal with a child caught in the aftermath of a murdered parent – but he also pauses over the connection itself (we shall return to this). And second, in an important document included in some posthumously published papers, *Ad me ipsum*, he notes cryptically:

> To act is to give oneself up. The Alkestis and Oedipus theme sublimated in *Elektra* (Elektra in relation to the deed treated with irony, it's true. Elektra–Hamlet).[9]

Here, a play of Sophocles – on Oedipus – is extended to include another by Euripides with the motivation specifically linked to an act of self-surrender (we shall also return to this). "To give oneself up" relates to unconscious motivation, and how Hofmannsthal's treatment of Elektra differs from that of Sophocles (and others) will be our central concern. Let us pause over these parallels.

In the *Interpretation of Dreams*, a copy of which Hofmannsthal kept in his library, Freud also connects Sophocles and Shakespeare. He begins his famous comparison of *Oedipus Rex* and *Hamlet* by addressing the plays' shared psychology: a son lives under the shadow of a murdered father and comes to term with a surviving mother who, unconsciously, he desires.[10] Yet, he continues,

> the changed treatment of the same material reveals the whole difference in the mental life of these two widely separated epochs of civilization: the secular advance of repression in the emotional life of mankind. In the *Oedipus* the child's wishful phantasy that underlies it is brought into the open and realised just as it would be in a dream. In *Hamlet* it remains repressed; and – just as in the case of a neurosis – we only learn of its existence from its inhibiting consequences.

And as for the dramatic impact of the two plays,

> strangely enough, the overwhelming effect produced by the more modern tragedy has turned out to be compatible with the fact that people have remained completely in the dark as to the hero's character.

To leave the core issues unspoken with the audience left in the dark thus holds the key to modern rhetorical power. Freud's thinking about *Hamlet* is consistent with his thinking about *Richard III*. With Hofmannsthal's *Elektra*, as we shall see, we likewise remain in the dark about Elektra's character as, indeed, she does herself, though the author does give us some useful leads.

But there is another, more burning issue that separates ancients and moderns. This relates to dramatic background. Here is the story as the ancients knew it. Agamemnon is heading for Troy to recapture Helen, the erring wife of his brother Menelāus. But he is becalmed. For he

> has caught a stag, then boasted that he was a better huntsman than Artemis, whereupon the offended goddess held the Greek fleet wind-bound at Aulis. [The diviner] Calchas told [the Greeks] to appease her by sacrificing Iphigenia [one of Agamemnon's daughters]. . . . [However,] Iphigenia is a child . . . and Agamemnon is her killer, for which Clytemnestra never forgave him [Clytemnestra is not only Agamemnon's wife and Iphigenia's mother, but also Helen's sister].[11]
>
> During Agamemnon's absence at Troy [Clytemnestra] took his cousin Aegisthus as a lover, and on Agamemnon's return after the ten-year war she murdered him.[12]

She also murdered Cassandra, the prophetess and spoil-of-war who returned with Agamemnon from Troy as his concubine. Yet Aegisthus also had his own grievance. For he was the only surviving son of Thyestēs, the brother of Atreus, who in turn was the father of Agamemnon. In a deed of extreme horror, Atreus had killed Thyestēs's two elder sons and served them up in a pie for Thyestēs to eat. So by killing Agamemnon, Aegisthus had avenged the killing and cooking of his brothers by Agamemnon's father. Then,

> years later Orestes [Agamemnon's son] avenged his father's murder by killing both Clytemnestra and Aegisthus.[13]

In these killings, he was ably supported and encouraged by one of the surviving sisters, Electra. Now, by killing Clytemnestra and Aegisthus, Orestes fulfilled the tyrannical command of Apollo, the presiding deity at Delphi. But by killing Clytemnestra he also committed matricide, thereby arousing the wrath of the Erinyes (the nocturnal female furies), later to be known as the Eumenides. He is eventually acquitted by a court on the Areopagus.

Though rooted in myth (via Homer), the story finds its locus classicus in six Greek dramas dating from the fifth century BC. In order of composition they are the three parts of Aeschylus's *Oresteia* (*Agamemnon, The Choephori* and *The Eumenides*); Sophocles' *Elektra*; and Euripides' *Elektra* and *Orestes*. Together, they offer a panoramic view of the kernel of the myth as it unfolds over three generations (as far as it concerns us here, for other plays deal with later events).

Within the story, Elektra clearly has a subordinate role. Yet each dramatist handles the role in his own way. With the *Oresteia*, Elektra appears in just the first half of *The Choephori*. We see her arrive at the grave of Agamemnon accompanied by a chorus of resentful libation-bearers and watched at a distance by Orestes and Pylades. She is grief-stricken, humiliated, vengeful and acutely mindful of the gods: she appeals to Mother Earth, and prays that her own ways and thoughts should in no way be like those of Clytemnestra, her own mother. When Orestes reveals himself, the stored-up love she bestows on him is enhanced by the memory of her murdered sister (Iphigenia). Thereafter she is nowhere to be seen. Her fatalism is expressed succinctly in a modern version of the play by Ted Hughes. She addresses the Chorus:

> Friends, we share the misery of the house
> And we share a hatred
> As if we were links in the one chain.
> The gods know our fate –
> Whether slave or free
> Neither you nor I can choose
> Or escape it.[14]

Yet after killing Aegisthus and Clytemnestra, Orestes finds his brain 'in a whirl', his heart 'crouching in terror': before him he sees "demons [who] are the decomposition of my mother's blood", whose whips he can feel.[15] It is this new and unexpected set of horrors betokening a ravaged conscience that prepares us for *The Eumenides*. There, both he and Apollo (and through him Zeus) will be put on trial against the furies (and through them Mother Earth). He will be acquitted by the casting vote of Athene, whose diplomacy, indeed, will reform Athenian justice. It is she who reinvents the furies as the Eumenides, 'the kindly ones'.

Next, Sophocles' *Elektra* rebalances the mix: about one-third of the play is devoted to the return of Orestes and the inexorable working out of his revenge (including the planting of the 'fake news' of his death); and the remaining two-thirds to the sufferings of the three women inside the house: Clytemnestra, who is tormented by a bad (and proleptic) dream; her daughter Elektra, who thirsts for Clytemnestra's blood; and another daughter, Chrysothemis, who by contrast is an appeaser. Since Agamemnon's death, the family home has been lived in and run by Clytemnestra and her severe lover Aegisthus. The play opens with Orestes along with his friend Pylades greeting the old family tutor; and, after Orestes has revealed himself to Elektra and killed Clytemnestra, closes with the pair driving Aegisthus to the slaughter. Elektra, who has prayed to Apollo for this moment, is desperate to silence Aegisthus: "Let him say nothing! For God's sake, brother, do not listen to him", she cries. For Aegisthus might persuade Orestes to think twice.

Finally, in Euripides's *Elektra*, we find that Aegisthus has betrothed Elektra to a farmer who, though of good stock, has fallen on hard times: "[Aegisthus's] aim was to weaken his own fear by giving her to one so weak as himself" – out of house and out of mind.[16] But the farmer retains his pride: he has never touched her. Although grateful for being left *intacta*, Elektra feels doubly humiliated: for Clytemnestra and Aegisthus, by having had children of their own, have further reduced her status. The main drama begins, as in Sophocles, with the arrival of Orestes and Pylades. As before, they slowly reveal their identity to Elektra. The three then hatch their murderous plot and pray to Zeus, with Elektra insisting that it should be for her to kill her mother. Orestes departs, and, in the course of a ritual sacrifice slaughters Aegisthus. He returns with the man's head, which Elektra duly upbraids. But Elektra has to steel Orestes to kill the approaching Clytemnestra: for, suddenly, he is assailed by doubt. Can he bring himself to matricide?, he asks himself; "I cannot believe this command from the oracle was well made", he wails. Clytemnestra arrives and engages Elektra in a fraught exchange, adding to her complaints that Agamemnon returned from Troy with a concubine (Cassandra). Elektra reciprocates by accusing Clytemnestra of acting the harlot in Agamemnon's absence. Clytemnestra observes acutely:

> My child, from birth you always have adored your father.
> This is part of life. Some children always love
> The male, some turn more closely to their mother than him.
> I know you and forgive you.[17]

She is then murdered. But now both Elektra and Orestes are struck with remorse. Clytemnestra's divine brothers, Castor and Pollux, appear ex machina, and, condemning Apollo for his 'lies', take matters into their own hands: Elektra is to wed Pylades, Orestes is to be tried (but acquitted), and both are to be banished and debarred from seeing each other again.

From the ancients, then, we learn, inter alia, that Elektra has an abnormal bond with her dead father that fuels her lethal hatred for Clytemnestra. This is established even before any of the plays begin, even before the murder of Agamemnon. It is more than what Freud calls "the general rule for a normally constituted girl to turn her affection towards her father in the first instance",[18] or what Jung calls the 'Electra complex' – a reverse Oedipus complex.[19] It is also the opposite of what Freud argues in "Psychopathic Characters on the Stage": Hamlet, he says, is not innately psychopathic, but merely becomes so during the course of the action – a becoming that is artistically vital by allowing the dramatist "to induce the same illness in us"[20] and thereby help us to identify with Hamlet's repressed impulse.[21] Rather, the plays of Sophocles and Euripides start in medias res: the mental situation of each protagonist is already firmly set. They allow us to observe the working out of Apollo's command through the actions of Orestes and the intense suffering endured by the women. In a Brechtian sense, it is a kind of 'epic' presentation. Only in Euripides is the ground of the revenge – Apollo's command – seriously probed.

All six Greek plays show mankind, not only in thrall to the gods, but also as defensively patriarchal. It is particularly clear from Aeschylus. In *Agamemnon*, the Chorus hail Clytemnestra's words as "like a man's", and Aegisthus's decision to stay at home, seduce the king's wife and plot his murder, as the action of a 'woman'; in response to Clytemnestra's defiant "Greatness wins hate", Agamemnon sneers "It does not suit a woman to be combative".[22] In *The Choephori*, Orestes refers to "Aegisthus the wolf-bitch, tail and ears down, cowering to the pack's boss, Clytemnestra".[23] And in *The Eumenides*, Pallas Athena, who famously had no mother but sprang fully armed from the head of Zeus, pre-empts the verdict of Orestes's trial with the following:

> In my reckoning,
> The death of a woman who killed her husband
> Weighs nothing
> Against the death of her victim.
> The father's right, prerogative of the male,
> Has my vote.[24]

That is to say, in ancient Greece 'the phallus rules, OK'. And in fin-de-siècle Vienna . . .?

Hofmannsthal's Elektra play

Hofmannsthal begins his play on *Elektra* quite differently from Sophocles (or his peers):[25] he 'follows' the Greek 'act' by rendering it freely. He no longer opens with Orestes and Pylades; there is no immediate invocation of the gods, no inexorable, framing strategy. Rather, he places us at once inside the palace and tells the story from the viewpoint of those who are in the dark. It is a remarkable start, with nothing of the gradualist approach Freud celebrated in *Hamlet*. Already the atmosphere is at fever pitch, though it will intensify. Five servants and their overseer – strikingly, all women – are talking about Elektra. From them, we learn about her neurosis – her Freudian 'wishful phantasy' – through its 'consequences': she may be a princess, but she howls for her father, spits like a wild cat, eats with the dogs and orders the maids to keep their distance, crying "I'm feeding a vulture in my flesh". In a brief, and surely unprecedented, first entry, she darts in and out "like an animal to its lair". When the fifth maid castigates the others for cruelty, claiming them unfit to breathe the same air as her royal mistress, she gets beaten. The tension in the household is a dramatic projection of the ferocious endopsychic war in which Elektra finds herself embroiled. On the one hand, she projects her impotence, her self-contempt, onto the maids, who return and feed it lavishly – and, as we shall see at the end, lethally; on the other, she hoards her pride with regal disdain. The disdain is also fuelled by envy. Elektra has become a solitary whose neurosis debars her from meaningful bonding or childbirth: "Creep into bed with your men", she reportedly shrieks at the maids. As the scene ends, the overseer remarks:

> And when she sees us with our children, she screams
> Nothing can be so accursed, nothing,

As children which, like animals, slithering about
In blood on the stairs, we have conceived and borne
Here in this house.

As in Sophocles, the next scene starts with Elektra alone.[26] But Hofmannsthal's version of her monologue is especially revealing. She no longer behaves 'like an animal', but holds herself as a woman. She has a fixation with Agamemnon that locks her into a quasi-libidinal childhood bond to her father – Freud's 'general rule' has now become a pathological state. Thanks to 'events', she has never been able to 'move on'. Her body has matured, but not her affective state. As Freud and Breuer had observed,

> ideas which have become pathological [persist] with such freshness and affective strength because they have been denied the normal wearing-way processes by means of abreaction and reproduction in states of uninhibited association.[27]

We hear her reliving the trauma of Agamemnon's murder as if she had been a witness, even though she would have known the murder only by report. It is the falseness of her memory that enhances her hysteria. In her phantasy she revels in 'blood' with a Wildean extravagance (the steaming bath, the running of blood over the father's eyes, the dragging of the corpse with splayed legs); and she craves an unsparing retributive bloodbath involving man and beast characteristic of an unyielding, infantile superego:

And we will slaughter the steeds for you
Which are in the house, we will drive them together
Before your grave, and they will sense their death
Beforehand and neigh into the wind of death
And die, and we will slaughter the dogs for you
Because they are the brood and the brood of the brood
Of those who have hunted with you, of those
Who licked your feet, to whom you flung
Morsels of meat, therefore their blood
Must go down to do you service.[28]

As this is the anniversary of Agamemnon's murder, her suffering is especially acute: she is at the peak of a repetitive cycle. And there is no surprise that she tries to summon up her father's ghost: for she is stuck at the familiar first stage of mourning where 'denial' of loss appears to restore the dead object – though in Elektra's supremacist phantasy, Agamemnon will return with a royal wreath of shining purple that sits on his brow and feeds off his open head wound. Her idealisation testifies to the power of a quasi-Oedipal attachment that has had no opportunity to work itself through. In the opera, Strauss goes further by having her utter the name 'Agamemnon' repeatedly – thus reinforcing a dramatic monologue with a tiny, obsessive 'refrain'.

Other factors, though, have reinforced the fixation. Elektra is acutely mindful that her mother Clytemnestra has profaned 'the royal bed' by marrying her partner-in-crime Aegisthus. Thus any attempt to come to terms with, or even ameliorate, her current situation has been blocked. Elektra cannot form any kind of surrogate attachment to her stepfather, an impediment that may aggravate her attitude to her mother who enjoys intimacy with him. The situation has made the 'hard act' that Elektra has had to follow an intolerable one. Indeed, her resentments find an outlet in triumphalism: she envisages herself dancing on the graves of both Clytemnestra and Aegisthus. True, she can count two 'good' people in her life: her sister Chrysothemis and her long-absent brother Orestes. This confidence is vital, and she trusts that, as family, they will join her in celebrating a bloody victory:[29]

> and we,
> Your blood, your son Orestes and your daughters,
> We three, when all this is done and purple tents
> Have been raised by the haze of the blood
> Which the sun sucks upward to itself, then
> We, your blood, will dance around your grave.

Yet, one of the functions of Hofmannsthal's narrative will be to destabilise even this trust.

That Hofmannsthal does not begin with the gods does not mean that he has eradicated them from the action: on the contrary, he has largely replaced and redirected them. He invites us to observe, not so much the inexorable will of Apollo coolly exercised by Orestes, but rather the unfettered urgings of Dionysus ruthlessly exercised by Elektra. It is as if Hofmannsthal is reading Sophocles in the spirit of Nietzsche.[30] Of course, throughout both play and opera, there are occasional references to the ancient gods. Elektra maliciously reminds Clytemnestra of her divine descent; in delivering the 'fake news' of his death, Orestes suggests the gods have been unable to countenance her brother's excessive joy; after revealing himself Orestes divulges he is on a divinely appointed mission; and, as she waits with extreme anxiety to hear evidence of Clytemnestra's murder, Elektra cries "there are no Gods in heaven!" Yet Hofmannsthal suppresses the passage in Sophocles where Elektra humbly prays to Apollo as Orestes enters the house to murder their mother. Rather, as it seems, he allows Orestes to follow her bidding, and her to sanctify him. It is as if their palace has become a shrine, and she its high priestess. In a frenzy, she cries:

> He is blessed [*selig*], he who comes to do his deed,
> Blessed he, who yearns for him,
> Blessed, who beholds him!

Blessed who knows him,
Blessed who touches him![31]
[*etc.*]

Whereas in Sophocles Elektra invokes "Hades, Persephone, Hermes, steward of death, Eternal Wrath and Furies", in Hofmannsthal she makes no such invocation. Divine authority and its attendant sacrifices are hers to bestow. As we shall see, there may be a reason for this.

There is a still more telling suppression. At the end of Elektra's first monologue in Sophocles, the women of Mycenae (the chorus) approach. Though sympathetic and maternal, they nevertheless ask her to face facts. Why weep when tears won't bring back the dead? Why not follow the example of her sisters Chrysothemis and Iphianassa, who have not given up on life? Why not relax her anger without forgetting the past? And why not trust in the supreme God? Elektra is riled: her role model is the distraught Niobe,[32] and as for God, may he reduce the pomp of Clytemnestra and Aegisthus to ashes! She will await Orestes. But the women persist. "Remember the harm you do yourself", they warn in a passage of remarkable insight, "the mischief is in your own self-torture. Hoarder of grief, your sullen soul breeds strife unending".[33] Elektra replies:

I know my passion all too well,
But I shan't cease
Plaguing them while I live.[34]

The chorus sees her commitment to just revenge as harbouring as much danger to herself as to others. She agrees – but she can only continue. Her stance reinforces the self-sacrificing role of woman to man among the ancients.

Hofmannsthal has suppressed Sophocles' chorus altogether – leaving it for us to configure its warnings, knowing Elektra would ignore them anyway. But he has also suppressed other things. Elektra neither makes nor will hear any criticism of Agamemnon. She will not debate the back history of the house of Atreus. Yet, as we know from myth, it was Agamemnon who started the fateful episode: though deemed a good ruler in Argos, he put strain on the community by setting sail for Troy following the abduction of Helen (Menelāus' wife and Clytemnestra's sister), hence abandoning his people and family for ten years; en route he aroused the wrath of Artemis for an impulsive killing for which he had to his sacrifice his daughter Iphigenia; he was later cold to the vanquished people of Troy and brought suffering to the newly widowed women of his own Argos; and he returned with a concubine, Cassandra, whom he asked his already aggrieved wife to treat well. Cassandra issued the starkest of warnings – a proleptic vision that also served as a projection of Agamemnon's turbulent unconscious – but he does not – and by Apollo's edict cannot – heed them. Both will die. By clinging to her infantile, idealised father-imago, Elektra resists adult debate, manifestly to her own detriment and that of those around her. We, as an informed audience, are left to act as our own chorus.

Elektra, Agamemnon and Alkestis

We learn more about Elektra from three separate meetings: first with her mother, then with her sister (a second meeting, in fact) and finally with Orestes. In all three, Hofmannsthal has far exceeded the content and decorum of Sophocles, and in all three Elektra acts as a 'space-invader'. The meeting with the mother stands at the centre of the drama. It is long and harrowing. Images of bestiality and sacrifice have emanated constantly from Elektra, but now we see how they have taken hold of her mother. Clytemnestra enters, bloated and ravaged by a (proleptic) nightmare, with a retinue of sacrificial cattle. It is a ritual she repeats compulsively and to no avail: the mental horror persists. She compares her "living body" to a "waste field", with "this nettle growing out of me".[35] When Elektra replies, with sadistic glee, that "your own neck must bleed / when the hunter has moved in for the kill", she envisages a slaughter of surpassing horror. Clytemnestra will die even more brutally than Iphigenia or Agamemnon. But for Elektra, the horror is the gateway to the highest triumph, though she may not consciously understand the import of her words: "Then you will dream no more, then I shall have / no further need of dreaming, and whoever still lives, / will exult, and can rejoice in his life". By annihilating dreams, death will restore the health of the body politic, but as mother and daughter are alike in sharing bad dreams, we are bound to ask, whose will be the death?

Elektra's second meeting with Chrysothemis occurs after she has received the startling 'fake news' of Orestes's death. (In the first meeting she had heard her sister's pleas for pity.) Elektra has two reactions: she recognises that she has not the physical strength to slaughter her mother on her own (her arms are "sad and dried") and asks her sister to be her accomplice. Indeed, she tries to invest Clytemnestra with a masculinity she previously associated with Orestes: "You could choke [either] me or a man in your arms. Everywhere you have such strength in you!" Elektra also yearns to invade her sister's being through some mental and physical metempsychosis into a blood-relative: "I want to wind myself around you, sink my roots into you and pollute your blood with my will!" She even hopes to recover her impeded sexuality through a vicarious identification with her sister in her nuptials:

> I shall sit with you faithfully in your room and wait for your bridegroom. For him I shall rub you with ointment and for me you must plunge into a fragrant bath like a cygnet, and hide your head on my breast before he takes you in his strong arms, glowing through your veil, to the wedding bed.

And so forth. Chrysothemis, who, as a contrast-figure to Elektra, is keen to 'move on', is rightly appalled. In due course, she flees. (Strauss defines her musically by the waltz, an icon of liberated sexuality.)

It is at this point, when Elektra thinks she is finally all alone, that the real Orestes appears. Their meeting is in three parts. First, Orestes brings the fake news of his own death. Elektra is initially inhospitable and contemptuous, not least when he comments on her pitiable condition. Then, as "the gloomy old servant" and three attendants advance (movingly) to kiss his hand, he reveals his true identity. In Sophocles she merely exclaims "O light! O joy!" and gradually adjusts to the changed situation; in Hofmannsthal, she utters his name ("Orest!") seven times, hailing his appearance as finer than any dream image. She begs him not to vanish, although, if he has been sent to carry her away, she concedes she will die more blest (*seliger*) than ever she lived. Here the life and death instincts converge – significantly, as we shall see. Hofmannsthal's ten lines are in the libretto but not in the play. Yet only music can convey the tone and force of Elektra's feeling: in his fictional *Letter* of 1902, Hofmannsthal has his Lord Chandos, 'writing' in 1603, renounce rhetoric in favour of a new kind of form that "creates poetry and truth all at once; a play of eternal forces, a thing as magnificent as music or algebra".[36] Strauss indeed reacts with one of the greatest passages in opera: a slow resolution of a massive dissonance at the point of recognition leading into a tender cradle-song that builds on the valedictory love-music of *Tristan und Isolde*: for Strauss, Wagner was always the act hardest to follow – but follow he did, and with a 'magnificent thing'.

After this passage of sublimated love, Elektra returns to matters in hand. In Sophocles, she tells Orestes –

> I can't stop crying.
> How could I? Today you returned and I saw you dead,
> And today I see you alive. It has been amazing.
> I shouldn't think it a miracle any more
> If Father came back to life. I'd believe my eyes.[37]

In Hofmannsthal, by contrast, Elektra abruptly resumes her position of concentrated self-deprecation. She repels Orestes and speaks without inhibition. Once she had

> Such hair, that made all men tremble
> This hair, unkempt, besmirched, denigrated.[38]

More still, she has sacrificed her precious 'shame' for her father. For whenever she has 'taken pleasure' in her body, Agamemnon's sighs, his groans have forced themselves into her bedroom. This is the epicentre of her suffering, the womanly sacrifice a daughter has been compelled to make in light of the 'hard act' committed by the mother against her father:

> Jealous are the dead: and he sent me hate,
> hollow-eyed hate, as my bridegroom.
> So I have always been a prophetess
> And from my life have brought forth
> Nothing other than curses and despair.[39]

The shape of this meeting, with its contempt, transient nobility and resumption of contempt, now enhanced, parallels that of the opening scene with the maids: there we saw just the consequences of Elektra's endopsychic war, here we come face to face with the war itself.

Like Chrysothemis before him, Orestes is appalled by what he hears. Yet he is determined to act. As he enters the palace, Elektra darts round in anticipation "like a caged beast". She hears the sounds of Clytemnestra's murder. Then Aegisthus returns, and after a sadistically arch exchange, and in a variation of Sophocles, she ushers him into the palace. She hears the sounds of his murder too. In Sophocles, the chorus, which has already sensed the presence of the wily Hermes, guide to the dead, sees the act of retribution driven by a shade:

> The deadly curse is now at work –
> Eye for eye, tooth for tooth.
> The dead below are rising up to life,
> And now the old slain
> Suck their killers' blood dry.[40]

In Hofmannsthal there is no chorus. So, in answer to Aegisthus's dying plea "does no-one hear me?", Elektra simply names the shade: "Agamemnon hears you". The lines to the underworld are now open.

Only the opera marks the celebrations that follow. First, in a duet, Chrysothemis and Elektra rejoice for opposite reasons – one for the promise of a new life, the other for the freedom to indulge her triumphalism. "Who can live without love?" cries Chrysothemis, "Love kills!" retorts Elektra menacingly (and, did she but know it, prophetically), "But no-one departs without having known love!" Then, as Chrysothemis rushes out to find Orestes, Elektra gives herself over to a Dionysian victory dance "of utmost intensity". At its height, she drops dead. We are stunned. It is Hofmannsthal's trump card: neither in myth nor in Sophocles does this happen. For Elektra, the 'hard act' of Agamemnon's murder has proved an act impossible to follow, her victory dance a dance of death.

How do we react to this apparently catastrophic reversal? Initially, we recall the observations of Freud from life: the shade of Agamemnon – the shadow of the object – has risen lethally to claim its victim; Elektra's critical ego has been fatally dethroned by identification with her father's. We then recall all we have learnt about Elektra: at first a girl intensely and uncritically bonded with her father, later a woman with adult sexual needs but an arrested affective development; a sullen soul with a vengeful, infantile superego and a febrile mind in which events and dreams feed upon each other; a female conscious of lacking male strength ravaged by an endopsychic war between pride and self-contempt; a hieratic personality who ruthlessly attempts to invade the space of others; a fighter who is forever caught between the demands of love and death; and so forth. Next, we wonder how Elektra would have coped had she lived: how would she adjust to the open space of joy after being confined for so long in the dark corners of vengeance? But, still to be Freudian, we have also to consider the demands of art.

Here we return to Hofmannsthal's parallel between his play and *Alkestis*. This is how Euripides tells the story.[41] After the turbulence among the gods that follows Zeus's punishment of his impulsive son Apollo, Admetus, a prince, finds, for some undisclosed reason, that he must die unless someone takes his place; to his fury, his old father refuses; only his wife, the adored Alkestis, accepts. She duly dies, to universal sorrow. But a visitor, the demi-god Heracles, is so taken by the selfless hospitality shown to him by Admetus at this time of extreme grief that he fights the demon Death and, in an outcome already predicted by Apollo, restores Alkestis to Admetus. In his own, youthful version of the play, Hofmannsthal believed that Alkestis sacrificed herself for the very principle of kingship, which is itself divinely approved. As Egon Wellesz, the Austrian composer who initially collaborated with Hofmannsthal on an operatic version of the play, writes:

> [Alkestis] is a woman capable of one great act, the sacrifice of her life . . . she prepares for death as for a great ceremony, in which her life is consummated.[42]

And with his *Elektra*, it seems, Hofmannsthal exceeded even his own 'hard act': for Elektra too puts herself on trial and, however unconsciously, sacrifices herself, not just for her father, but for the blessed order he – and subsequently Orestes – represents. It is her 'one great act', a manifestly female triumph. Only, unlike Alkestis she is not brought back to life. From a musical perspective, Strauss also had to 'follow' the triumph of his own 'decadent' one-act opera on Oscar Wilde's *Salome* (1905): Salome not only performs the Dance of the Seven Veils, but is later crushed to death for lavishly kissing the severed head of Jokanaan (John the Baptist). Strauss would have been disappointed if the climax of *Elektra* was perceived as any less shocking.

These perspectives complicate our evaluation of Elektra's death: is it a disaster, or is it a triumph? Has Elektra shown her incapacity to rise to a great test in life, or has she revealed her heroism by resolutely holding out for justice, even at the expense of her life? If the questions are unanswerable, then the power of both play and opera lies in the impasse they create. Even more than with *Hamlet* in Freud's reading, the rhetoric of *Elektra* 'persuades' us through its very inscrutability.[43]

Notes

In the text I have adhered wherever possible to the German spellings Elektra and Alkestis, though, especially in these notes, I follow the English spelling Electra for accuracy of reference. On the other hand, I use throughout the English Clytemnestra rather than the German Klytämnestra.

* Hilary Finch, former music critic at The Times of London clearly agrees, adding to the editor that this rhetorical power, albeit inscrutable, in turn "empowers us to continue an ever-creative intellectual response to the work".

1 Julia Cresswell, *The Cat's Pyjamas: The Penguin Book of Clichés*, London: Penguin, 2007, p. 53.
2 Christopher Wintle, *Metapoetics: Aphorisms, Thoughts and Maxims on Life, Art and Music*, London: Plumbago, 2010, pp. 43–46. See 'A talent for magic – the capacity to release transfiguring fantasy – is our first criterion in assessing an artist', p. 44.
3 *The New Oxford Dictionary of English*, Oxford: OUP, 1998, p. 2048.
4 Wintle, 2010, p. 50.
5 Sigmund Freud, 'Einige Charaktertypen aus der psychoanalytischen Arbeit' (1916), *S.E.*, Vol. 14, pp. 309–333, especially pp. 314–315. The translation of the title is by me, but that of the text by E. C. Mayne.
6 Ibid., p. 315.
7 For an overview of the poet's life see: 'Hofmannsthal', in *The Oxford Companion to German Literature*, ed. Henry Garland and Mary Garland, Oxford: OUP, 1976, pp. 394–395.
8 *The Correspondence between Richard Strauss and Hugo von Hofmannsthal* (1952), London: Collins, 1961, pp. 135–136. The translation is by Hanns Hammelmann and Ewald Osers.
9 Hugo von Hofmannsthal, *Selected Plays and Libretti*, ed. and intro. Michael Hamburger, London: Routledge and Kegan Paul, 1963, pp. xxxiv–xxxv. *Ad me ipsum* appears in the posthumous *Aufzeichnungen* of 1959.
10 Sigmund Freud, *The Interpretation of Dreams: An Entirely New Translation by James Strachey* (1900), London: George Allen and Unwin, 1954/67, pp. 264–266. Bryan Gilliam, writing that "Scholars have addressed the issue of Freudian elements in *Elektra*", points to an account of the sources in: Lorna Martens, 'The Theme of the Repressed Memory in Hofmannsthal's *Elektra*', *German Quarterly*, Vol. 60, No. 1, 1987. Brian Gilliam, *Richard Strauss's 'Elektra'*, Oxford: Clarendon Press, 1991, p. 28.
11 'Agamemnon', in *Oxford Dictionary of the Classical World*, ed. John Roberts, Oxford: OUP, 2005, pp. 15–16. This is not the only account of the fate of Iphigenia. In another, she is saved at the last moment by Artemis, who replaces her in the sacrifice with a hind. Iphigenia then becomes a priestess of Artemis. See ibid., 'Iphigenia', p. 373.
12 'Clytemnestra', ibid., p. 162.
13 Ibid.
14 Ted Hughes, *Aeschylus: The Oresteia*, London: Faber and Faber, 1999, p. 93. Aeschylus also tells how Clytemnestra "mutilated the body of Agamemnon / As Atreus butchered / The two brothers of Aegisthus", making her killing into a compound revenge on behalf of herself and Aegisthus, pp. 111–112.
15 Ibid., pp. 140–143.
16 Euripides, *Elektra*, trans. John Davey (1998), London: Penguin, 2004, p. 137, lines 38–40.
17 Euripides V, *Elektra*, trans. Emily Townsend Vermeule, Chicago: University of Chicago Press, 1959, p. 55, lines 1102 ff.
18 Quoted in: 'Delusions and Dreams in Jensen's Gradiva', in *Sigmund Freud, Art and Literature*, London: Pelican, 1985, Vol. 14, p. 58. The translation is by James Strachey. (Originally: Sigmund Freud, 'Der Wahn und die Träume in W. Jensens *Gradiva*' (1907), *S.E.*, Vol. 9, pp. 1–95.)
19 Carl Jung describes the 'Elektra Complex', in his *Collected Works*, Vol. 4, London: Routledge, 1961, pp. 151–156. In his writings Freud reacted to the concept three or four times, but basically thought it unnecessary, if not downright misleading.
20 Sigmund Freud, 'Psychopathische Personen auf der Bühne' (1905–6), *S.E.*, Vol. 7, pp. 303–310. The translation is by James Strachey.
21 Cf. Sigmund Freud, 'Der Dichter und das Phantasieren' ('The Creator and His Phantasy', 1907/8), *S.E.*, Vol. 9, pp. 141–153. Freud suggests that "how the writer accomplishes this is his innermost secret; the essential *ars poetica* lies in the technique of overcoming the feeling of repulsion in us which is undoubtedly connected with the

barriers that rise between each single ego and the others". He further suggests that there may be two ways for an author to overcome such repulsion: by altering and disguising the character (a softening, or taking of poetic license), and by 'bribing us' with the formal, or 'aesthetic', yield of pleasure offered in the way he presents 'his phantasies'. By calling these ways the "*incentive bonus* or *fore-pleasure*", Freud sexualises the relation of writer to audience, and implicitly casts the experience of the art-work as a sublimated act of *coitus*, albeit one that involves body, mind and spirit. (The translation of the title is by me, but that of the text by I. F. Grant Duff.)

22 Aeschylus, *The Oresteian Trilogy* (1956), trans. Philip Vellacott, London: Penguin, 1966, pp. 55, 98–99 and 75.

23 Aeschylus/Hughes, 1999, p. 105. Elektra takes up the same imagery as, later, she says of Clytemnestra to the Chorus and Orestes, 'The She-Wolf Suckles a Wolf / That Will Rip Out Her Throat.' Ibid., p. 111.

24 Ibid., p. 181.

25 Hugo von Hofmannsthal, *Selected Plays and Libretti*, ed. Michael Hamburger (*Electra. A Tragedy in One Act freely rendered after Sophocles*, trans. Alfred Schwartz), London: Routledge & Kegan Paul, 1963, pp. 1–77. Hamburger's introduction is richly informative. For a discussion of the transformation of 'From Play to Libretto', see: Gilliam, 1991, pp. 18–48. Gilliam, noted (on p. 18) that Strauss did most of the cutting down of the play to libretto size: "Hofmannsthal's only significant contribution . . . was the additional text for Elektra's aria in the Recognition Scene, and the text for the duet between Elektra and Chrysothemis in the final scene". A parallel English/German translation of the final libretto appears in: *Salome/Elektra. Strauss*, ENO/RO Guide 37, ed. Nicholas John, London: Calder, 1988, pp. 87–126; my own discussion of the music for *Elektra* appears on pp. 63–86.

26 Strikingly, the staging also reflects Elektra's mind-set: "*Elektra comes out of the house. She is alone with the patches of red light which fall like bloodstains from the branches of the fig tree obliquely across the ground and upon the walls.*" Hofmannsthal/Hamburger, 1963, p. 11.

27 From 'On the Psychical Mechanism of Hysterical Phenomena', in Sigmund Freud and Joseph Breuer, *Studies in Hysteria* (1893–5), trans. James Strachey and Alix Strachey, London: Penguin, 1974, pp. 53–69, especially p. 62; *S.E.* Vol. 2, 'Über den psychischen Mechanismus hysterischer Phänomene (Vorläufige Mitteilung)', pp. 3–17. The book was in Hofmannsthal's library.

28 Hofmannsthal/Hamburger, 1963, p. 12.

29 A further sister, Iphianassa, though mentioned by Sophocles, plays no part in any of the 'Elektra' plays.

30 The dichotomy between the characters of Apollo and Dionysus, and the need to worship both, was introduced in Friedrich Nietzsche, *The Birth of Tragedy from the Spirit of Music* (1872). It was through the Dionysiac, the author argued, that the spirit of music revealed itself, notably in the work of Richard Wagner.

31 *Salome/Elektra* ENO/RO Guide (1988), p. 119. The translation is mine. (Here the opera libretto is more succinct than the play.)

32 Niobe, daughter of Tantalus and granddaughter of Jupiter, gave birth to seven sons and seven daughters by Amphion, King of Thebes. She proclaimed herself superior to Latona, who had just two children, Apollo and Artemis. The two ruthlessly punished her for hubris by shooting dead (with arrows) her 14 children. Amphion took his own life, while the frantic Niobe wept before turning into a rock, literally petrified.

33 *Sophocles: Electra and Other Plays*, trans. E. F. Watling, London: Penguin, 1953, p. 75.

34 *Sophocles: Electra and Other Plays*, trans. David Raeburn, London: Penguin, 2008, p. 143.

35 *Salome/Elektra* ENO/RO Guide (1988) for the German libretto. However, the translations here and hereafter are by me.

36 Hugo von Hofmannsthal, *The Lord Chandos Letter and Other Writings*, trans. Joel Rotenberg, New York: NYRB, 2005, pp. 117–128, especially pp. 118–119.
37 *Sophocles: Electra and Other Plays*, 2008, p. 181.
38 *Salome/Elektra* ENO/RO Guide (1988), p. 118 in my translation.
39 Ibid.
40 *Sophocles: Electra and Other Plays*, 2008, p. 185.
41 In the following summary, I am indebted to James Morwood's notes in Euripides, *Heracles and Other Plays*, Oxford: OUP, 2003, pp. 125 ff.
42 Egon Wellesz, *Essays in Opera*, London: Dobson, 1950, pp. 145–152, especially p. 148. The 19-year-old Hofmannsthal freely adapted Euripides's play into a 'tragedy' of his own, which Wellesz in turn adapted for his one-act opera *Alkestis* (Op. 35). This was first performed in Mannheim in 1924. For the text and music (in vocal score), see: Hugo von Hofmannsthal and Egon Wellesz, *Alkestis, Drama in einem Aufzuge nach Euripides* (UE, 1923), Leopold Classic Library/Amazon, n.d. [2017].
43 Adding to the inscrutability is the fact that none of the Greek dramatists consider the powerful motive Aegisthus has for revenge on Agamemnon in light of the Thyestēs episode, a motive that would have cemented his union with Clytemnestra. Nor even does Melanie Klein in her otherwise percipient study of the House of Atreus, 'Some Reflections on *The Oresteia*'. See: Melanie Klein, *Envy and Gratitude and Other Works 1946–1963* (1975), London: Hogarth Press, 1984, pp. 275–299. For her striking account of Orestes's manic-depressive personality, see p. 286. In a thoughtful introduction to his *Orest* (2011), a modernist opera derived from Euripides, Manfred Trojahn describes Orestes as "utterly spineless" yet nevertheless gifted with a vision "that saps the strength of certain influences which might otherwise easily turn him into a puppet, a tool in the hands of third parties".

In Shakespeare

Chapter 3

Under the shadow of silence

On speechless love in *King Lear*

Steven Groarke

I must admit that reading Steven Groarke's chapter that follows has left me, well, speechless. *Indeed, it is this – the emphasis on speechlessness – on silence that is, in so many ways, the very thrust of this paper – specifically Cordelia's silence in Shakespeare's* King Lear *which, as the author writes, "leaves 'nothing' (as it were) to speak for itself".*

Groarke's is certainly a complex and demanding paper, but then again so is the subject matter – Cordelia's "broken speech of a love unutterable" which stands as silent/compassionate witness to her father's suffering. Hers is a 'gratuitous' love in the most transcendent or religious sense of the word. Drawing on the significance of this gesture, the author lends new meaning to the title of our preface as he writes, "Together, witness and response remain a hard act to follow".

> . . . love is not love
> Which alters when it alteration finds.
>
> Shakespeare, *Sonnets*, 116, ll. 2–3

Cordelia is the hard act to follow in *King Lear*.[1] Lear's purgation stands in all its tumultuous magnificence as among Shakespeare's greatest achievements. The redemptive force of the play, however, derives explicitly from the ordeal of Cordelia's silent witness. We sense that Cordelia is in touch with something other than what we are able to make of her, precisely at the point where she falls silent. In developing and demonstrating this claim, I shall focus on an underlying conflict of interpretation in Shakespearean criticism, a conflict that has far-reaching implications for our understanding of literature and its value. In particular, I propose to consider the conflict between psychological (Freudian) and poetical interpretations of Cordelia. The serious challenge that her character poses for the contemporary reader, subject under the conditions of modernity to a secular worldview, is directed first and foremost at her father, the aged and dying king. The challenge consists in weighing the various existential and ethical possibilities evoked by Cordelia's silence. Lear expects to be loved, and he certainly doesn't want to hear his favourite daughter telling him what she cannot say. In the event, silence stages a catastrophic misrecognition based on incommensurable understandings of love. Lear's insistence on being fêted by devoted daughters, coupled with his youngest daughter's refusal to play the pander for the old man, proves disastrous.

The tragedy is of course open to different readings, even as Cordelia's silence admits various meanings. There is no doubt about the 'unhappy ending'. The tragic catastrophe at the heart of Shakespeare's darkest play is ineradicable; further to the shattering of their bond by the old man's folly, father and daughter are reunited only in death. Lear realises too late that he has failed to recognise his daughter's love. But does this mean that the play is ultimately pessimistic? Love isn't necessarily triumphant at the end of the play; but nor is it completely destroyed or ruined. On the contrary, it seems to me that Cordelia's restrictive speech is a sign of unrestricted love, that her silent witness is continuous with her compassionate response to her father's suffering. As such, her silence touches on the transcendent dimension in our ordinary capacity for love, indeed a love that begins in acts of kindness (Everett, 1989, p. 60).

I present this affirmative reading of the play against the background of a central philosophical problem. Paul Ricoeur, in his magisterial *Freud and Philosophy* (1970), sought to identify two opposing directions in our reach for meaning. I am certainly not suggesting that 'critical hermeneutics' is a generally agreed definition of psychoanalysis. Nonetheless, my reading of *Lear* takes its bearings from Ricoeur's (1970, p. 460, passim) account of the Freudian interpretation on the one hand and, on the other, restorative hermeneutics, understood as 'a recollection of the sacred'. The important point is that these interpretative perspectives aren't necessarily incompatible. An interpretation that attempts to 'demystify religion' may be seen as complementary to one that "tries to grasp, in the symbols of faith, a possible call or kerygma" (1970, p. 343). Together, critical and restorative hermeneutics provide a comprehensive understanding of the reach for meaning, including, our anticipation of the future (hope) as well as our sense of the past.

To outline my argument, I begin by locating the general distinction between disenchanted and redemptive readings of *Lear* in terms of Cordelia's gratuitous love. I don't intend to rehearse the long-standing debate about Lear and the reconciled life. Aside from the perennial wrangle concerning spiritualised interpretations of the play and its tragic hero, I contend that Cordelia's speechless love evokes feelings of hope in a situation that is otherwise subject to despair. The identification of an excess (gratuitous love) beyond disaster sets the scene for a more detailed reading of the conflict of interpretations, starting with Freud and the idea of Cordelia as a figure of death. Freud saw reality as inherently tragic and, in his "The Theme of the Three Caskets" (1913), he advanced a reading of *Lear* along the lines of what we might call tragic, if not ruined love.

A. C. Bradley, on the other hand, was the authoritative source throughout the first half of the twentieth century for the redemptive *King Lear*. Bradley, in his 1904 lectures *Shakespearean Tragedy*, comes to the conclusion that there is indeed "nothing more noble and beautiful in literature than Shakespeare's exposition of the effect of suffering in reviving the greatness and eliciting the sweetness of Lear's nature" (1905, p. 284). However, together with the Bradleyan approach to character, the redemptive reading remains fundamentally out of step with modern literary theory and the all-pervasive scepticism of contemporary critical thought. I accept that the affirmative reading of the play as a journey on Lear's part from power to love needs qualifying (Everett, 1989, p. 60). And yet while Lear himself doesn't reach as far as Cordelia when it comes to an understanding of love, the tragedy is nonetheless replete with unyielding acts of kindness and their redemptive reach. I remain indebted to Bradley, then, for his understanding of the religious and moral dimensions of Shakespearean tragedy.

One

Shakespeare presents us with a portrait of various extremes in *Lear*. The old man wants to be told, as Rowan Williams (2016, p. 37) puts it, that "he is loved immeasurably beyond debt and duty, beyond the ordinary finite exchanges of 'due' affection and loyalty". Cordelia also renders love excessive, but in an entirely different way to her father. In contrast to Lear's self-destructiveness, the gratuitousness of her love, understood as a sign of the sacred, is the starting point for my reflections on Cordelia as a hard act to follow. Whereas the old man hankers after public displays of love and gratitude, Cordelia bears witness to a gratuitous love that is, I suggest, rooted in the affective archaism of the infant's aggressive love coupled with a growing sense of concern.

This is a necessarily personal starting point based on my own experience of the play. I have never come away from a performance of *Lear* over the past 40-odd years, or completed a reading of the text during this period, believing that Cordelia was no more than a corpse in the final scene. I have always felt that there is more at the end of the play, more to come, than the blank pain of her death. Her reduction to "silence for ever" (Everett, 1989, p. 78) strikes me as a difficult, rather than a conclusive, proposition. Leaving aside the symptomatic reading of my own wishful thinking, like Williams (2016, p. 1), I found my first encounter with *Lear* at senior school "something of a watershed moment". I remain particularly grateful to my English schoolmaster for this piece of good fortune; in fact, I don't recall a comparable literary experience either before or since. And I agree with Williams that the play as a whole is shocking, precisely because it doesn't promise consolation or a straightforward palliative vision. We are shocked by something other than sense issuing from the heart of the human situation.

Cordelia's profound and compelling silence has nonetheless continued to haunt me as a *lesson* of sorts. Instructive in its very severity, her silence seems to me to raise important questions about the role of the religious and moral imagination in Shakespearean tragedy. I don't believe that Lear's daughter keeps silent in order to teach her father something, nor that she undertakes to do without her father in a display of righteous arrogance – although I can see how these proposals would find favour in a culture excited by the twin enticements of iconoclasm and the ablation of parental authority. But Cordelia doesn't scorn her father. She loves him unreservedly. At the same time, she undergoes an ordeal herself, an experience of speechlessness interior to the meaning and value of her character.

In approaching the play, we find ourselves in much the same position as her father – that is, under pressure to make sense of her silence. What does she bring about by keeping silent? What does the silence make of her and of those around her? And to underline the religious aspect of Cordelia's witness: does the silence admit the breath (*spīritus*) of her life even beyond the end? Anthony Nuttall (2007, p. 312), one of Shakespeare's most astute readers, poses the problem at its most fundamental: Does Cordelia represent an 'infinite sweetness' beyond mundane comprehension? Note the critical transposition of the word 'sweetness' from Lear's nature to Cordelia's in the readings of Bradley and Nuttall, respectively. The overarching distinction between redemptive and disillusioned readings of the play comes to the fore with the evocation of nothingness in Cordelia's silent witness. The distinction continues to guide readers, theatregoers and critics alike in their approach to the problem of tragic love. Broadly speaking, we find ourselves attempting to make sense of the love between Cordelia and her father from one or other of these two interpretative perspectives.

Two

Disenchantment has become something of a modern dogma not only in the sociological tradition of Weber after Nietzsche; but more importantly, perhaps, in light of the Freudian interpretation. The mythological philosophy of Freudian thought rests on the conjunction of tragedy and reality. This is evident in Freud's recourse to the figure of *'Ανάγκη* (Necessity): "If we are to die ourselves . . . it is easier to submit to a remorseless law of nature, to the sublime *'Ανάγκη*, than to a chance which might perhaps have been escaped" (Freud, 1920, p. 45). The reformulation of the 'reality principle' (Freud, 1911) as a mythic figure of necessity provided Freud with a general vantage point from which to view the illusions of human narcissism. The excoriation of illusion is integral to the Freudian interpretation and, approaching *Lear* along these lines, Freud (1913, p. 299) interprets the tragedy with reference to the psychic mechanism of 'wishful reversal' or substitution. By concentrating on Lear's love-test, his fateful whim to divide his inheritance among his three daughters, "in proportion to the amount of love that each of them expresses for him", Freud (1913, p. 292) aims to understand the father's choice as well as the third daughter's identity.

We are considerably advanced in our understanding by Freud's findings regarding the psychological depths of the play. The choice between the three sisters, according to Freud (1913, p. 300), isn't a choice at all, but a matter of necessity: "The free choice between the three sisters is, properly speaking, no free choice, for it must necessarily fall on the third if every kind of evil is not to come about, as it does in *King Lear*". Here, as elsewhere, the Freudian interpretation is unflaggingly comprehensive: whenever the theme of the choice between three women occurs in literature, as it does with the three sisters in *Lear*, "the choice between the women is free, and yet it falls on death" (1913, p. 298). On this reading, Lear's ill-fated choice reveals the degree to which his freedom was underwritten by necessity from the beginning. There was only one viable option open to him, which, with tragic consequences, he failed to realise.

The Freudian interpretation underwrites a tragic 'worldview' that admits no consolation; nothing is reconciled into 'sweetness'. Rather, the essential *un*kindness of life is yoked together with the renunciation or acceptance demanded by reality. As a symbol of a *Weltanschauung*, and not merely the symbol of a "principle of mental functioning", necessity is precisely "the symbol of disillusion" (Ricoeur, 1970, pp. 327–328). On Freud's (1915, p. 299) reckoning "the first duty of all living beings" consists in "tolerating life", and insofar as "it makes this harder for us", illusion is seen to have little or no value. Thus, in Lear's case, Freud emphasises the shattering of illusion in terms of the old man's struggle towards the acceptance of reality with resignation.

What does this make Cordelia? Essentially, Freud sees Lear's daughter – indeed, as "the fairest and most desirable" of the three sisters – as a representation of death. She appears as such, according to Freud, in a twofold disguise – namely, as the object of her father's so-called free choice and, second, as a comparable figure to the Aphrodite of the Judgement of Paris, the Goddess of Love, in her role as his "one loyal daughter" (1913, p. 298), the only one of his three daughters who really loved him. The detail as well as the method of Freud's interpretation rests on an analogy in which dreams and works of literature are seen as capable of fulfilling wishes in fantasised form. Freud (1913, p. 295) 'transposes' his interpretation of the choice between three sisters from "the language of dreams" to "the mode of expression" used in a primaeval myth that Shakespeare reworks in his play. Consequently, for Freud the wishful reversal of choice and necessity is played out in Shakespeare's tragedy alongside the reversal of love and death.

Three

Freud (1913, pp. 294–295) interprets the conjunction of love and silence, in its wider mythological context, as a defining characteristic of the 'excellent third' woman or sister. Moreover, drawing on the symbolism of death in Stekel's *Die Sprache des Traumes* (1911), he proposes that 'dumbness' so defined is "a common representation of death". Having arrived at these basic propositions (on the strength of the analogy between dreams and scenes from myths and fairy tales), Freud (1913, p. 296) is confident that he knows who the three sisters are and why the choice must fall on the third:

> the third one of the sisters between whom the choice is made is . . . Death itself, the Goddess of Death . . . the sisters are [therefore] known to us. They are the Fates, the Moerae, the Parcae or the Norns [cf. the virgin goddesses of fate in Norse mythology], the third of whom is called Atropos, the inexorable.

Lear and Cordelia (father and daughter) are thus bound together, at the very heart of the tragedy, through resignation to the inexorable.

Crucially, the necessity of death is revealed in the guise of Cordelia's "speechless love" (1913, p. 293). In saying what cannot be said, Cordelia falls silent. At this point, driven by an analytic imperative aimed at exposing our susceptibility to illusion, Freud bases his interpretation on the underlying mechanism of wishful substitution. He interprets the silence as a symbol of death, where the "fairest and best of women . . . has taken the place of the Death-goddess" (1913, p. 300) in the same way that choice stands in place of necessity. The two aspects of Freud's interpretation (i.e. regarding the father's fateful decision and the daughter's real identity) come together in and through the play of illusion-disillusionment. Freud argues that our wishes substitute for death its contrary (i.e. love and beauty) in accordance with the primaeval identity of life and death in the myth of the Great Goddess. The most beautiful woman is seen as the substitute for death, in particular, as the figure of death for the aged patriarch who adamantly refuses "to renounce the love of women" and, indeed, insists to the extreme point of madness "on hearing how much he is loved" (1913, p. 301).

Freud proposes that the third figure of woman, who comes after both the mother and the partner modelled on the pattern of the mother, appears as the figure of Death itself. Under the heading of pitiless realism, the final verdict of the Freudian interpretation is unequivocal: "the third of the Fates alone, the silent Goddess of Death, will take [us] into her arms" (1913, p. 301). And yet Freud leaves a crucial question unanswered here, concerning the 'regressive revision' that he attributes to the primaeval myth of the Death-goddess – disguised and distorted by wishful illusion. Should this obscurity be counted as a lapse? It certainly points to a matter of some psychological significance. Does the aged and dying father "renounce love, choose death and make friends with the necessity of dying" (1913, p. 301) through regression to the primordial figure of the mother? Are we meant to understand the figure of Mother Earth in these terms? Is this the figure that Lear has to acknowledge, the lesson he has to learn? Is the old man supposed to come to terms with reality at the hands of the mother who receives him at the end? Are we meant to understand Cordelia as a hard act to follow in these terms?

In one sense, Freud would have us extend the meaning of the 'common mother' (cf. *Timon of Athens*, IV. iii. 178) to death itself. Alternatively, his interpretation allows for the possibility that the illusion of primary love shatters, that the regressive tendency towards imaginary infantile love is subject to a violent and transformative disillusioning – precisely, at the point where woman becomes the figure of death for man. The ambiguity is left unresolved in Freud's text. There may be no other way of approaching the matter, insofar as the absent mother, necessarily disguised, haunts Freud's interpretation no less than the play itself. In any event, Freud (1913, p. 301) posits a formidable figure in the guise of Cordelia, where the old man's wish to be loved as he was in his mother's arms comes to nothing – "Thou'lt come no more. / Never, never, never, never, never" (V. iii. 283–284). In the name of reality, the Freudian interpretation thus emphasises what *King Lear* records at its most pessimistic – "No, no, no life" (V. iii. 281). Silence is seen as a figure of absolute tragedy.

Four

The Shakespearean discrimination of course isn't confined to negative evaluations and speechless despair. Whether or not Freud opts for tragic fatalism is a moot point; the option, however, is definitively ruled out in Shakespearean tragedy by the possibility of "a consciousness . . . of solemnity in the mystery we cannot fathom" (Bradley, 1905, p. 279). Rowan Williams (2016, p. 26) comes to much the same conclusion, regarding the reach of the 'tragic imagination' and its liturgical setting – it must repeatedly show us "what we do not know and cannot know . . . reconnecting us with whatever possibility we still possess of building the sacred into our politics". For Williams, as for Bradley, *Lear* performs the essential work of tragedy, classical and modern, as the affirmation of a future (an inner future) beyond the enactment of catastrophic collapse. There is no question that pain matters, and matters profoundly, in the evaluation of human life. Freud was right about that. But tragedy also provokes us to work through loss and, thereby to learn, by means of a decidedly difficult love, what pain does *not* take away from the world.

Turning to restoration and the reclamation of the sacred, Bradley (1905, p. 317) is the canonical source not only for the redemptive *King Lear*, but also for the reading of Cordelia as "a thing enskyed and sainted" (cf. *Measure for Measure*, I. iv. 33). Where does this reading take us? In particular, what does it tell us about Cordelia's capacity for love? Shakespeare presents us with a difficulty in the form of a paradox, when it comes to Cordelia's excessive speechlessness. Bradley (1905, p. 316), with characteristic critical acumen, suggests 'paucity of expression' as both the form and function of Cordelia's speech, which he sees as commensurate with the 'infinite beauty' of her character. This strikes me as a strong and indispensable reading. While she is undoubtedly expressive and fluent as the occasion demands; we would, I think, be wrong to approach Cordelia as eloquent by nature (Everett, 1989, p. 78). Indeed, I wish to retain the idea of restrictive speech as a signifier of unrestricted love. At the same time, I should like to suggest something more than a deliberate avoidance of 'expansive speech' on Shakespeare's part. My argument is that Cordelia *holds her tongue*, beyond both internal and external restrictions, as a positive enactment of gratuitous love.

The conflict of interpretations pivots on the idea of *speechlessness* – indeed, Lear unwittingly homes in with prophetic accuracy on the nature of his daughter's silence, instructing her with foolhardy imperiousness to 'mend' her speech (I. i. 97). How right and wrong the old man is in issuing his patriarchal injunction. Alongside his obsessive preoccupation with ingratitude, the king proves himself ungracious with his own misplaced talk of mending. Reparation is clearly wide of the mark. Cordelia's silence does amount to a kind of broken speech. And yet far from the want of mending, her speechlessness stands in its very brokenness as an irreducible manifestation of love. She isn't confined to no more than "a stubborn stammering" (Everett, 1989, p. 78). On the contrary, by 'broken speech' I mean a kind of distress, a speech that is always replete with agony and, in keeping with its function as a significant sign, a simultaneously confident and vulnerable mode of address.

The paradox of broken speech is apparent from the opening scene of the play, where Cordelia's symbolic standing is determined by what cannot be said. The play effectively takes its bearings from this inaugural manifestation of speechlessness. Something breaks out at the beginning, which constitutes the beginning itself as an excess, an interruption of the closed system of exchange that Lear would have his daughters re-enact in the name of love and gratitude. Like Antigone, in this respect at least, Cordelia stands by what exceeds her. As such, she evokes a relation to the law that is no longer or primarily tragic. Her announcement of love *for nothing* exceeds her father's patriarchal embrace; it falls towards or away from the 'broken middle' in the form – implicit but actual – of what Gillian Rose (1996) called "inaugurated mourning". To put it more simply, *Lear* reveals the extent to which the work of mourning overruns the tragic imagination; not everything in the play comes under the heading of ruined love.

Based on this inaugural enactment of speechlessness, silence subsequently assumes both positive and negative value as the central dilemma of *Lear* – indeed, where the worst is yet to come: "And worse I may be yet. The worst is not / So long as we can say 'This is the worst'" (IV. ii. 27–28). The work of the negative continues to haunt the action of the drama with its relentless emptying and undoing. Accordingly, the action proceeds towards the "dread summit" of England's "chalky bourn" (IV. v. 57), where Gloucester gropes in unraised darkness on the threshold of Milton's "void profound" (*Paradise Lost*, II. 438). The worst – "th' extreme verge" (IV. v. 26) – remains always no more than a step away; negation and cessation are a constant threat, alongside the horror of an empty end.

Nevertheless, the forces of good hold up not only in Cordelia, but also in Edgar, Kent, and the Fool. Following Lear's death, Albany, in a final attempt to stay the negative, assigns the order of things to Edgar and Kent. He does so in the name of the "gored state" (V. iii. 296) and its future. It turns out that Kent has had enough and, in any case, appears to be otherwise obligated – by what or to whom isn't entirely clear. Although of course the king had been his raison d'être; more than a feeling for authority, Kent is motivated by love of his sovereign: "My life I never held but as a pawn / To wage against thine [Lear's] enemies" (I. i. 155–156). And it is, he tells us at the end, his "master" who calls him (V. iii. 298). It is down to Edgar, then, to assume the obligation of the future as a burden of "this sad time" (V. ii. 299), and we rely on his feel for life – his natural buoyancy and religious soul (Bradley, 1905, pp. 306–307) – in taking on this task.

The watchword for the play, I suggest, is contained in the variously defined and contested meanings of 'not-yet', or what Ricoeur (1970, p. 551) calls "the evocation of possibility". Consequently, we can compare the modern Freudian education to reality with the more expansive reach of the Shakespearean imagination. The latter calls for a philosophical frame of reference that is adequate not only to what is possible (*kata to dynaton*), but also to what might become possible (*dyná-mei on*). What failure doesn't break, what is yet-to-come, is at least as important as the breakdown that occurs under the weight of failure and loss. Thus, further to the idea of tragedy as resignation to cruel necessity (an idea common to Freud and Schopenhauer), the evocation of possibility presupposes a determined use of language in which "I leave off all demands and listen" (1970, p. 551). Cordelia enacts this way of listening more fully than anyone else in the play. While there is no guarantee of educative consolation, nonetheless, her silent witness is attentive to that which is yet-to-come (the inner future), to the potentiality as well as the antecedents of "this sad time".

The temporal burden of past and present ("this time . . ."), which is weighed in the activity of listening under the sign of the future, issues essentially from Cordelia's initial insistence on "Nothing" (I. i. 89). In effect, Cordelia appropriates Lear's 'nothing' at its most brutal, the dreadful casting off of "paternal care" (I. i. 113) and the reduction of his daughter to non-existence: "Better thou / Had'st not been born than not t'have pleased me better" (V. i. 233–234). Whereas Lear's destructive love makes 'nothing' of his daughter; her 'nothing' in turn remains integral to her love. Nothingness, therefore, isn't simply privative, but functions in the wider context of the play as the condition for the possibility of anticipation. Lear is of course immediately impatient with the situation in which he finds himself placed by the calling up of nothingness; he demonstrates a passion for *not* listening: "Nothing will come of nothing. Speak again" (I. i. 90). Impatience as an obstacle to grace returns, most notably by way of Kafka,[2] as among the most trenchant themes of modernism. Cordelia, for her part, promises a more tolerant, less persecuted attitude towards nothingness which, in the context of the play, allows for the future-to-come.

Five

Cordelia's attentive, inner stillness is, I suggest, consistent with the phenomenon of prayer. Prayer is always a reach beyond merely privative silence towards a presence of some kind. As an enactment of inwardness, in which one is taught by what cannot be said, listening and keeping silent go together with speech. Once again, speechlessness isn't a figure of "absolute tragedy" (Steiner, 1990) or irredeemable negation. This is certainly true of Shakespearean tragedy, where speech and silence are never simple opposites. The fact is that speech alone can (by the enactment of what doesn't go into words) "transform silence into an act of presence, and not into privation" (Chrétien, 2000, p. 160). Cordelia says what she can: "Good my lord, / You have begot me, bred me, loved me. / I return those duties back as are right fit – / Obey you, love you, and most honour you" (I. i. 95–98). The repetition of 'you' frames a genuine expression of sentiment towards paternal authority, even as it places Cordelia in "the Court complex of power, love and honour" (Everett, 1989, p. 75). At which point, the princess falls silent, leaving 'nothing' (as it were) to speak for itself.

The broken speech of a love unutterable is open to any number of readings. I wish to emphasise the religious meaning of this gesture and, moreover, to point out that Lear follows his daughter's example only in extremis with his pivotal prayer for "Poor naked wretches" (III. iv. 28). Even as his daughter falls silent, Lear prays for the wretched of the earth. This seems to me a viable reading of Cordelia's silence: continuous with her compassionate response to her father's suffering, her silent witness represents an austere and binding expression of loving relatedness. Together, witness and response remain a hard act to follow. In stark contrast to the idle speech of Lear's two ungrateful daughters, Cordelia's prayerful silence betokens a gratuitous love. As a mark of respect, adoration and thanksgiving, in accordance with the *favete linguis* (the facilitation of the ritual acts by keeping silent), silence appears before the other and for him. How, exactly, does this differ from idle speech? Chrétien (2000) describes the interior dialogue of prayer, understood as the religious phenomenon par excellence, in terms of what he calls "destined speech". Comparable to my understanding of broken speech, he posits the "wounded word" of prayer in terms of "a silence before You" – "The silence of prayer is here a silence *heard* by God; it is still and always dialogue, and can be so only because a first silence, different and purely privative, was broken" (2000, p. 160).

Similarly, the audience 'hears' Cordelia's love in the silence. The silence of broken speech is a breaking out of itself towards compassionate response, what Williams (2916, p. 26) describes as "a showing of the sacred". Compare if you will Iago's recourse to silence with Cordelia's broken speech: "Demand me nothing. What you know, you know. / From this time forth I never will speak word" (V. ii. 309–310). Notwithstanding the profusion of unalloyed evil in *Lear*, indeed, to a greater degree than in any of Shakespeare's other tragedies; Coleridge's celebrated annotation on Iago's "motiveless malignity" (i.e. the thoroughly ineffable evil of Othello's perverse opponent) denotes a nihilism unsurpassed in Shakespeare. Nothingness thus repeats itself *ad nauseam* in a decidedly privative silence. In this case, Lear's proclamation that nothing will come of nothing proves dreadfully accurate, and as such is echoed in Regan's cruel-hearted calculation: "What need one?" (II. ii. 437). The comparison makes the point in the most extreme terms: Iago's solipsistic collapse into nihilism counts alongside the hideous brutality of Regan's destructive narcissism, which voids life and has nothing to pass on.

By contrast, broken speech issues from the call (*ekklēsia*) of prayerfulness, its address to 'You' – "whereso'er you are" (III. iv. 28) – is inscribed in the ecclesiology of Our Father (Chrétien, 2000, p. 155). To underline my main argument, Cordelia's love is imbued with a transcendent meaning by virtue of its gratuitousness. This is certainly an excessive gesture, but one that evokes nothingness at the opposite end of the spectrum to nihilism. Williams (2007, p. 68) lends weight to this argument by drawing attention to the way in which we show God's love to one another in a boundless way – "God never *starts* being in loving relationship; it's an aspect of what he is eternally". Cordelia effectively stakes her claim on these uncompromising grounds. Together with the broken speech ('wounded word') of prayerful silence, the traditional Aristotelian distinction between *kata to dynaton* and *dynámei on* illuminates the meaning of the inner future in *Lear*.

None of the survivors achieves a comparable quality of inwardness to Cordelia, who, by the end of the play, bestows an essential vitality on the ambivalent future as it appears in the gap opened up by Edgar and Albany. Lear remains confined to the end by his "monolithic inwardness" (Everett, 1989, p. 63); whereas Cordelia, beyond Kent's "promised end" (V. iii. 38), confirms the positive evaluation of what is yet to come. The latter is bequeathed through the conjunction of love and silence: "What shall Cordelia speak? Love and be silent" (I. i. 62). A hard act to follow indeed. On this stern reckoning, a silence surrounds us where we live, love and work – which presents a daunting prospect from any perspective.

Six

By holding her tongue, Cordelia exposes her father as morally and psychologically immature; but he is also a gullible and soft-hearted old man. Lear wishes to be loved even as he loves himself. This doesn't make him corrupt, and nothing leads us to think of him as a base or disgraceful figure. Nevertheless, his imperious demand turns on a basic fault and, in hankering after his own narcissistic image in the eyes of his daughters, vanity gets the better of the old man with disastrous results. Importantly, Lear is in conflict with himself before the violent collision with his daughters irrupts and drives him mad. He is undone, the calamities and catastrophe ensue, on condition that he acts from an inward sense of inconsolability prior to his madness. We can speculate about his deep-seated incapacity to mourn; in any case, something troubles Lear who, even at his best, is given to "hideous rashness" (I. i. 151). This raises an important question. It isn't clear what order of necessity connects inward and outward reality in Lear's case. We don't know what motivates his fatal decision to divide Britain between two hypocritical daughters and, at the same time, to banish Cordelia, his abiding third daughter, and faithful Kent.

Furthermore, we are no clearer to begin with about the direction of the play than we are about the motive forces – by the end of the First Act, we have yet to discover the consequences of Lear's actions. In fact, the inner conflict (which represents the hero's tragic character) is revealed, in retrospect, by the calamities and complications of the external conflict – including, the dramatic doings of Lear's daughters and Kent (incognito) as regards the main plot, and of Gloucester and his two sons regarding the secondary plot. The doubling of the action along these lines, at the primordial level of what we might call deep family relations, drives home the impression of a bleak, irredeemable world. Dramatically speaking, at least, the play turns upon the appalling characters of Goneril, Regan and Edmund, all of whom are intent on causing harm or doing evil. Lear's internal reactions, the passions of his tormented soul, continue to unfold in relation to those around him whose outward actions signify their monstrous cruelty. To be clear, the tragedy rests on Lear's decision to divide the kingdom, and to make the division dependent on public displays of love from his three daughters: who loves best gets most. As the action unfolds, however, Lear suffers as much as he acts, and his suffering comes about on account of enormous cruelty.

The representation of inner and outer conflict is different in Cordelia's case. Most importantly, unlike Lear she recognises helplessness itself – her own and her father's fallibility – from the standpoint of mature and restorative consolation: "O my dear father, restoration hang / Thy medicine on my lips, and let this kiss / Repair those violent harms that my two sisters / Have in thy reverence made" (IV. vi. 22–25). As a symbol of love rooted in kind-heartedness, this singular metaphor of reparation is turned towards her father's tyrannical destructiveness – as well as the depravity of the "unnatural hags" (II. ii. 452), Cordial's two sisters – without the least trace of vengeful intent. She is simply more mature and kinder than her father. In what seems to me the most decisive of the many reversals that structure Shakespeare's central poetic work, the difficulty of living up to his daughter's *exemplum* is the existential proof of Lear's breakdown. He fails to see love for what it is, and whether this failure is the consequence or condition of his impatience – either way, it is only when he has learnt patience (and unlearned hatred) that the old man can take a proper measure of his daughter's maturity.

In a sense, we are all in the old man's shoes; we share Lear's central dilemma in having to repeatedly sort out the difference between regressive imaginary love (i.e. how one would like to be seen and to see oneself) and the symbolic import of mature love. Shakespeare sharpens the distinction between the imaginary and symbolic registers by emphasising the conjunction of love and silence, or what Freud (1913, p. 293) called "speechless love". As the immediate catalyst of Lear's catastrophic disappointment, his daughter's unswerving silence takes love beyond the reflection of a narcissistic image. Exactly how far 'beyond', and in what direction, Cordelia's love extends is my theme in this chapter. Lear is put under pressure by his daughter's steadfast gesture; without degenerating into debilitating inhibition or hysterical misery, the young woman's evocation of nothingness haunts the action of the drama from beginning to end. We can sympathise with her father's bewilderment. There is I think something almost incomprehensible, an ungraspable excess, in Cordelia's singular tolerance of nothingness. On the basis of a certain "intertwining of the human and divine calls" (Chrétien, 2000, p. 164), her response, from beginning to end, presupposes a call that continues to reverberate in excess of whatever it is thought to mean.

Seven

The play is framed by Cordelia's silence as the action moves from her "Nothing" at the beginning to her death at the end. To begin with, she admits that her love is "More ponderous than [her] tongue" (I. i. 78), that she "cannot heave / [Her] heart into [her] mouth" (I. i. 91–92). Announcing her love in terms of what cannot be said, she supports her claim to this effect with reference to what is right and fit, refusing to say anything more than her filial "bond" (I. i. 93) dictates. Together with the mutual ties of blood, the symbolic meaning of love is thus acknowledged by means of the rhetorical figure of apophasis (i.e. saying something by stating that you will not mention it). The young woman knows that she owes herself to her father, even in ways she cannot express or that he cannot fathom. She owes him "a debt of unreserved attention and love, and an excess of involvement, care, disregarding calculation altogether" (Williams, 2016, p. 51). She says as much at the point where speech falls silent. And the paradox of silent witness deepens with her death. The sudden entrance of Lear, with his daughter's dead body in his arms, leaves us at a loss on so many levels, faced with what Freud (1913, p. 301) described as "one of the culminating points of tragedy in modern drama". No matter how often one has seen or read the play, this harrowing image remains thoroughly shocking. The old man dies in turn and, seemingly in a state of joy, commands the onlookers to "Look on her. Look, her lips. / Look there, look there" (V. iii. 286–287).

What are we supposed to be looking at? Opposing worldviews come sharply into focus here. Does the old man believe his daughter is still alive? Are we meant to read apprehensions of hope in his command? Or is this a last defence against blank pain? It is worth pursuing Freud's interpretation a little further. *Lear* is a play about paternal hubris as much as filial ingratitude, in which Gloucester's torment on muddling good and evil (Edgar and Edmund) mirrors Lear's suffering as a consequence of his own misguided judgement. At the same time, it stages the father's death as resignation to necessity. In following the action of the drama (Lear's belated realisation of Cordelia's irrefutable love), we find ourselves witness to the inner workings of a seemingly inexorable order of reality. Lear is purged, but dies enfeebled nonetheless; similarly, Gloucester is blinded in a grotesque display of brutality that cannot be undone. Adversity, at this level of extremity, seems irredeemable. The Freudian interpretation proves itself on the grounds that catastrophe marks the *terminus ad quem* of Shakespearean tragedy. Kent thus pronounces, in an appropriately solemn tone, on the old man's departing spirit – "let him pass. He hates him / That would upon the rack of this tough world / Stretch him out longer" (V. iii. 289–291). In Kent's thoroughly trustworthy estimation, the end requires only as much time as it takes for the ruined sovereign to be gone. There is no call for an aftermath, no reprise, nothing to reclaim in compensation.

And yet if we allow for the "unbearable joy" (Bradley, 1905, p. 291) of Lear's last speech (as I think we should), this creates a very different impression of the old man. We see him now illuminated in his daughter's radiance. This isn't a sign of madness. Lear is finally drawn towards Cordelia's evocation of nothingness. Once again, I don't mean to say that things end happily. The play turns out to be immensely sad. Nevertheless, we do, I believe, feel somehow enlivened at the end, or as Bradley (1905, p. 292) puts it, that "everything external has become nothing to [Lear], and that what remains is 'the thing itself', the soul in its bare greatness". One need not necessarily draw an analogy here to the narrative of

Christian redemption, but the humiliation that issues from the very ignobility of Cordelia's death by hanging is lifted up through a combined sense of joy and bare humanity. As he lays his daughter's body down, the mention of her "breath" (V. iii. 237) allows for the possibility of a vital link beyond the old man's delusions. In the humane vision of the tragic imagination, the breath of life anticipates the future to come. This is how I read the end of the play: Cordelia has managed to turn her father's "offices of nature" and "dues of gratitude" (II. ii. 351–352) profoundly inward, embodying the silence without reserve in a religious atmosphere of spiritual grace.

This suggests a very different kind of boundary concerning the father–daughter relationship in conjunction with 'the mystery of resurrection' (Josipovici, 2016, p. 119) and the restoration of love. *Lear* thus announces and inaugurates a preoccupation that marks Shakespeare's final period, the period of *Pericles, Cymbeline, The Winter's Tale*, and *The Tempest*. As we have seen, there is an aspect of prayerfulness in Cordelia's falling silent to begin with, a quality which extends its reach through her compassionate response to her father's suffering – "For thee, oppressed King, I am cast down, / Myself could else outfrown false fortune's frown" (V. iii. 5–6) – to the symbol of her death at the end of the play. In this respect, Shakespeare presents us with a character who, in the profound continuity of her witness and response, calls for something more restorative than the Freudian dispossession of consciousness. At once silent and compassionate, Cordelia lights the path of bare humanity that Lear painfully works his way towards throughout the course of the play. Shakespeare, in other words, presents us with someone whose capacity for love reaches her father in a final agony of ecstasy, and who may yet open "the door to a future even when we can see no hope" (Williams, 2007, p. 44).

In conclusion, the Freudian interpretation of the Death-goddess gets us only so far in our appreciation of *Lear*. Further to the critique of illusion, a vital belief in the world announces itself in a love that falls silent to begin with. What cannot be said, in this case, speaks of our situation in the sacred. No less daunting than Lear's "O without a figure" (I. iv. 174–175), Cordelia's transcendent rendering of "Nothing" (I. i. 89) goes beyond words (she stands by what cannot be said), but also beyond the eloquence of silence. She cannot, nor would she wish to, put words to her father's worldly demand for repayment, a return for *his* generosity towards her and her two sisters. And yet for all that, I don't think Shakespeare means to turn silence into a rhetorical ploy. Cordelia doesn't credit Lear's notion of gratitude, even while he remains insanely blind to hers. Averse to considerations of reciprocity or repayment, in matters of the 'heart' at least (I. i. 104), the child embodies a deeper sense of grace, and a more profound understanding of kindness than her father is able to reach in his person. In this respect, far from a type of persuasive speech, her broken restrictive speech interrupts the exchange of gifts. Cordelia thus defers the catastrophic collapse of meaning that is otherwise all-pervasive in this darkest of Shakespeare's poems.

Notes

1 Quotations from Shakespeare in this chapter are based upon the edition of Stanley Wells and Gary Taylor (1987); and I refer throughout to its numeration of acts, scenes and lines.
2 See Chapter 10 of this book.

References

Bradley, A. C. (1905). *Shakespearean Tragedy: Lectures on Hamlet, Othello, King Lear, Macbeth*. Second Edition. London: Macmillan.
Chrétien, J.-L. (2000). 'The Wounded Word: The Phenomenology of Prayer'. In D. Janicaud, et al. (eds.) *Phenomenology and the "Theological Turn": The French Debate*. New York: Fordham University Press.
Everett, B. (1989). *Young Hamlet: Essays on Shakespeare's Tragedies*. Oxford: Clarendon Press.
Freud, S. (1911). 'Formulations on the Two Principles of Mental Functioning'. *Standard Edition* 12: 218–226.
Freud, S. (1913). 'The Theme of the Three Caskets'. *Standard Edition* 12: 291–301.
Freud, S. (1915). 'Thoughts for the Times on War and Death'. *Standard Edition* 14: 275–302.
Freud, S. (1920). 'Beyond the Pleasure Principle'. *Standard Edition* 18: 7–64.
Josipovici, G. (2016). 'Two Resurrections'. In *The Teller and the Tale: Essays on Literature and Culture 1990–2015*. Manchester: Carcanet, pp. 114–124.
Milton, J. (1998). *Paradise Lost*. Second Edition. Edited by A. Fowler. Essex: Longman.
Nuttall, A. D. (2007). *Shakespeare the Thinker*. New Haven: Yale University Press.
Ricoeur, P. (1970). *Freud and Philosophy: An Essay on Interpretation*. Translated by D. Savage. New Haven: Yale University Press.
Rose, G. (1996). *Mourning Becomes the Law: Philosophy and Representation*. Cambridge: Cambridge University Press.
Steiner, G. (1990). 'Absolute Tragedy'. In *No Passion Spent: Essays 1978–1996*. London: Faber and Faber.
Stekel, W. (1911). *Die Sprache des Traumes. Eine Darstellung der Symbolik und Deutung des Traumes in ihren Beziehungen zur kranken und gesunden Seele für Ärzte und Psychologen*. Wiesbaden: Verlag von J. F. Bergmann
Wells, S. and G. Taylor (eds.) (1987). *The Complete Oxford Shakespeare*. Oxford: Oxford University Press.
Williams, R. (2007). *Tokens of Trust: An Introduction to Christian Belief*. Norwich: Canterbury Press.
Williams, R. (2016). *The Tragic Imagination*. Oxford: Oxford University Press.

Chapter 4

"Madness, yet there's method in it"

The shadow of the doctor in Hamlet's mirror

Paul Heritage

Like our last contribution, the paper that follows also references Shakespeare – but in a way that could hardly be more different.

Here, Professor Paul Heritage analyses different aspects of Hamlet and he does so with the help of Vitor Pordeus who is a medical doctor, psychiatrist, public health official, scientist, teacher, director and therapist.

But Heritage goes beyond Shakespeare, extending his exploration of madness and its treatment to Vitor Pordeus's own experience both in his work at the theatre and treating patients in a clinical setting.

From the initial question it poses to the final reply, we learn both how the Shakespearean theatre has found its place on the psychiatric ward: how 'sombre ancestral shadows' may well hang over both the characters played by the actors and the actors themselves. Might similar, albeit not identical ancestral shadows, hang over us all?

PAUL HERITAGE: You are a medical doctor, psychiatrist, scientist, teacher and therapist. Each role might, in some way, be considered that of a substitute father. How do you perform these different roles in a clinical setting? And what happens when you invite Shakespeare to join you?

VITOR PORDEUS: Those roles were so complicated for me for so many years. I used to just put on my white coat and hang a stethoscope around my neck along with my hospital identification pass. As I passed through the corridors everyone could see that I was a medical student, then a doctor and later a medical researcher. But the doctor became ill: I got sick and was diagnosed with depression. I started on the pharma-therapeutic path. I was prescribed lithium, fluoxetine and other antidepressants but continued my medical research. I worked in hospital labs and clinics from São Paulo to Tel Aviv and then Rio de Janeiro, all the time getting more and more sick. Eventually I was diagnosed with a major depressive disorder.

But in Rio I began to resist the pharmaceutical interventions that other doctors were making in my life. I had an intuition, at some point in 2006, that I needed theatre not pills, because I was beginning to understand that medicine and science were themselves chronically ill. Theatre was a distant memory that I still carried with me from my childhood in Realengo, a poor neighbourhood on the western outskirts of Rio de Janeiro. I began to look for somewhere I could learn to make theatre again.

So I sought out Dionysus and, entering the tumbled and tumultuous rehearsal room of *Tá na rua* (It's in the street) under the direction of Amir Haddad, an inspired and inspiring theatre maker. I hung up my white coat and wrapped myself in the glittered, sequined and patched parade of costumes in which Haddad has adorned his actors for the last 37 years as he created Latin America's most distinguishably bohemian street theatre company. *Tá na rua* is still there today, occupying an abandoned ruin of a once-glorious nineteenth-century townhouse that is a relic of Rio de Janeiro's imperial past, in the central district of Lapa. Today whenever I visit, I can still see my white coat dancing, 11 years after I had thrown it into their costume hampers, put on a skirt and began to dance, to act, to wear a wig, to explore different mechanisms of treating my own mental health. I joined the company and made theatre in the street. I went forth with the actors and lay down with the homeless who are always with us, playing their part in our urban theatre. It was there I learnt to change masks.

When I began working as a public health coordinator at Rio de Janeiro's municipal Secretariat of Health in 2009, I was still a street performer – the actor who is constantly putting on different masks. I set up a Cultural Centre of Health and Science, which eventually we named the *Hotel and Spa of Madness*. It was based at Rio's largest psychiatric hospital, named in honour of Nise da Silveira, the pioneering doctor who established Brazil's first clinical programme of art therapy there in the 1940s. At the *Hotel and Spa of Madness* I carried on working with theatre, and began to train psychiatric patients as actors. If you visit today you will find our actors – many of them hospitalised for decades – not only performing in public spaces in the local community of Engenho de Dentro but also training other patients.

I use theatre with people when they are suffering their most severe crises. The same people who rolled on the floor in our workshops and who went to the extremes of our theatrical processes are today training others from the same hospital wards.

Theatre is about masks. The father, the son, the brother, the doctor, the scientist, the director, the president and the policeman are all just the *masks* we wear. We can learn to swap those masks: to play others and live differently. When Shakespeare says that the purpose of theatre is "to hold, as 'twere, the mirror up to nature",[1] I hear him saying that we have to expose our own image to the possibility of ridicule. As Hamlet instructs the actors who have arrived at Elsinore, we too must learn to "show virtue her own feature, scorn her own image, and the very age and body of the time his form and pressure"[2] in the way in which we make our theatre. What I think Shakespeare is saying to the players and to us today is that we have to know how to adapt ourselves to each moment. We need to be ready to hold ourselves up to ridicule at one moment and to present our virtues at another – but above all we must hold up that mirror. What is most significant in Hamlet's speech to the players is that we discover that we are all mirrors for each other. We can only really see ourselves in the other. That possibility of recognition is what psychotherapy offers.

PH: Before we speak further about Shakespeare in general or *Hamlet* in particular, I want to go back to that moment when you first walked through the doors of the Nise da Silveira Institute in 2009. You discover over 200 chronically psychotic patients living at the edge of society and in the shadow of members of their families who, in many cases, they have not seen for years.

VP: Severe mental illness is so often traced back to absence or rejection by fathers and/or mothers: to a lack of parental love, to sexual abuse, violence, negligence, etc. We live in a society of shadowy abusers, of violent parents who mercilessly prey, in almost *vampire-like* ways, on their own children.

When I arrived at the psychiatric hospital[3] that now bears the name of Dr Nise da Silveira, I found the most severely psychotic patients, all from the most vulnerable social class or background. The treatment offered – which is not exclusive to Brazil but appears to have become an international 'standard' – was custody and drugs. When patients didn't respond they were given electro-convulsive therapy: the politics of annihilation, of de-structuring the individual or wiping out memory. Instead of restoring memories, which is what the Hippocratic tradition teaches us to do, we destroy what people remember, making them accustomed to a lethal situation in which they are always at risk. People die in these hospitals. They die at weekends, die suddenly. They die and no one notices. These patients become dead bodies that are then sold for use in anatomy classes in medical schools. We all know the authoritarian shadow cast by health professionals invested in a symbolic power imposed using a coercive treatment of patients with mental illness – a 'care' in which brute force, rather than dialogue is used.

Hippocrates said that it is dialogue that restores mental health. It is the recollection of memories (anamnesis) and telling of a person's history – the remembrance of things past – that brings a diagnosis. Today we are moving in the opposite direction from the Hippocratic tradition: using the shadows of authoritarianism and violence to invade the 'other' rather than respecting their limits. This is a profound psychological issue rooted in our patriarchal civilisation. It comes from god who is a man, and from the demonisation of all that is feminine. Women became devils and then witches and then mentally ill. Madness is the pathologising of the feminine through the patriarchy of men. The men that burnt millions of women on the fires of the Inquisition. Four centuries of men burning women – wise women, curers, herbalists, midwives – and then taking over medicine themselves. For the last 200 years we have lived in medicine's patriarchal shadow. It's the medicine of the father who wants to control nature. It's Faustian.

PH: So we are all living in this shadow? Not just those with mental illness?

VP: It is a shadow cast over us all – the Western shadow where, to use the Jungian perception, *the vampire* lurks. But to have shadows, we must have light. The light of consciousness. We have at least 5,000 years of consciousness, of individuality, of ego, of the development of our own inner universe, of subjectivity, of our own autonomy. The individual psychological evolution, according to the Jungian psychiatrist John Weir Perry,[4] is associated with the appearance of Solar Gods and related kings, wise and skilful men who helped the human species develop the notion of the individual. This Solar God, however, may become a vampire, and that is when tyranny and violence begins.

So we have our shadow and our light, and it is the light of our consciousness by which we are all linked. It is the light by which we dance with our bodies, paint images, recite poetry and sing songs. Absolute rationality may well come in the form of the written word – those first laws and codes that prescribe misogyny, that advocate imperialism, and that today we see as threatening women, nature and the planet. As *the word* became sacred, truth became singular and any level of death and destruction could be wreaked in the name of that same truth which, as Jung has indicated, we find repeated in myths and archetypes.

The archetype of God the Vampire is the archetype of a god who instead of nurturing his children destroys them in his mad desire for control and domination. Donald Trump is the latest manifestation of this process. He is Marduk, the Babylonian King of the Gods, carrying his nuclear lightening in his fists. The patriarchal shadows have stretched out over us creating an excess of masculinisation. "Unsex me here", we hear Lady Macbeth cry.[5] Take away the milk of my breasts because I want to kill, to destroy. There is both an excess and a crisis of masculinity as Macbeth himself waivers in his intent, so it will be his unsexed wife who thrusts him towards violence again.

PH: How does the therapeutic doctor take the stage?

VP: I think the male doctor must be the *feminine father*. The father who knows how to cure and care, and does not need to punish or control. Instead he develops his healing powers. When I read Freud, I am struck by his sensitivity not only to what the patients say but also to their vocal variations. He was as attentive to what his patients did not say as to what they did say. He listened to their silences, and would speak about them alongside the stories of their dreams.

What are we doing today? Prescribing drugs – rather than listening to the stories of most patients. We are not interested in what they have to say or how they say it. In their own ways, Freud and Jung can be considered *ultra-feminine*. They paid attention to the minimal details that the patient was producing: the variations, the emotions, the affects, the posture, the gesture, the dreams, the images instead of just the words.

Hippocrates, writing 2,500 years before them, was saying the same thing: "you have to look at what a patient says and doesn't say. You have to look at where and how they drink water, and who gives them that water. What foods are they eating? Who serves that food and how do they eat? This is all important. Does the sickness come in Springtime, Autumn, Winter or Summer?" It seems that Hippocrates was much better informed than many of our doctors today, whose measures feel *anti-pedagogic:* holding people back instead of making them better. Rather than enabling patients to become more active and autonomous, we make them more fragmented and ragged. How could Medicine have changed like this? How is it that we are destroying people rather than strengthening and sustaining them?

Of course this is not everywhere but it is particularly clear in the psychiatric population. Whether I am working in Rio de Janeiro or in Montreal, the situation is the same: rapid deterioration of health, low quality of life, diminished life expectancy, unexpected deaths. Is this story being told? Are doctors looking at the food psychiatric patients are eating? At the houses or communities in which they are living? What sort of records do we really have of the history of the patient's illness?

As doctors in the Western tradition, we swear the Hippocratic oath which requires us to pay attention to patient's memories (anamnesis) and to believe that a patient's illness – their delirium, their manias – must come from somewhere.[6] Yet we have allowed the shadow of rationality to grow over us all. It is the shadow of the father who claims absolute wisdom, who has no fear or doubt, but relies on rationality as he relates to patients and to himself; not collecting memories but imposing worldviews. This goes completely against the Hippocratic tradition. As doctors we display a form of schizophrenic behaviour that leads to the epidemic of legal and illegal drug overdoses.

PH: In whose shadow do you feel you were living when you first entered the psychiatric hospital to practice as a doctor – that of Freud? Jung? Nise da Silveira? Shakespeare? I ask you this because when I visited you at the hospital – in the *Hotel and Spa of Madness* there were graffiti images of all four of them. Their images dominated the wards and corridors. Why did you want to live in their shadows?

VP: Art makes everything possible. Art works in the shadows. Art works with the manifestation of the shadows. I was working in the same place where Nise da Silveira revolutionised Brazilian psychotherapy. The territory held ideas and traditions. It had ancestry and a rich collection of latent characters. So I decided to transform a disused psychiatric wing into a cultural centre dedicated to the history and memories of people who had lived and worked there. For the years that followed, it not only opened its doors to the psychiatric patients still resident or being treated at the hospital but it also provided a residency space for artists and arts collectives from across the city. Eight years on from when I started, the work is stronger and clearer than ever, even though the project was expelled from the hospital last year and the actors were sent hither (although many of them remain as patients). They have re-formed as a company supported by and working in the local community of Engenho de Dentro.

Over the years, the patients, staff and artists who worked with us have created and performed hundreds of plays about Nise da Silveira; but the one we produced this year[7] in a public square was, in my mind, the most powerful to date. We not only brought Nise to the streets, but also Adelina Gomes, Fernando Diniz, Emílio de Barros and Carlos Pertuis – patients with whom Dr Nise worked at the hospital during the 1950s and '60s and who went on to establish themselves as leading figures in Brazilian modernist art. Their work was seen by Carl Jung in Zurich and at Biennales and exhibitions all over Europe and Brazil. Our actors didn't have Jung as a witness, but we felt his presence when performing in the street. When I invited one of our spectators to play Carl Jung, an old man stepped forward and suddenly the Swiss founder of analytical psychology was with us in Engenho de Dentro. Our actor-patients know how to work with the stories that are in that territory because for eight years we have been training together. That is what I do. I train psychiatric patients as actors because it is as actors that they make manifest the forces amongst them as a community.

For me the question is always how to train the patients as actors in a methodological, clear way. "Madness, yes, but there is a method in it". That's what I am looking for – a method of working. Indeed Euripedes' Dionysus insists that the city has to dance, to sing, to honour its ancestors if it is to have mental health, wellbeing and strength to move forward.

So what we are doing is to generate a culture that is public and in the streets, one that nurtures communities. We have to open *theatre-clinics* everywhere and begin to work with those who are most severely mentally ill in each community. Because that is how we will open new ways forward: finding the ghosts that are there and that need to come out. Just like Hamlet does.

PH: Does theatre cure?

VP: When I look at our cast for *Hamlet*, and see the way in which Reginaldo, Miriam, Pelezinho, Zezé, Karina and all the others are evolving, I can see that there is a force. They are engaged. They are active. They are getting better. What they do develops them in a thousand different ways. They were all in a situation of extreme social vulnerability before, yet now they are working. In their own ways they are doing what they can to get on with their lives.

These actor-patients recognise each other and work together collectively. They discuss and decide things in a group. All this gives them a different experience of life. Together we have been discovering the role of 'characters' in the process of psychiatric healing. In the theatrical process, the characters are born, die and born again for every show. That's how it is when the work is well done. It is the characters who transport us, so when you play one of them, they take you with them. You see that autonomous forces are involved and that your own 'self' is in fact made up of various, interconnected characters. Health comes as we make contact with these entities for they are all elements of our collective unconscious. They are the shadows we all carry with us.

PH: In addition to being a medical doctor and a trained psychiatrist, you are also a biomedical researcher specialising in immunology. Does the body cast a shadow over our minds?

VP: I spent ten years in the research laboratories of Tel Aviv University and still work with Nelson Vaz, the Brazilian scientist who has made such an important contribution to our understanding of immunology. That research is the basis for everything I do today because it is how I learnt how to look at medicine and disease. In researching our gut I learnt about autoimmune diseases, infections and allergies.

It was laboratory-based research that taught me how an organism works and how it is affected by culture, ecology, air quality, seasonal changes, food and diet. Vaz's research has shown how the mucosal immune system (the collection of microscopic species that live in us) profoundly affects our overall wellbeing. It was an ecological vision that looks for a dynamic equilibrium between nature and culture which guided how we set up the Centre of Culture, Science and Health for severely psychotic patients in Rio de Janeiro.

Nise da Silveira was what today we might call an *ecological doctor* because she was influenced by the images of emotions of disease. Diseases are controlled by emotions, as she knew from her reading of the Dutch philosopher Spinoza who I would describe as a 'seventeenth-century ecologist'. It is Spinoza who insisted that mechanical thinking will not give us the solution to life. We have to understand **affect** if we are ever to understand the human mind. We need to know what we mean by freedom and by culture. We need to know the importance of symbols and words, of everything that makes up the normal functioning of our psyche. There – in the hospital with the severely disturbed patients – I understood how the theatre that I had learnt to make in the streets was linked to the work that Nise da Silveira had initiated in the same hospital over 70 years ago.

The basis of street theatre is improvisation. Dr Nise, citing Kandiski, showed that the images of the unconscious emerge through improvisation. As a doctor, one has to learn to work with images as they emerge, just as Hamlet has to learn to deal with the ghost of his father and Macbeth must conduct a dialogue with the witches. Ghosts and witches are archetypal images. With these images you can start to make connections: as you simulate a family in the circle of the theatre, you can start plugging up 'the holes', i.e. those traumas that each patient carries in their memories. In our competitive world what we are missing is for people to find ways to be in neighbourhoods, in families. As you heal the traumas, then pleasurable, creative ways of being together become possible. We stimulate communal awareness to create a celebratory gathering, a collective ritual of theatre, which restores memory and builds the patrimony of a community. That's the cure. That's how people make advances.

PH: When Hamlet improvises and says he wants the players to present a play that "will catch the conscience of the King", he and Shakespeare seem to have an absolute faith in theatre's irresistible power over an audience. Is that what you mean by a cure?

VP: Theatre provides its own "biomedical laboratory for immunological research". In the *theatre laboratory* we are dealing with affective reactions, revelations, surprises, the removal of masks, conflicts and confrontations with aggression, hate and the instincts that can lead to murder. Great plays take us through that process. The best actor is the one who can liberate all these things by letting energies flow. And the psychotic is the best actor of all because psychosis is a flux and flow of characters. We stage what John Weir Perry[8] might describe as a cascade of images, a ritual drama of renewal.

Theatre brings the constant promise of change: the metamorphosis of Dionysus who transforms himself into different characters. I work in a way that doesn't specify or fix roles. We have actors who lead or dominate certain roles, but generally the cast play all the characters. Everyone gets to play Dionysus one day and Hamlet the next, including the schizophrenics who learn their words by group declamation and repetition. As we are reciting the text, they are learning the words.

After all these years we have a number of ex-patients, still actors with our group, who 'speak Shakespeare' in their everyday lives. They all begin by speaking act 3, scene 2 of *Hamlet*, which for two years we presented every Wednesday afternoon as the sun set on the rocks that frame the beach at Ipanema in Rio de Janeiro. They have a ritual theatrical language that has immense power to generate meaningful memories.

PH: *Hamlet* is more than just a play about a son confronting his father, but about sombre ancestral shadows that hang heavy over all the characters. You often talk about the importance of ancestral roots of trauma for your patients that go beyond their particular family context. How does this evolve through your use of Shakespeare in a clinical context?

VP: The wards of all psychiatric hospitals are full of poor people. Poverty makes mental illness more prevalent and much more severe, just as it does all disorders whether cancer or heart disease. The poorer a person is, the worse their clinical state, the more morbid is the evolution of their disease and the greater risk of mortality. In Brazil we are witness to a genocide of the poor that, from a psychological perspective, is a paternal betrayal. Our fathers invaded this land, raped the indigenous women they found here and the black women they brought as slaves but refused to recognise their own offspring. We were brought up by the strength of our mothers. Brazil is a matriarchal society. We have the African religions of Candomblé and Umbanda – kingdoms where women reign – that are being destroyed for the practice of witch-hunt all over again by the same patriarchs that are repeating the traumas of the Inquisition.

Brazil as a country is like a child without its father, seeking an identity that can overcome the traumas and unite us around a project of citizenship that includes at least the minimal respect for children. Brazil is guilty of national infanticide. We are abusing our children. Young people live on the street. You don't see that anywhere else in the world: children abandoned on the street, being brought up on the street. What sort of future will that give us? I see this as a psychological defect, because we want to grow but we don't want to do the necessary work. We have to address the fundamental issues of how the 'House of Brazil' has been built. The basic psychology of our country is so disturbed that we are faced with ever-increasing violence. It is Hamlet's dilemma.

PH: Colonialism is 'a hard act to follow'?

VP: We always live in its shadow. There is something in Brazil's ancestry that strengthens us today, but there is also a permanent trauma of our history of slavery which saw over five million Africans forcibly moved to this country. We still live with the legacy of 385 years of ideological persecution by the Holy Inquisition of the Catholic Church. The Inquisition was state-sponsored psychological and ideological terrorism. A rule of fear reigned in which anyone could be denounced, and you had to have money to buy yourself a legal defence against being prosecuted and losing everything. Imagine living under the terror of being burnt alive in the public square? This has traumatised generations who still live in fear. It is one of our greatest traumas. The genocide continues and we continue to live with murderous fathers. As Macbeth says:

> Blood hath been shed ere now, i' th' olden time,
> Ere human statute purged the gentle weal;
> Ay, and since too, murders have been performed
> Too terrible for the ear. The times have been
> That, when the brains were out, the man would die,
> And there an end. But now they rise again
> With twenty mortal murders on their crowns
> And push us from our stools. This is more strange
> Than such a murder is.[9]

There is a "smell of blood" in Brazil as there is on Lady Macbeth's hands, and not all the perfumes of Arabia will remove it until we learn to deal with this shadow. Denial doesn't work. Denying the violence of our past makes it worse in the present and for the future.

Theatre, poetry, music, dance, visual images can re-signify the shadows and the cycles of death and rebirth that we cross and re-cross in such disturbed ways. It shouldn't be like this. We have to learn to deal with our birth and our death and to find some sort of harmony between them. Mental health and wellbeing is found in the ways in which we ritualise who we are and who our ancestors are: our history and our community. We find our common humanity in dance and song. In the vowels of our words.

PH: As when Othello incants "Blood, blood, blood" to Iago? Shakespeare knew that the actor needs all three words. The repetition of those long vowels will connect deep with the ancestry of his audience whose fathers and grandfathers had been soaked in the blood of the Battle of the Roses.

VP: It is this ritual which binds us in the theatre. Over the eight years of the Hotel and Spa of Madness, the actor-patients at the Nise da Silveira Institute began to speak of their joy. Joy is the sacred force of healing. Spinoza says that joy increases our capacity to engage with the world. Joy is a recognition of your moment, of the greater potential in your destiny.

PH: Did you find Denmark inside the hospital?

VP: The psychiatric hospital is ruled by King Claudius, the vampire. As Hamlet says,

> For my uncle is King of Denmark and those that would make mouths at him while my father lives give twenty, forty, fifty, a hundred ducats apiece for his picture in little. 'Sblood, there is something in this more than natural, if philosophy could find it out.[10]

In a psychiatric hospital you see corruption, misuse of money, deaths of patients who don't need to die. If you work at a weekend or at nights as I did, then you see how the patients are abandoned to their fate. They are given appalling food, then drugged up with psychotropic drugs, to be locked up and immobilised. What result can we expect? Acute heart attacks. Sudden deaths. An electric shot to the heart. They have turned the place where Nise da Silveira worked into a concentration camp with her name above the gate. If you use drugs as your principal treatment method, and no one believes that painting or theatre can help resolve a patient's problems, then we are just going backwards. Those of us who work with Shakespeare and theatre know what is an act, what is a scene, what is a prologue and an epilogue. We have to know these things to be able to organise narratives, to be able to position characters.

PH: You propose the ritual of theatre as an opposition to the rites of the medical profession but it is not just the act of making theatre that fascinates you. You are discovering how Shakespeare's characters and his narratives affect your patients. The opening scene of *Hamlet* sets up what might be described as the ultimate 'hard act to follow' when Hamlet sees the ghost of his father. How did you use the relation of Hamlet with his father in your work?

VP: The actor who has played Hamlet for over eight years at the Hotel and Spa of Madness is Reginaldo Terra. A survivor of the Brazilian psychiatric system where he has been incarcerated since he was 11 years old, Reginaldo himself is a living shadow. He carries all the ills, all the abuses, all the violence of the system. Over four decades he has lost one leg and all of his teeth, yet he is a great actor. He is infallible. He has never missed one workshop, rehearsal or performance. Even today, he still participates every Tuesday and Thursday with the group that now performs outside the hospital in the local neighbourhood. Reginaldo is the archetypal sun king who we found on the wards, and he always plays the king in our productions. As Nise da Silveira demonstrated, in patients diagnosed with chronic psychosis, we frequently see them manifest archetypes in a more abundant, dramatic and even poetic way. As Reginaldo plays the ghost of Hamlet's father (the former king) who is "doomed for a certain time to walk the night", he must tell us in every performance that "the serpent that did sting thy father's life, now wears his crown".[11] We hear his urgent plea for justice. It is the cry we must hear in that hospital. He is the ghost of the murdered father, which is the shadow of our positive psychological energy assassinated by our negative psychological energy. Just as in a psychotic crisis or a schizophrenic syndrome. It is a broken, corrupt state of being – a deep social crisis, like the agitation that we have heard is breaking out in Denmark. The state itself is fragile and may fall at any moment. A coup d'état is in the air. Our actors bring all that uncertainty in their very bodies. They are explosive forces that need to be heard above the acute, violent psychic crises.

Shakespeare's theatre has found its place on the psychiatric ward. Reginaldo is an actor who is always on stage. He has critical distance and is never defeated or bowed. He is always good humoured and always playing, drawing in everyone with his performance. He is a true actor who, as Shakespeare says at the end of *The Tempest*, is set free by the applause of the audience.

The world of Shakespeare – of dreams, madness, murders, traumas, tragedies, comedies – is the material world of these patients. As they teach us about their chaotic and closed world through these plays, they also teach us about the plays themselves. They show us what a ghost really is. They show us that a terrible mother can sometimes be a seductive goddess. They show us the devil himself. With their help, we see that character is a projected, archetypical shadow, and this is an acknowledgement of our ancestry.

Knowledge comes to us in the form of shadows and in the shape of masks. In the language of Yoruba, 'mask' indicates a spiritual ancestor. Without our spiritual ancestors we cannot know ourselves and are condemned to suffer the high seas of mental illness, tossed from side to side. To know our masks is to know our history, our ancestral roots and to recognise our shadows. It is to know Shakespeare.

Notes

1 *Hamlet* act 3, scene 2.
2 Ibid.
3 In Engenho de Dentro, one of Rio de Janeiro's northern suburbs.
4 Weir Perry, J., *The Lord of the Four Quarters: Myths of the Royal Father* (New York: G. Brazilier, 1966).

5 *Macbeth* act 1, scene 5.
6 See Pordeus, V. and Rosenberg, L., The Disease as Oracle: Anamnesis, Diagnosis and Prognosis: Past, Present and Future, *EC Psychology and Psychiatry Review*, www.ecronicon.com/ecpp/pdf/ECPP-05-00158.pdf.
7 2017.
8 Weir Perry, *The Lord of the Four Quarters*.
9 *Macbeth* act 3, scene 2.
10 *Hamlet* act 2, scene 2.
11 *Hamlet* act 1, scene 5.

Part II

‘I’-witness accounts

In psychoanalysis

Chapter 5

'Derealization'

In the shadow of *the son*

Faye Carey

Why would the earliest, grandiose feelings we all have at the start of life accompany us unconsciously to its very end? How and why did these vestiges of infantile omnipotence accompany Freud on his trip to the Acropolis, age 48? The chapter that follows focuses on the uncanny sense of timelessness – indeed, immediacy – of our unconscious and the exciting yet disturbing feelings it may occasion.

Why this disturbance in Freud? As Faye Carey emphasises below, there was more to Freud's experience in Greece than a sense of triumph over the father through worldly achievement – an Oedipal fantasy certainly – but perhaps a denial of even the need for a father – the fantasy of the self-made baby, or one borne solely of the mother, that is at play here, or what the author has described as "parthenogenesis on the Parthenon". In this context, who is the hard act to follow? Let's read on.

Introduction

In his classic work, 'Cognitive Development', Roger Money-Kyrle (1968) states, 'What actually seems to happen is that, while part of the developing personality does learn to understand the facts of life, suffers the pains of an Oedipus complex, discards it from guilt, becomes reconciled to the parental relation, internalises it and achieves maturity, other parts remain ignorant and retarded.'

One way of thinking about the psychoanalytic project is to consider three common and rarely entirely relinquished misconceptions, often encountered clinically, and succinctly summarised by Roger Money-Kyrle (1968, 1971) as the mistaken belief – regardless of logic and evidence to the contrary – that we have created ourselves, that we have nurtured ourselves, and that we are immortal. Freud's (1936) account of his strange experience on the Athenian Acropolis touches on these ordinary delusions – significantly those to do with conception and mortality. The event itself took place when Freud was 48, and perplexed him well into his later years, lending credence to Money-Kyrle's insight that these earliest, necessarily grandiose, fantasies –inevitable at the start of life – often accompany even the most self-reflective of us, however unconsciously, to its very end.

I see vestiges of this infantile omnipotence evident in those feelings described by Freud as the 'derealization' that characterises the story of his visit to Athens, written in response to an invitation to contribute to the 70th birthday celebrations honouring a distinguished friend, the French philosopher Romain Rolland. The account that Freud describes as "a disturbance of memory" (Freud, 1936) then unfolds as a first-hand example of the timelessness and immediacy of the unconscious that treats historical events as current.

The phenomenon that Freud describes has a distinctly uncanny character that I trace back to the earliest defences against separation, loss and the consequent intimations of mortality, alongside fear of the return of something that has been repressed. Such experiences seem to take the subject by surprise – both back to the womb, and forward to the tomb – which may contribute to the characteristically vertiginous feelings and associated compression or distortion of time, wherein a deep, sensual memory of the first alarming experiences of severance both within the self (splitting) and from the other (separation) provide a premonition of an end to life that touches on the mortal terror implied in Bion's (1962) "nameless dread".

Freud described the experience of 'derealization' as being akin to, but in some ways the obverse of, 'déjà vu', that is to say, an experience of something that *should* be familiar, yet is unexpectedly strange: in fact, the quintessence of estrangement, standing unexpectedly outside of one's sense of self. In his eventual but, in my view, incomplete analysis of this incident (at any rate, in the published version of the memory), Freud recognised this as a psychological event containing elements that were both defensive, evasive and deeply rooted in early emotional and sensual experience. His analysis focused primarily on Oedipal anxieties, but here I want to suggest a complementary and extended approach to that understanding. I use Freud's account of his unexpected visit to Athens as a point of departure, to explore these ideas. But to do this, I begin with another city: Rome.

Rome – the *internal* city

In 'Civilization and its Discontents' (1930) Freud uses Rome to illustrate his concept of the structure of the mind, stating,

> in mental life nothing which has once been formed can perish – that everything is somehow preserved and that in suitable circumstances . . . it can once more be brought to light.
>
> (p. 69)

Evidence of Rome's continuing existence from her earliest foundations to the present day is visible in the traces and ruins of the modern city, where

> there is certainly not a little that is ancient still buried in the soil of the city or beneath its modern buildings. This is the manner in which the past is preserved in historical sites like Rome.
>
> (p. 70)

If this were the description not of the archaeological strata of an excavated, yet still living city, but of a "psychical entity", it would effectively describe a system 'in which nothing that has once come into existence will have passed away and all the earlier phases of development continue to exist alongside the latest one such that everything that has once been, continues to be' and,

> In the place occupied by the Palazzo Caffarelli would once more stand – without the Palazzo having to be removed – the Temple of Jupiter Capitolinus; and this not only in its latest shape . . . but also in its earliest one, when it still showed Etruscan forms and was ornamented with terracotta antefixes. . . . And the observer would perhaps only have to change the direction of his glance or his position in order to call up the one view or the other,
>
> (p. 69)

an analogy that accurately expresses not only the tenacity of the contents of the mind, even those that should not, logically, coexist but also, a strategy for discovering those contents by "changing the direction of one's glance", for example, through psychoanalysis.

For many, Rome, like Athens, is at once mythical and real. Both cities, and iconic sites like them, exist in (at least) three registers. The current place (mapped, measured, visible, visitable), the historical site (mapped, measured, recorded) and the mythical, bequeathed and inherited through tales and legends, some of which can be seen to have a basis in scientific fact – a category, therefore, that accommodates a continuous, at times imperceptible, slippage between fantasy and reality, such as Freud's lifelong perception of Athens. Here, first impressions may predate the actual experience of Rome itself, the imagined city constructed from fables, histories, maps, and images. Early accounts may then be superseded by a visit, the physical experience underpinning or possibly contradicting first impressions, but in any event generating a mental album of impressions floating one above the other, neither reinforcing nor supplanting, but creating an internal visual, sensual and narrative palimpsest. With a longer stay, the city may become more concretely familiar through walking, working, living, loving, learning the language. This version may come to dominate the conscious perception of Rome, but – just as Freud describes – the others still survive, silently, secretly, in dreams, unwilling to surrender their position in some part of the mind, as if there is a part of the psyche that insists on retaining the original or earlier Rome(s), however fantastical or contradictory, as equally authentic, refusing to yield their place to succeeding accounts, however verifiable.

This sequence could apply as well to objects, spaces, ideas and relationships – including the relationship with the self – where the original, and subsequent impressions are never wholly relinquished, with the consequence that we may hold several – often conflicting – 'Romes' (or self-identities) within us at any one time, reminiscent of the Venice that Italo Calvino (1974) is compelled to describe repeatedly, obsessively, as separate cities, since no one description, however accurate, can ever encapsulate the elusive whole. Further, each version evokes, and is identified with, a distinct, at times separate and split-off self – so that while we appear to sustain a seemingly integrated and continuous sense of self, that continuity is also an illusion. The later versions do not entirely displace the earlier, possibly unrealised, versions, still waiting, not as memories exactly, but more as ghosts of unfulfilled expectations, only partially aware – and unwilling to accept – that they have been supplanted, perhaps many times over. Although these expectant and subtly influential selves remain mostly dormant, from time to time we catch a glimpse of them, a nostalgic flicker, and it is just such a backward glimpse that I believe Freud caught on the Athenian Acropolis.

In *The Psychopathology of Everyday Life*, Freud writes that one must not be ignorant of the "complicated . . . emotional impulses of which a child of some four years is capable", adding that these "same forgotten childhood achievements . . . have exercised a determining influence for the whole of his later life" (Freud, 1901, p. 46).[1]

Disturbing memories

It was in 1927, while reflecting on his thoughts on religion, that Freud, then aged 71, first alluded to a "remarkable experience" (1927, p. 25) which took place on a visit to Athens 23 years before, in 1904, when he was 48. The event remained indelible in his mind, but in the background of his thinking, only to come forward in more detailed clarity a further nine years on from that first recorded account, and fully 32 years after the actual event, in the open letter to Rolland. It is here that the word "derealization" appears uniquely in Freud's published writings (1936, p. 244), where he uses the term to illustrate this uncanny experience – not in relation to his clinical practice, but deriving from personal experience. In the earlier (1927) account, Freud remembers standing on the hill of the Acropolis in Athens, "between the temple ruins, looking out over the blue sea", when "a feeling of astonishment mingled with my joy"[2] (p. 25). Freud initially attributes the incredulous feeling to the "shallow and weak" (ibid.) nature of his belief that such a place could really exist beyond myth. He traces a linear perception of himself: incredulous schoolboy, bedazzled middle-aged man and, finally, the world-renowned – yet still bemused – octogenarian. In that later, fuller, account (1936), we see a man still grappling with the uncanny experience, still unassimilated, over this span of 60 or so years between the first and last decades of his life. Here, he returns to the exploration of this phenomenon, determined now to pin it down, which he does in the form of the open letter celebrating his friend's birthday.

Freud and Rolland

Freud had been corresponding for some years with Rolland, the French philosopher and Nobel laureate who – as it happens – introduced the term 'oceanic' to Freud in describing the sensation of religious experience, feelings that Freud either could not, or would not, recognise within himself (Freud, 1930).

The two men met only once, in 1924, but were respectful admirers of each other's work, with Rolland – having read *Interpretation of Dreams*, in 1900 – dubbing Freud "the Christopher Columbus of the new continent of the spirit".[3] Equally, Freud admired Rolland's work, referring to him as the "Artist and the Apostle of the love of man". In 1927 he sent him a copy of 'The Future of an Illusion', which provoked Rolland to enquire into Freud's position regarding "spontaneous religious feelings". Freud responded that his "remarks on the feeling which you name 'oceanic' leave me no respite" (Freud, 1929, p. 388). He maintained, nevertheless, that he was as "closed to mysticism as to music", and that Rolland should not look for any note of conversion in his forthcoming volume, 'Civilization and Its Discontents', in which he does, indeed, analyse 'oceanic feelings'.

Still wrestling with the subject, in response to the celebratory invitation almost 10 years on, Freud revisited the unresolved puzzle of the enigmatic feelings that overcame him on the Acropolis, and set out his thoughts, describing in some detail the journey that took place many years before, the memory of which had remained elusive and disturbing over these many decades.

A disturbance of memory

> *"What I see here is not real." Such a feeling is known as a "feeling of derealization".*
>
> (Freud, 1936, p. 244)

The open letter recounts the summer of 1904 when, aged 48, Freud was holidaying with his only surviving brother, Alexander, younger by 10 years, and planning at this point to travel from Trieste to Corfu. However, while in Trieste the brothers were advised by an acquaintance that a visit to Athens would be a better choice at that time of year, and, although apprehensive, they duly set off the following day for Athens with uncharacteristic spontaneity. Arriving in Athens, Freud reports,

> As I stood on the Acropolis and cast my eyes around upon the landscape, a surprising thought suddenly entered my mind: "So all this really *does* exist, just as we learnt at school!" To describe the situation more accurately, the person who gave expression to the remark was divided, far more sharply than was usually noticeable, from another person who took cognizance of the remark; and both were astonished, though not by the same thing. . . . The second person on the other hand was justifiably astonished, because he had been unaware that the real existence of Athens, the Acropolis, and the landscape around it had ever been objects of doubt. What he had been expecting was rather some expression of delight or admiration.
>
> (Freud, 1936, p. 241)

Here Freud appears to be describing an emerging awareness of a splitting or fragmenting of the self, where the mind is at once holding a number of perceptions that are both complementary and contradictory: the present actual experience of the middle-aged man on the Acropolis, bears within him the long-held multiple perceptions of the schoolboy, that Athens was only a myth / that it was a real historic site / that it was a city existing in real time. Both the child, and the man, understood that it was of course all of these, but somewhat less aware that they were also held as separate, contradictory, perceptions. It is the very strangeness of the experience at the time that moves him to set aside the more pragmatic, seemingly logical explanation for this response – the wonder at finally seeing what had only ever been imagined since childhood, whether as myth or reality – and turns instead to an interpretation that acknowledges something more elusive, enigmatic, suggesting an element of repression that may perhaps contribute to the uncanny quality of the event.

He discerns two distinct reactions: the first is incredulity – how could it be that this long held desire has finally been realised, and seemingly so unexpectedly – as if transported there by wishful thinking. The second is a disturbed and somewhat depressive feeling, the antithesis of excitement, more a sense of disquiet. Freud is aware that these responses – incredulity, excitement and depression that had begun to take shape in Trieste, and culminated on the Acropolis – are at once mutually contradictory and yet somehow intimately connected. The joy of achievement is overshadowed by apprehension, the simple has become complex, pleasure trails anxiety in its wake. The sensation is, indeed, disturbing.

In his incredulity at actually being there, Freud recognises that something like the defence of repudiation is at work – but why? The fulfilment of a wish should, surely, be gratifying. He is reminded of patients who are ruined by success, who "go entirely to pieces, because an overwhelmingly powerful wish of theirs has been fulfilled" (ibid., p. 242), and he sees this as essentially a consequence of a severe or punitive superego, the notorious "heir to the Oedipus complex".

Freud considers that the enormity of the wish, and the subsequent disquiet at its fulfilment, contributes to the uniqueness of the feeling. He reasons: "I could really not have imagined it possible that I should ever be granted the sight of Athens with my own eyes – as is now indubitably the case!" (p. 243). But as the ambition had remained alive, although dormant, for some 40 years, its sudden achievement felt overwhelming. So the further question arises as to why such a thought should remain quiescent, in such a dynamically suppressed form. The core feeling is incredulity, which Freud says, has been "doubly displaced"; first, it is transposed from the present to the past, and second, "from my relation to the Acropolis on to the very existence of the Acropolis" (ibid.).

How have these transpositions come about? He reasons that there must first have been something of the 'unbelievable and the unreal' in the current situation. The existence of the Acropolis cannot be doubted, so the sense of uncertainty must be associated to the past, specifically, the wonder that so mythical a place really exists. This deeply ingrained incredulity seems to have been transferred to the present and, in spite of the actuality of the place being now undeniable, he thinks: "What I see here is not real" (p. 244). It is this ineffable, complex and little understood phenomenon that Freud defines as "derealization" (*Entfremdungsgefühl*) and that, while not so unusual, has nonetheless something of an abnormal structure about it.

Freud distinguishes between derealisation and other similarly somewhat delusional experiences – such as 'depersonalisation', 'fausse reconnaissance', 'déjà vu', 'déjà raconté' – by noting that these latter are all expressions of a wish to bring something into the ego, whereas the former, uniquely, strives to keep something out.

He also notes the condition of 'double conscience' or 'split personality' that is characteristic of depersonalisation and this, I believe, is where the two similar but nonetheless contradictory sensations most dynamically overlap: not in the pathological sense of 'split personality' as it has come to be understood, but in the sense of being both indicative and evocative of the earliest site(s) of the splitting of the self.

In both derealisation and depersonalisation there is a sense of distancing or alienation from the familiar self, characteristically accompanied by apprehension or anxiety. Often described as feeling 'out of place', it is as if the place that one is in, though objectively familiar, seems subjectively strange. There may also be a distortion in the sense of time, as in '*déja*' experiences.

But if *déjà vu* can be described as an experience that is 'strangely familiar', then derealisation may be described as one wherein the familiar has become perplexingly strange, whereby something that should be recognisable is now inexplicably alien. Freud characterises the phenomenon as both defensive, harnessing denial and disavowal, and as drawing on the store of repressed memory. He then deconstructs the elements contributing to the strangeness of the experience. As we have seen, he first considers the possibility that his present incredulity is retrograde, belonging to or deriving from his schoolboy past. But he rejects this hypothesis in favour of another. Walking through Athens and up the hill to the Acropolis, he had just remarked to his brother of being reminded of their long walks in Vienna, being impressed at 'how far they had come'. It is just then that the clue to what he understands as the possible source of his anxiety appears in the form of a sudden association to an anecdote regarding Napoleon at his coronation, turning to *his* brother, Joseph, saying, "What would *Monsieur notre Père* have said to this, if he could have been here to-day?" and seen 'how far' his sons had come (ibid., p. 247).

Here, the memory that is 'disturbed', meaning both agitated and uncomfortable, does not refer to a schoolboy confusion between myth and reality, but to the anxiety surrounding unconscious wishes with regard to overtaking the father – who had not 'come so far'. Here, Freud specifically identifies the disturbance as emanating from a feeling of anxiety and guilt over betrayal, not only of his background, and his secret wish to distance himself from it. But further, the more deeply rooted Oedipal wish to triumph over the father, to have outdistanced him. Freud says,

> there was something about it that was wrong, that from earliest times had been forbidden. It was something to do with a child's criticism of his father,

> with the undervaluation which took the place of the overvaluation of earlier childhood. It seems as though the essence of success was to have got further than one's father, and as though to excel one's father was still something forbidden.
>
> (Freud, 1936, p. 247)

Here, Freud is specifically referring to the anxiety connected to overtaking the father in terms of worldly achievement. However, curiously, he does not discuss such triumph – whether Napoleon's or his own – in terms of its fundamental and physical source, the underlying triumph that is (the fantasy of) the (exclusive) possession of (the body of) the mother.

While his initial attribution to the schoolboy confusion is understandable – a form of 'screen memory' (Freud, 1899) simultaneously revealing and concealing the repressed Oedipal feelings of boyhood – of equal, if not greater significance is the reference to an even more deeply repressed wish relating to yet earlier, pre-Oedipal experiences – those more intimately connected to the mother, of whom no mention is made in this letter. Indeed, the word 'mother' does not appear in the account – other than by implication, hidden as she is, in both the Oedipal triangle, and within the Acropolis itself, a space where the mother is also disavowed, Athena having sprung 'fully armed' from the mind of her father, Zeus. (Interestingly, Greek legend does state that the mother was already hidden in the father, having been swallowed by him, unnoticed (Graves, 1960), evocative of Melanie Klein's concept of the phallus embodied in the mother (Klein, 1924).)

The body of the mother

H. Slochower (1970), who regards this work of "psychoanalytic self-revelation" as a "literary gem", describes it as an account of a journey to both the "'mother' of Western culture" and the "sacred temple standing on the mountain", that includes a significant detail of a specific repressed memory: that of Freud, aged four, having seen his mother's naked body. The Oedipal links he ascribes to the experience on the Acropolis would certainly be amplified by this voyeuristic association (if such exists, as Freud himself does not mention it in the letter). But such an association, however unconscious, could indeed contribute to his anxiety at the thought of the journey to Athens, rather than to Corfu as originally arranged, and a result of the "conflict between the desire to 'see' and the defence against this desire" (p. 90). Slochower also refers to Freud's regard for Athens and Rome as the "parents of European civilization" (p. 95) and that ideas of both mother and father are inextricably linked to both cities. It is the mother-image, however, that dominates in relation to both the city and the temple on the Acropolis (both devoted to the goddess Athena) and it is the ascent of this mount that is the source of the anxiety whereby, I suggest, the child has indeed triumphed over the father, not only by 'overtaking' him, and not only by symbolically gaining possession of the body of the mother, but connecting to the even earlier disavowal of the role of the father in the generative process, a fantasy – strikingly, here on the Parthenon – of parthenogenesis, somewhat as suggested by Money-Kyrle, above.

So, it is not only the (castration) anxiety that would be expected to accompany wishes and feelings of triumph, but those wishes and feelings relating to the actual earliest pre-Oedipal experience of truly possessing, and being possessed by, the body of the mother. In that case, the source of the feelings of alienation that Freud is describing predates classical Oedipal wishes and fears, and refers to the moment, or moments of a much earlier separation, at a more primitive developmental stage (and may perhaps be understood as 'proto-castration anxiety'). Such feelings would be associated to the moment of splitting from the embedded, 'oceanic' feeling of being symbiotically fused with the mother and the shock of recognition that the self may be a separate entity, split off, detached, isolated or abandoned. This would coincide with the moment that introduces a split in the unified self and alongside – or subsequent to – birth itself, the original psychic trauma.[4] Thus, it is not only, or not necessarily, guilt that accounts for these feelings – that is a further development – but shock, at the first awareness of such schismatic feelings as absence, loss and betrayal that give birth to at times inexplicable longing.

For Freud, then, this event was more than the unexpected fulfilment of an early ambition, but something more complex – a feeling against which he had been long defending himself – that included a sense of having over-reached himself, and that put him in immediate touch with the grandiose or omnipotent self that is part of the eternal (as well as normal and universal), delusional system described by Money-Kyrle. This feeling was both dazzling, dizzying and, indeed, disturbing.

Freud asks why it had taken him so long to fulfil this long-held ambition. Why had the unconscious 'taboo' against visiting Athens been so persistent as to prevent him from doing something he had always wanted to do and, practically, was perfectly able to do? These questions are not merely matters of curiosity for him, but also of regret since the awareness of this unconscious paralysis draws attention to other wishes and ambitions that may remain unfulfilled, that occupy the same space of repression as this one that has now come to light and, in particular, that never-to-be-fulfilled desire that is the prototype of all future frustration and disappointment, that lies at the heart of this story: the longing to return to the time before separation, and its sister wish, namely the desire for – or at least the resistance to giving up the belief in – one's own immortality.

Although in the illustration of Rome, Freud memorably compared the unconscious to buried ruins, and the task of the analyst to that of the archaeologist uncovering ever deeper strata for clues to the construction of a civilisation, in 'A Disturbance of Memory on the Acropolis', he appears to describe what might almost be seen as the reverse of this process: here, the ruins are entirely visible and yet the evidence of one's eyes is difficult to credit.

This incident puzzled Freud for 32 years. It is not until he is coming towards the end of his life that he manages to find the words to describe this mysterious event in appropriately, although uncharacteristically, elusive language (and to the man who donated the term 'oceanic' to his vocabulary) to describe the sort of mystical experience that Freud felt eluded him personally, but believed could be traced back precisely, according to Jones, "to the earliest stage of infancy, to a time when no distinction is made between the self and the outer world" (Jones, 1957, p. 340).

Freud here, aged 80, now also laments his own waning powers. He too can now be overtaken by those who are younger, stronger and more vigorous: his own daughter, Anna, for example (Zeus-and-Athena-like, as it is not difficult to imagine Anna having sprung "fully armed" from the mind of her father, congruent with the theme of parthenogenesis). She has in fact already been mentioned in the letter with regard to her then current work on defence mechanisms, and is destined to take up not only Freud's mantle – but the cudgels as well, for there is at this time an ongoing battle, on the field of psychoanalysis, for its future and its fate.

The core theme of *that* conflict is perhaps significant in relation to Freud's 'disturbance of memory'. This centred on the controversies – and the potential for both loyalties and betrayals – that had been recently taking place in the psychoanalytic world concerning the differences in approach exemplified in the disagreements between Anna Freud and Melanie Klein, that included inter alia their divergent attitudes towards the analysis of the Oedipus complex. In effect, Klein's approach places greater emphasis on the symbolic role of the mother in her formidable power and position in the fantasy world of the infant.

These ideas, with regard to rivalry and conflict seem to find unconscious expression in the letter, as manifest in the Oedipal anxiety of surpassing the father. What is missing explicitly, but nonetheless detectable in Freud's letter, is the embedded memory (more emphatically Kleinian) of the earlier experience, the infant's pre-Oedipal, pre-separation fusion with the mother, and the consequent ineradicable fantasy of that conjoined power. Freud, at the temple of Athena, on the mound of the Acropolis – as if now reunited with the body and mind of the mother – *marginalises* this central element in the story that is, it seems to me, at the very heart of the matter, being so physically close as he now, in Greece, to the actual realm of the Oedipal conflict to which he attributes the disturbance. His account acknowledges that his disturbance derives from having superseded his father in worldly terms but he specifically does not mention the key concept of the Oedipal conflict, that of displacing the father sexually. But further, it is as if the child has bypassed the father utterly, and returned to a time prior to the onset of the fear of the father, with its attendant castration anxiety and the burden of the superego; in the womb, or just out of it, it is as if there is no father and, furthermore, no need for one. This links directly with the persistent fantasy, identified by Money-Kyrle, that the infant has created himself or, at the very most, has been generated 'parthenogenically' by the body of the mother. This sensation of going back to the source, and therefore back in time – which, in any case, is intrinsic to the experience of visiting such historic sites – would also contribute to the vertiginous quality of such events.

If the role of the mother is implicit in the letter, it is more as the incidental object of rivalry and not as the source of the feeling itself. Freud does not take up this relationship overtly, but concentrates on the later struggle with the father almost as if to do otherwise would be to concede to the new directions that were taking place in psychoanalysis, with the less Freudian (both Sigmund and Anna), more Kleinian, emphasis on the centrality of the dominance of the mother in the psyche.

Haunting memories

Freud's 1936 account of his experience on the Acropolis immediately caught the attention of D. Feigenbaum (1937), who commented on the communication that same year – in fact, at the same time that Anna Freud was engaged with her major work on defence mechanisms (1938) – and reinforces Freud's (*père*'s) observation that such states are indeed defensive, rather than pathological. Feigenbaum is particularly interested in the psychological setting that produces the transient feelings of depersonalisation, locating these, as did Freud, primarily in the sphere of guilt and attendant castration anxiety, always marked by projective mechanisms. He critiques Freud's reasoning his way through those aspects of the memory that betray internal conflict, such that "he projected this denial into the past. It is a retroactive doubt originating in a momentary feeling of estrangement, against which he protected himself by this very memory falsification", the resistance, discomfort and estrangement all being manifestations of the feeling that it was "too good to be true" (Feigenbaum, 1937, p. 4).

The feeling that is being defended against, however, is not only the castration anxiety that attaches to the Oedipal situation, but its precursor – object loss – that Paul Federn (1926, 1928) sees as a generative source of derealisation. He suggests that such states may arise if a sense of the unity of the ego in time is absent. Such a fracture in a sense of self-continuity that may occur when an event is perceived suddenly or unexpectedly, leads to a sensation that the 'present' is constantly restarting, boundaries in time and space become uncertain, leading to such vertiginous feelings as panic, or a sense of alienation and isolation. In agreement with Nunberg (1923), who first identified the characteristics of depersonalisation in psychoanalytic terms, Federn traces this feeling back to an experience of the unexpected loss of the object. He emphasises the point that "the first alienation in childhood is due in most cases to a shock" in which "the ego loses its narcissistic boundary-cathexis. Every shock is accompanied by the feeling of alienation" (Federn, 1928, p. 408).

The theme of object loss appears in many commentaries on these uncanny states (Anna Freud, 1938; Selinsky, 1957; Bird, 1957; Sarlin, 1962). Bird (1957) states that the shock of separation consequent upon any loss may subsequently be experienced as a loss of reality, often expressed as denial or disavowal, as exemplified by Freud's reaction on the Acropolis. He suggests that eventual distinction comes about not through the awareness of the existence of objects but "through, and is entirely dependent upon, the infant's recognition and delineation of the outlines, configurations, and boundaries of *his own body* – and, as an extension of the body, the ego. The important thing is the body, not the object". So the first thing he must do in finding out about reality is 'to learn how far he himself goes in every direction – to learn, as it were, all his own edges'. And it therefore follows that conversely, a sense of unreality, "represents a partial return to an undifferentiated state when such boundaries did not exist" (p. 260).

Further, the sequence of separations compounds the trauma: the new-born infant from the womb; the baby from breast; the relinquishing of the mother to the father; the separation from home into the world. Each natural, inevitable, progression harbours within it the actual or vestigial traces of anxious associations to these earliest psychical events, cataclysmic to the infant ego, however inevitable. As one becomes progressively accustomed to each state, it replaces the original at best idyllic, or at least comfortable, state and the cycle of separation begins again. Each state takes on the familiar contours of a protective boundary, before yielding to the next threat: the unfamiliar and inconsolable space. In this way, the experience of derealisation is essentially a form of regression to a particular moment – albeit one that is repeated in successive new versions – which is the moment of the shock of separation from the sense of self that is, or has become, familiar, into one that is once again alien.

In all these experiences, what is essentially lost is the sense of a 'self' or a part thereof, as much as the 'object', suggesting that the uncanny nature of the experience is due to being 'haunted' by that part of the self that has been split off, yet lives on as a kind of 'ghost' twin, separated from but still attached to the part that survives, generating a sense of an eternal echo chamber such as Freud experienced on the Acropolis.

The uncanny nature of the experience

Freud says that "an uncanny experience occurs either when infantile complexes which have been repressed are once more revived by some impression, or when primitive beliefs which have been surmounted seem once more to be confirmed" (Freud, 1919, p. 249). Further, the uncanny is often characterised as that which can metamorphose into its opposite: from comfortable to menacing, homey to sinister ('heimlich' to 'unheimlich').

J. A. Arlow (1959) contrasts the weird experience of 'déja vu' with that of derealisation, and suggests that in both distortions of perception, the elusive, diverting discomfort of such experiences may take preference over a more specific form of anxiety, the very one described earlier as embedded in the conflict between wish and fear, that is both the fear of dying, and its counterpart wish to return to the womb that equates with the longing for quiescence. This evokes Freud's 'death wish', certainly, but here understood not in the vague sense of 'quiescence', but more specifically as the forbidden longing to return to the body of the mother.

Bearing in mind that Freud's 'uncanny' signified the return of the repressed within the dynamics of the Oedipus complex, the strangeness of these experiences would appear to emanate from the same source, that is, repressed memories – particularly those that predate the triangularity of the Oedipal conflict, and belong to earlier developmental states. Further, the early infantile confusion regarding the mother who holds and nourishes alongside the mother who spurns and deprives, lays the foundation for such contradictory experiences that are at once awe-inspiring and terrifying, as the unexpectedness of the moment temporarily breaches the defences that are normally in place to protect against such assaults on the sense of continuity of self.

The awesome and the sublime

I. B. Harrison's (1966) clinical research bears out aspects of Freud's 'Oedipal' conclusion, and sees the ascent to the Acropolis as analogous (in scale) to the infant in relation to the body of the mother, including a thrilling, but forbidden, trespassing or voyeuristic element. Harrison therefore suggests that the thought, "What I see here is not real", may be a form of talismanic disavowal of the evidence of one's senses, to deflect the retaliation of the father.

But it is more complex than that, since Freud's Acropolis experience suggests a feeling of awe that, as well as being disturbing, includes a powerful element of beauty and ecstasy, having something of the transcendent quality of the 'sublime', at once grandiose and humbling. Harrison draws attention to the fact that such experiences often occur in relation to iconic or historic sites such as Rome or the Athenian Acropolis but also awesome geological or archaeological features. These will often be places that have a scale, presence and significance in a collective awareness thereby evoking also a sense of group identification. Compelling and conflictual Oedipal and pre-Oedipal experience, alongside maternal awe, are common to all. It is this sense of overwhelming engulfment that may be understood as the sensation that underpins the feeling described as 'oceanic', the signature term within Freud's discourse with Rolland.

Freud did indeed trace such feelings to those moments of earliest differentiation made by the infant between itself and the mother, connecting oceanic feelings to those of "limitless narcissism" (Freud, 1930, p. 72); however, he did not appear to regard the consequences of this separation as having equal significance as those that follow from the later Oedipal conflicts consequent upon the "need for a father's protection" (ibid.). Seen in this light, it may be that this relegation of the earliest loving and fearful feelings that the infant has for the 'awesome' mother is the true subject of repression, that comes back to haunt, when defences are down, and that this was the nature of Freud's 'disturbance' on the Acropolis, in the presence of both the Parthenon and the sea, evocative and symbolic of both womb and tomb.

Harrison suggests that distortions in early development "tend to skew the awe experience in the direction of anxiety or fear" and such uncanny feelings as "horror, terror, or dread". Where the source is anxiety related to these very early stages of development, the symptom may manifest more as fear of smothering or engulfment rather than to the feelings related to the fear of the paternal phallus.[5]

Harrison (1975) links Freud's overwhelming experience on the Acropolis to such an association, particularly in view of the Parthenon's significance as a temple sacred to the goddess, and the element of wonder being associated to the body of the mother – and in more disturbed associations, to being either claustrophobically trapped within that body, or agoraphobically overwhelmed by the enormity of its power, wherein "there are no boundaries or limits" (p. 192), leading potentially to vertiginous states such as dizziness, fainting, disorientation, not unlike Freud's own experience. Separation implies loss, including a loss of identification of self. Awe, perhaps by way of compensation, involves superego or ego-ideal identification and, Harrison says, "such identifications are re-emphasized by the aesthetic – often architectural – qualities of the stimuli" (p. 193), a common characteristic of sacred buildings or those designed to symbolise power and authority.

The description of some aspects of the experience on the Acropolis evoke Donald Meltzer's (1973) observations regarding the processes of idealisation and splitting in his explorations into the apprehension of beauty, that he says has its roots in the infant's sensual perception of the elusive beauty of the mother, and the consequent pain of loss. He writes,

> What the fragile ego of the child cannot sustain and is riven by, the lifetime of development strives to restore, so that the beauty of the object may be looked upon directly, without doing "damage to the soul", as Socrates feared.
>
> (Meltzer, p. 229)

In Bion's terms, the present object is seen to contain the shadow of its absence which may account for its, at times, persecutory character, similar to the conflictual feelings of which Freud speaks in his account.

With this construction in mind, we can better understand the uncanny nature of Freud's experience, certainly as the outcome of a repressed wish, but the wish that has returned is not only the Oedipal fantasy of triumphing over the father through the symbolism of worldly achievement, or even the actual sexual rivalry that underlies it, but also denying the necessity for the father at all: the baby is at best self-made, or at least, borne solely of the mother, the result of parthenogenesis. It seems only apt that the experience takes place in Greece, Oedipus territory, where the elation of achieving this god-like status is at the same time accompanied by the castrative anxiety of hubris. All these factors appear to be simultaneously at play in Freud's experience in 'classical' Athens.

Summary

Freud's father, Jacob, had not 'come so far' as his illustrious son, and in that sense was not a 'hard act to follow'. However, Jacob was the husband of a very attractive young wife, his third, and 20 years his junior, with whom he had eight children (of whom Sigmund was the eldest), following the two older sons he had already had with his first wife, so in that sense he was indeed 'a hard act

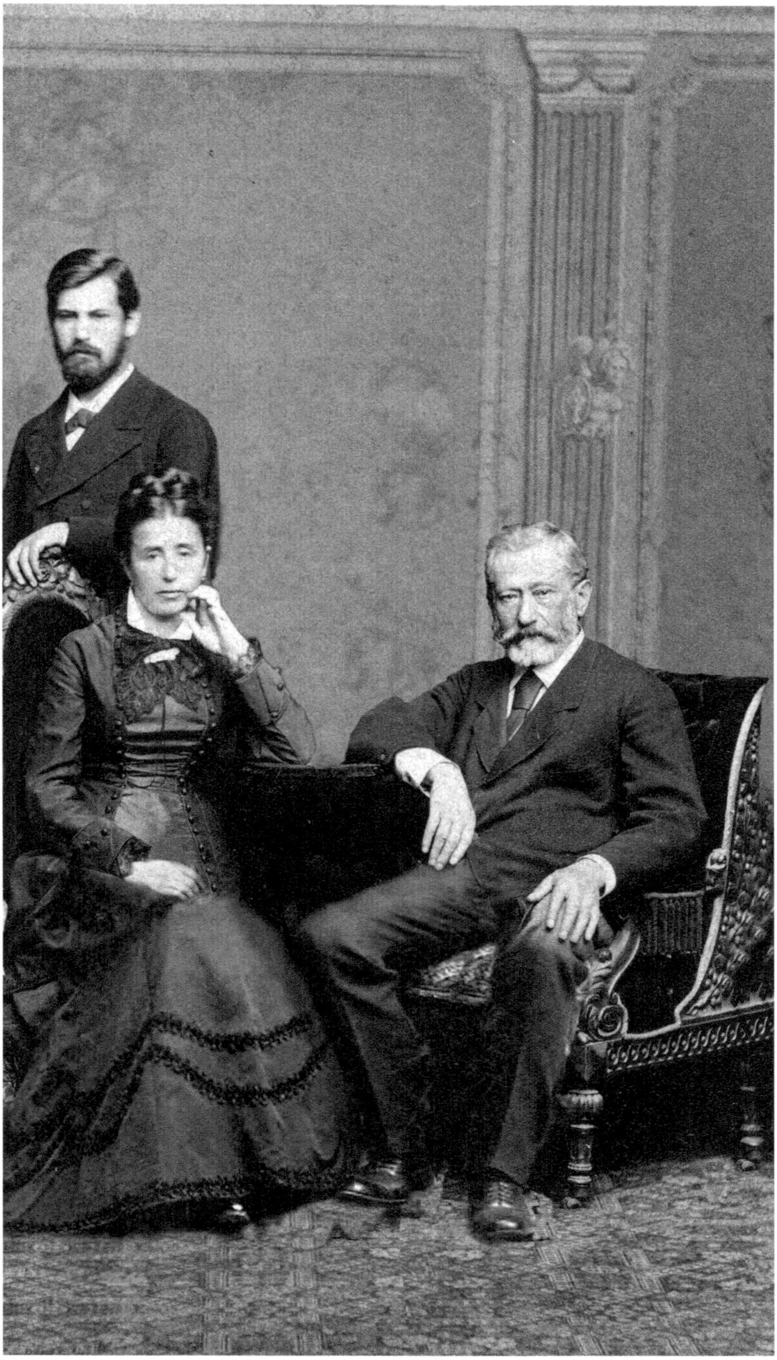

Figure 5.1 Sigmund Freud and his parents, Amalia and Jacob

Source: Based on an original image, courtesy Freud Museum, London.

to follow': Freud's mother would have been pregnant every one of the first ten years of his life. Peter Gay (1988) tells us that Freud would write warmly of "his father's characteristic mixture of deep wisdom and fantastic lightheartedness" (p. 88), but that he was also uncomfortable about his meekness in the face of the anti-Semitism that plagued the lives of Austria's Jews at the time. But whether in spite, or because of, the external reality, Jacob Freud represented for his precocious son a boundary that could not be crossed due to an internal barrier, a taboo. Freud acknowledges that barrier mainly in worldly terms in his open letter, but he does not fully address the underlying sensual element that is the hallmark of the experience of derealisation: that physical connection to the mother that takes precedence over the experience of the father, or any other form of interference. His unexpected visit to the Acropolis evoked in Freud, in one overwhelming moment, feelings linked intimately to these bonds, boundaries, separations and taboos. What needed to be defended against was both the longing and the terror of returning to the body of the mother, alongside the Oedipal triumph over the father. The defences at work were denial and disavowal that then gave rise to the anxiety, depression and disenchantment that Freud goes on to describe so vividly and so poignantly.

However, he does not expand on that aspect of Oedipal anxiety that goes beyond overtaking the father in worldly matters, that touches on not only the rivalry for the mother's love, but on denying the father's part in the generative process itself, as if there were no father, and no need of one.

The deep resistance against mother–infant separation by both mother and infant (that is to say, by everyone) is central to the experience that Freud describes in his open letter. The tendency to deny its reality is persistent, and recurs in different forms throughout life. However, separation is inevitable, and so both mother and infant (that is to say, everyone) unconsciously invent compensations for that painful, universal loss with fantasies of endless potential, deferral, revisions, repetitions, superstitions, inventive denials of mortality and persistent fantasies of everlasting life, at times readable in man-made monuments to gods and emperors such as those found in Athens, in Rome or experienced in the awesome power and wonder of the natural world.

Notes

1 Then, 30 years later, when Freud's hometown of Freiberg was marking his 75th birthday with a plaque, he wrote to the mayor saying, "of one thing I am certain: deep within me, although deeply overlaid, there continues to live the happy child of Freiberg, the first-born of a youthful mother". From Ernest, L., *Freud's Letters of Sigmund Freud*, New York: Basic Books, Inc., 1960.

2 In this connection I am reminded of another, very remarkable, experience. I was already a man of mature years when I stood for the first time on the hill of the Acropolis in Athens, between the temple ruins, looking out over the blue sea. A feeling of astonishment mingled with my joy. It seemed to say: "So it really is true, just as we learnt at school!" How shallow and weak must have been the belief I then acquired in the real truth of what I heard if I could be so astonished now! But I will not lay too much stress on the

significance of this experience; for my astonishment could have had another explanation, which did not occur to me at the time and which is of a wholly subjective nature and has to do with the special character of the place.

3 Notes on the relationship between Freud and Rolland are taken from I. B. Harrison's (1979) translation of C. Cornubert's (1966) doctoral thesis, 'Freud et Romain Rolland. These #453, pour le Doctorat en Médicine Paris: Faculté de Médecine de Paris'.

4 Otto Rank, *Die Analyse Des Analytikers*, Leipzig und Wien: Franz Deuticke, 1930 writes, "The inner fear, which the child experiences with the birth process (or perhaps brings with it?) has in it already both elements, fear of life and fear of death, since birth on the one hand means the end of life (former life), on the other hand brings with it the fear of the new life . . . The fear in birth seems to me actually the fear of having to live as an isolated individual. . . . That would mean that primary fear corresponds to a fear of separation from the whole, therefore a therefore a fear of individuation on account of which I should like to call it fear of life; that it can also come in later as fear of the loss of this dearly bought individuality as fear of death, of being dissolved again into the whole. Between these two fear possibilities, these poles of fear, the individual is thrown back and forth all his life".

5 Greenacre's research on 'phallic awe' suggests that such an experience can only occur once body-ego boundaries have been established and a sense of separateness between self and other is in place. However, in the experience of awe, there is always some regressive loss of such ego boundaries (Greenacre, 1956, p. 9) in the direction of the early infantile relationship with the mother.

References

Arlow, J. A. (1959) The Structure of the Déjà Vu Experience. *Journal of the American Psychoanalytic Association*, 107:611–631.

Bion, W. R. (1962) *Learning from Experience*. (published 1984) London: Karnac Books Ltd.

Bird, B. (1957) Feelings of Unreality. *International Journal of Psycho-Analysis*, 38:256–265.

Calvino, I. (1974) *Invisible Cities*. London: Secker and Warburg.

Federn, P. (1926) Some Variations in Ego-Feeling. *International Journal of Psycho-Analysis*, 7:434–444.

Federn, P. (1928) Narcissism in the Structure of the Ego. *International Journal of Psycho-Analysis*, 9:401–419.

Feigenbaum, D. (1937) Depersonalization as a Defense Mechanism. *Psychoanalytic Quarterly*, 6:4–11.

Freud, A. (1938) *The Ego and the Mechanisms of Defence*. International Psycho-Analytical Library. Hogarth Press, London, 1937. *International Journal of Psycho-Analysis*, 19:115–146.

Freud, S. (1899) Screen Memories. *SE* III (1893–1899): Early Psycho-Analytic Publications, 299–322.

Freud, S. (1901) The Psychopathology of Everyday Life. *SE* VI.

Freud, S. (1919) The Uncanny. *SE* XVII (1917–1919): An Infantile Neurosis and Other Works, 217–256.

Freud, S. (1927) The Future of an Illusion. *SE* XXI (1927–1931): The Future of an Illusion, Civilization and Its Discontents, and Other Works, 1–56.

Freud, S. (1929) Letter from Sigmund Freud to Romain Rolland, July 14, 1929. Letters of Sigmund Freud 1873–1939, 388.

Freud, S. (1930) Civilization and its Discontents. *SE* XXI (1927–1931): The Future of an Illusion, Civilization and Its Discontents, and Other Works, 57–146.

Freud, S. (1936) A Disturbance of Memory on the Acropolis. *SE* XXII (1932–1936): New Introductory Lectures on Psycho-Analysis and Other Works, 237–248.

Gay, P. (1988) *Freud: A Life for Our Time*. United Kingdom: J.M.Dent.

Graves, R. (1960) *The Greek Myths: I*. London: Penguin Books, 44–45.

Greenacre, P. (1956) Experiences of Awe in Childhood. *The Psychoanalytic Study of the Child*, 11:9–30.

Harrison, I. B. (1966) A Reconsideration of Freud's "a Disturbance of Memory on the Acropolis" in Relation to Identity Disturbance. *Journal of the American Psychoanalytic Association*, 14:518–527.

Harrison, I. B. (1975) On the Maternal Origins of Awe. *Psychoanalytic Study of the Child*, 30:181–195.

Harrison, I. B. (1979) On Freud's View of the Infant-Mother Relationship and of the Oceanic Feeling: Some Subjective Influences. *Journal of the American Psychoanalytic Association*, 27:399–421.

Jones, E. (1957) *The Life and Work of Sigmund Freud*. Vol. 3. New York: Basic Books, Inc.

Klein, M. (1924) The Role of the School in the Libidinal Development of the Child. *The International Journal of Psycho-Analysis*, 5:312–331.

Meltzer, D. (1973) On the Apprehension of Beauty. *Contemporary Psychoanalysis*, 9:224–229.

Money-Kyrle, R. E. (1968) Cognitive Development. *International Journal of Psycho-Analysis*, 49:691–698.

Money-Kyrle, R.E. (1971) The Aim of Psychoanalysis. *International Journal of Psycho-Analysis*, 52:103–106.

Nunberg, Dr H. (1923) Depersonalization in the Light of the Libido-Theory. Report of the International Psycho-Analytical Congress in Berlin September 25–27, 1922. *Bulletin of the International Psycho-Analytic Association*, 4:358–381.

Sarlin, C. N. (1962) Depersonalization and Derealization. *Journal of the American Psychoanalytic Association*, 10:784–804.

Selinsky, H. (1957) On Depersonalization and Derealization. *Psychosomatic Medicine*, 19: 402–415.

Slochower, H. (1970) Freud's Déjà Vu on the Acropolis: A Symbolic Relic of "Mater Nuda". *Psychoanalytic Quarterly*, 39:90.

Chapter 6

Her mother's footsteps

Marion Bower

It seems clear to me that the story of Melanie Klein and her daughter Melitta could never escape notice when pondering our theme. Psychotherapist Marion Bower sets the scene:

> *Clever and beautiful, Melitta Schmideberg was the eldest of Klein's three children. By age 15 she had already been invited by her mother's psychoanalyst, Sandor Ferenczi, to join the meetings of the Hungarian Psychoanalytic Society. Forced to leave Budapest by a 'white terror', Melitta eventually followed her mother to Berlin where she qualified both as a doctor and as a psychoanalyst.*
>
> *As Klein's work had been met by a hostile reception in Berlin, with the help of friends Alix Strachey and Joan Riviere she settled in England where her work was warmly received. Melitta joined her mother in 1930, leaving her husband Walter in Berlin for two years while he awaited a visa. In no time Melitta became fluent in English and, like her mother, began seeing child patients. By 1933 she won a prize for a clinical paper describing her work with a three-year-old girl. Indeed Melitta's output of papers was formidable and she seemed set to be her mother's crown princess. But in 1945 she abandoned her husband and her mother and sailed for New York, not returning to England until her mother died in 1960. What went wrong?*

> Last but not least, let me very heartily thank my daughter, Dr Melitta Schmideberg, for the devoted and valuable help which she has given me in the preparation of this book.
>
> London, July 1932

These are the last words of the preface to Melanie Klein's *The Psychoanalysis of Children*. What they show above all else is that Klein wanted to be on good terms with her daughter. The anxious note they strike suggest Klein's awareness that she was dealing with an unexploded bomb. Twelve years later Melitta was tearing her mother's and her own reputation to pieces.

Where did it all go wrong?

Melitta was born on 19 January 1904. In an autobiographical fragment written in the 1950s Klein paints a rosy picture of Melitta's infancy:

> I was very happy with her. I gave her much of my time and attention, and she was very attached to me and her nannie [sic].
>
> (Sayers and Forrester, 2013)

Klein adds proudly that Melitta was very intelligent.

There was a darker side to this picture: Klein was probably depressed at that time. Her beloved older brother had recently died, and Klein had taken on the responsibility of arranging his funeral. Meanwhile the work of her husband Arthur, an engineer, was taking them around various dreary towns in Silesia.

Following the death of Melanie's father, her mother Libussa came to live with her and Arthur – managing the house and caring for the children whenever Melanie was away. Two more children were born: Hans in 1907 and Erich in 1914. Whilst Melanie and Arthur enjoyed travelling together, there were tensions in the marriage – tensions that were eventually to lead to its breakdown.

In 1910, however, life for the Kleins was looking distinctly good – with Arthur having secured a job in Budapest, a city that was then very much the glittering fin de siècle capital, with café life, concerts and opera. All this culture was a magnet for Melanie. At the same time her most important discovery was clearly a copy of *The Interpretation of Dreams* by Freud. Never shy, she approached Sandor Ferenczi, then president of the Budapest Psychoanalytic Society, and asked him to take her into analysis, which he did. It was not a minute too soon, as around this time, Libussa died.

Although Ferenczi was president of the Budapest Society, his methods were becoming increasingly unorthodox. He was beginning to exchange demonstrations of affection with his patients, for example, and in later life, according to Klein, he would only work with the positive transference. It was probably this experience that later drew Klein to Abraham, whose method was more rigorous.

For his part, Ferenczi was sensitive to Klein's affinity for children and encouraged her to take up this work. Klein's first patient was in fact her young son Erich (in the early days of psychoanalysis, the parent was thought to be the best person to psychoanalyse a child; Freud analysed his adult daughter). Though unable to free-associate like an adult, Klein found Erich best able to communicate through his play. Accordingly she gave him a regular 'analytic hour'. One can only assume that it would have been difficult for Melitta and Hans to have their mother so focused on their younger brother.

Klein wrote her membership paper for the Budapest Society based on her work with Erich, and qualified in 1919 when Melitta was 15. According to Melitta, around this time she too was invited by Ferenczi to attend the Budapest Society meetings. This was the beginning of a pattern in which Melitta could get close to her mother by following in her footsteps.

This somewhat happier period did not, however, last. The political upheavals in Budapest led to an intensely anti-Semitic 'white terror'. Ferenczi was forcibly removed from his university post. This must have been frightening for Melitta, and for her parents as well. Yet 20 years later Melitta was to liken her mother to Dr Goebbels, the Nazi minister for propaganda.

Initially Klein took the children to Ruzomberok in Slovakia, to Arthur's parents with whom she shared a friendly relationship. With difficulties between Arthur and Melanie increasing, however, the couple used this opportunity to separate, with Arthur moving to Sweden – whilst the marriage as yet continued. Klein also wanted her analytic work to continue and soon decided to move to Berlin, at that time very much considered the cutting edge of psychoanalytic work. This was partly due to the president of the Berlin Society, Karl Abraham, who was both rigorously Freudian and an independent thinker.

The society also had a purpose-built clinic[1] financed by Max Eitingon, where free or low-cost analysis was offered. In the aftermath of the First World War the clinic had been flooded with patients, including children who referred themselves. In addition it offered the first formal training in psychoanalysis, which Melitta was later to follow. At this time, however, Melitta was to stay with her grandparents and study for her matriculation examinations (learning Slovak in the process). It may not have been particularly easy to be left behind while Klein went to exciting Berlin with the boys; but in the event Melitta passed her examinations, then joined her mother and brothers in Berlin where she enrolled at university.

Initially Melitta decided to study philosophy but switched to medicine. It is likely that her mother had had a hand in this, as Klein's own ambition to study Medicine had been cut short by her early engagement and marriage. It seemed Melanie wanted Melitta to have what she herself could not have.

In time Melanie and Arthur decided to try and patch up their marriage. They rented a handsome house in Dahlen, a suburb of Berlin. (Erich remembers Melitta placing a star atop the Christmas tree there.) As Klein's consulting room was in the house, the children were expected to tiptoe around while their mother was seeing patients. A picture gradually emerges of a mother preoccupied with her own concerns: when Melitta was young Klein was preoccupied with the two younger boys; later it would be her work with other people's children. The German psychoanalyst Karen Horney, for example, sent her two daughters to Klein; later, sceptical of Klein's theories, Horney would become Melitta's analyst.

Despite their efforts, the relationship between Arthur and Melanie eventually broke down permanently. Klein had a passionate affair with a journalist, C. V. Kloetzel, and Arthur was probably also having an affair. After the separation Klein had to move to new albeit shabbier accommodation, taking Melitta and Erich with her, while Hans, who was planning to follow Arthur's profession and become an engineer, went with his father.

In the field of psychoanalysis Karl Abraham, the president of the Berlin Society, was considered the analysts' analyst. Some thought him better than Freud. He was certainly strict with analytic boundaries, something that Klein was to follow – whilst Melitta was to flout (by giving a young patient a birthday present, for example).

Klein wanted analysis with Abraham, but he did not believe in analysing colleagues. In 1924, however, Klein gave a presentation of her work, after which Abraham exclaimed "the future of analysis lies in the play technique" (Grosskurth, 1986). After this Abraham could not refuse Klein as a patient. Still he was right about colleagues who were patients. These *analytical sibling* relationships were to lead to some very thorny relationships later in England, particularly between Klein and Edward Glover, who had also been a patient of Abraham.

Not everyone was enthusiastic about Klein's work. Some of her colleagues in Berlin thought children would faint with horror at Klein's interpretations. However Alix Strachey, who had come from England at the time, along with the brothers James and Edward Glover, found Klein's work entirely convincing, and wrote to her husband James (fellow translator of Freud) about it. James Strachey suggested to Alix that she write a letter describing Klein's work for the British Society. This letter would change the course of Melanie Klein's and her daughter Melitta's lives forever.

Meanwhile Klein and Alix found another interest in common: dance halls. While the two roamed the dance halls in search of suitable partners, Melitta conscientiously pursued her studies. (It is hard to know what she thought of her mother dressed up as a *décolleté* Cleopatra for a fancy dress ball!)

With the help of James and Alix Strachey, Klein wrote to Ernest Jones, president of the British Society, offering to give six lectures on child analysis. Jones accepted immediately. Alix worried about Klein's English – she did not have Melitta's gift for language – while Klein herself seemed to have worried about what hat to wear (she chose a yellow one trimmed with swags of flowers)! As usual, Melitta and Erich were left behind. It is likely that Melitta felt excluded from all of this gaiety. Unlike her mother, she did not seem to have had a capacity for making friends and at this point in her life seems to have buried herself in her studies. Her *revenge* was to come later.

As for Klein herself, she felt that the three weeks she spent in England were the happiest of her life. She met analysts who would become important in both hers and Melitta's lives: Joan Riviere, Susan Isaacs, Edward Glover and Ella Sharpe. Both Glover and Sharpe were to become Melitta's analysts.

When Klein returned to Berlin the situation in the Berlin Society was bleak. Abraham was suffering from the illness from which he would soon die. Without Abraham's protection, Rado, Alexander and others did not hesitate to attack Klein's work. After Abraham's death, Alix Strachey returned to England. Meanwhile in desperate need of support, Klein turned to her friend Joan Riviere. Riviere was perfectly situated to help Klein. Tall, brilliant and beautiful, her second analysis had been with Freud (following a rocky start with Ernest Jones). She was a fluent German speaker and was also Freud's favourite translator. It was Riviere who explained Klein's plight to Jones who responded by asking Klein to come to England to analyse both of his children, as his wife had been struggling to bring them up. Emboldened by Jones's response and encouraged by Riviere, Klein wrote to ask what Jones would think of her settling permanently in England.

Within a short time Klein was in England building up her psychoanalytic practice. She had, however, opened a Pandora's box with her work with young children: indeed wherever she went, there would be people wanting to put her disturbing findings *back in the box*. While her English colleagues welcomed Klein who was very soon made a member of the British Society, a training analyst and a member of the training committee, a hostile response was brewing in Vienna. Freud's daughter, Anna, who had trained as a teacher, had begun working as a psychoanalyst with children. Her approach was entirely different to that of Klein. She only worked with older children who had clear neurotic symptoms, and only with the positive transference. In order to attach children to herself, she was prepared to knit clothes for their dolls and apologise for their bad behaviour to their parents. Anna's approach was not surprising as it seems likely that Freud only worked with the positive transference with her.

In 1927 Anna published *The Psychoanalytical Treatment of Children*. From the very first page it is hostile and critical of Klein's work. Rado, Klein's old *enemy*, so to speak, refused to publish a British response in the *Zeitschrift für Psychoanalyse*. This outraged Ernest Jones's sense of fair play. The British Society soon put on their own seminars on child analysis, which included some trenchant criticism of Anna Freud's technique.[2] Ella Sharpe commented:

> The problem of child analysis seems subtly implicated with the analyst's own deepest unexplored repressions . . . rationalisations that the child is too young are built upon the alarms of that same infantile superego in the analyst that he has to deal with in the child before him.
>
> (Sharpe, 1927)

These seminars were published in the *International Journal of Psychoanalysis* (1927) of which Jones was the editor, and were now in the public arena.

At that time Melitta was busy training as a psychoanalyst in Berlin, but the climate there was hostile to her mother, as the Berliners sided with Anna Freud. This may have played a part in Melitta's decision to come to England, but this may also have planted a poisonous seed in Melitta. As a young woman Melitta was very beautiful and, like her mother, she married early. Her husband, Walter Schmideberg was in fact 14 years older than her. A chance encounter with the psychoanalyst Max Eitingon when he was in the army had led Schmideberg to an introduction and friendship with Sigmund Freud. It is not clear where Walter Schmideberg received his psychoanalytic training or personal analysis from, but friendship with Max Eitingon, the founder and financier of the Berlin Clinic, suggests he trained in Berlin and met Melitta there. Phyllis Grosskurth, Klein's biographer, thought Klein was jealous of Melitta's medical degree and aristocratic husband. Subsequent events showed that Walter was very much in Melitta's shadow. He had a drug and alcohol problem and Erich remembered visiting him in a clinic where he had gone to be treated.

Melitta came to England on a permanent basis in 1930. She was now a psychoanalyst in her own right. Klein had turned her patients' waiting room into a bedroom for Melitta when she and Erich moved in. This seems to have symbolised Melitta's *on the edge* position in her mother's life. Being the daughter of Melanie Klein, however, appears to have smoothed the way for Melitta to acquire a visa. Still it took Ernest Jones, usually a 'whiz' with visas, two years to access one for Walter. It is interesting that Melitta chose to remain with her mother rather than her husband during this period.

While Klein was now surrounded by a group of loyal supporters, the abrupt and humourless Melitta found it difficult to fit in and make friends. She began an analysis with Klein's supporter, Ella Sharpe. Melitta's motives for this second analysis are not clear, although second analyses were very common in an era when a year would count as a long analysis. This time Melitta would be experiencing an analyst who admired her mother rather than one who disliked her ideas, as Horney had.

In 1929 an incident at the Oxford Congress clearly seems to have hurt Melitta's feelings: Joan Riviere's daughter, Diana, was studying at Oxford at the time, and Melitta had been packed off with her for a tour around the colleges. Not surprisingly, Melitta was not grateful to be seen as one of the younger generation. "It was interesting, but not scientific" was her response. Fortunately three years later Ernest Jones succeeded in getting a visa for Walter Schmideberg so that Melitta, now 28 years of age, could live with her husband. In the event, Schmideberg's arrival coincided with the publication of Klein's own *The Psychoanalysis of Children*, translated by Alix Strachey. Walter Schmideberg organised a dinner for Klein and her supporters at the Mayfair Hotel. The guests included James and Alix Strachey, Joan and Evelyn Riviere, along with Edward Glover and his wife Gladys. Edward Glover was at this stage one of Klein's staunch supporters, and he designed a birth certificate for the book. Later Glover was to become one of Klein's bitterest enemies.

During this honeymoon phase, Klein together with the Schmidebergs bought a Sunbeam car which they christened, hopefully, 'Sunny'. At weekends they went touring around England. After a while, however, Melitta put a stop to this symbiotic relationship, and the Schmidebergs bought out Klein's share of the car. On the surface this sounds a very healthy move by Melitta. However, the mental processes behind it were more sinister. By this time Melitta had decided to give up her analysis with Ella Sharpe and go into analysis with Edward Glover, who was then one of the most powerful figures in the British Society. As things were organised at the time, it was possible to accumulate senior positions for indefinite periods of time – as did Edward Glover, as indeed Ernest Jones had done. Glover was chair of the Training Committee, director of the London Clinic, and scientific secretary.

Glover's private life, however, was sad. His first wife had died in childbirth. His second wife had recently given birth to a baby with Down syndrome. This must have been particularly painful for Glover. He and his older brother James had also had a bitter rivalry about who was the cleverer. Their father considered James the intellectual star of the family. Both men were doctors, and James had persuaded Edward to follow him into analysis with Karl Abraham. Edward Glover, James Glover and Melanie Klein were all in analysis with Karl Abraham, and Abraham made no secret of his admiration of Klein. James Glover died of the effects of diabetes in 1926, leaving Klein as Glover's successful analytic sibling.

When Glover took Melitta into analysis, it was suggested that she was a replacement for his daughter with Down syndrome. Certainly Melitta's intellectual brilliance was not in doubt. My own view is that Melitta and Glover shared a feeling of being overshadowed by a more talented family member: Melitta by her mother, and Edward Glover by both his brother James, and by his *analytic sibling*, Klein. Melitta and Glover did not have the usual analyst/patient relationship, but a folie à deux, with an outcome that would be tragic.

At first Melitta seemed to be following in Klein's footsteps. She too worked with very young children. In 1933 she won the clinical essay prize at the British Society for an account of an analysis of a three-year-old girl (Schmideberg, 1934). Melitta's clear prose shows her command of English. Vivian, the patient, had difficulties eating, hysterical vomiting, and she wanted what she could not have. She thought that her mother only gave her bad things, but pretended they were good. Melitta suggests "Her mistrust of her mother was due to envy arising from oral-sadistic sources" (Schmideberg, 1934). This envious attitude affected her eating. Melitta's description of envy predates Klein's book on the topic by more than 20 years. Was this Melitta's original idea or did she derive it from a paper by Joan Riviere? Riviere, after all, had written about envy in an adult woman in a 1932 paper, of which Melitta must have been aware, given that Klein and Riviere were close, and that Riviere probably presented it at a scientific meeting at the institute.

At this time in her life, Melitta could acknowledge the influence of her mother whose book is in her list of references (Klein, 1932). Within a few years, however, Melitta's work had the aim of disproving her mother's work and that of other analysts. What changed? What I would suggest is that nothing had changed, but something had been revealed, and that something was *envy*. Ever since Freud, psychoanalysts have used themselves as clinical material or written about cases which resonate with themselves and their own life experiences. Melitta's three-year-old patient, Vivian, wants things from her mother but rejects them because they are experienced as bad. This is part of her envious attitude. Vivian's mother is Jewish and Melitta holds her responsible for some of Vivian's difficulties. This mother–daughter scenario in Melitta's patient has echoes of herself and her own mother. A family tragedy, described below, gave Melitta a weapon to attack her mother.

When Melanie and Arthur divorced, it was agreed that Hans, the middle child, destined to be an engineer, would stay with his father, and Erich would go to his mother. Melitta, the eldest of Klein's children, was independent, and chose to follow her mother to England. As the acrimony from the divorce died down,

Hans met his mother in Europe. A photograph, taken in 1930 shows Hans and his mother together. Klein is wearing fashionable beach pyjamas and Hans has his arm around her shoulders. Meanwhile Arthur wrote friendly letters to Erich. Then in 1934 the devastating news came to Klein that Hans had died in a climbing accident. Melitta immediately declared that it was suicide and blamed her mother. In fact the report was that the path he was on had given way. Klein had also received a letter from a Czech woman whom Hans had intended to marry. These factors would make suicide less likely. Rob Hale, a contemporary English analyst and expert in suicide, has suggested that in all cases of suicide there is a wish to live and a wish to die (Hale, personal communication). This is possibly reflected in the uncertainties surrounding Hans's death. But Melitta seemed to want to twist the knife into Klein. In a paper on suicide written in 1936 Melitta states:

> excessive feelings of disgust brought about by deep disappointments in loved persons or by the breakdown of idealisations prove frequently an incentive towards suicide.
>
> (Schmideberg, 1936)

No doubt Klein got the message. Melitta's idealisation of her mother had certainly broken down. There is no way we can know Hans's state of mind, but over the next few years Melitta committed psychoanalytic suicide. Her public proclamations were so crazy that it is hard to think of anyone referring patients to her.

The situation for Klein must have been unbearably painful. Not only had she lost Hans but, in a different way, she had lost Melitta. Melitta no longer followed in Klein's footsteps, but rather in Glover's. She had even taken on Glover's interest in treating delinquents and criminals.

Klein did not respond to Melitta's attacks, which she regarded as an 'illness'. What was the nature of Melitta's illness? It does not seem to have been a depressive one. However, as we shall see, from 1935 Klein entered on an intense period of creativity. Melitta, who had no children could not bear her mother to be pregnant with so many new ideas. Melitta may also have been expressing the envy felt by some of Klein's other colleagues, which may be one reason than no one took her to one side and helped her see that she was damaging herself.

As Klein emerged from mourning Hans's death she produced a series of highly original papers. In 1935 she wrote what is probably her most famous paper, 'The Psychogenesis of Manic-Depressive States'. In this paper she finally broke away from Freud's theory of libidinal stages – oral, anal and genital – to a theory of object relations. She identifies a sequence of paranoid, depressive and manic positions. This was not only a new theory of developmental stages but also an explanatory model of manic depression. This paper incensed Glover and Melitta. It has been suggested that Glover felt Klein was straying into the territory of psychiatry. The question of whether or not analysts should be medically qualified was hotly debated at the time, but never became a requirement in England, as it did in America. As for Melitta, she seemed simply affronted that her mother had produced a new idea, and she moved quickly to counter it. In 1935 Melitta wrote a paper on asocial children. In it she presents herself as an expert. She quotes Abraham's theories of libidinal development, as if to remind her mother that she had strayed from her analyst's path.

Melitta's productivity outstripped that of her mother, even if her creativity did not. In the same year she wrote a second paper, 'Reassurance as a Means of Analytic Technique' (Schmideberg, 1935b). This would have provoked many analysts who believed reassurance should be kept to a minimum. Melitta's examples do not inspire confidence in her ideas. She approvingly describes her husband Walter Schmideberg giving pills to an analytic patient of his who had a headache. To those familiar with Schmideberg's own drug problem this may have seemed more in keeping with his character, than a clever technique. Melitta's coup de grace came in 1937 when she read a paper to the British Society called 'After the Analysis', in which she accused unnamed analysts of unscrupulously promoting idealisation of themselves and psychoanalysis. In case the object of her attacks was not clear enough, Melitta included a specific jab at Klein and her new concept of the depressive position, writing:

> other analysts think that no analysis is satisfactory or deep-going enough if the patient has omitted to pass through a phase of depression.
>
> (Schmideberg, 1938)

In this paper Melitta undermines herself, because any reasonable points she makes are coloured by the hatred of her mother and her colleagues. Joan Riviere, who had a fiery temper herself, wrote to James Strachey that Melitta was accusing them all of being bad analysts. Klein herself did not respond.

At that time British analysts appeared so absorbed by their internal conflicts that they barely seemed to register the rise of Hitler in Germany and the worsening situation for the Jews. Many Jewish analysts went to America; a few came to England. This was partly because Jones did not offer encouragement, as Klein had changed the climate of the British Society. There was now a proper training in child analysis on which Klein taught, and many British analysts subscribed to some of Klein's ideas.

At this time, Freud, old and suffering from cancer, was reluctant to leave Austria. However the arrest of Anna by the Gestapo (she was subsequently released) persuaded him to change his mind. Jones rose heroically to the occasion. With the help of Princess Marie Bonaparte, Jones arranged for the Freud family and some of his entourage to be transported to safety in England. Unable to resist a jab at the Nazis, Freud resorted to humour. When asked to sign a form confirming that he had been well treated, Freud added that he could heartily recommend the Gestapo to anyone. Freud was forced to leave his elderly sisters behind, apparently unaware of the full extent of the Nazi machine. They all died in concentration camps.

Klein was horrified by the arrival of the Freuds. Her chief rival, Anna Freud, was now located in the heart of the British Society. Melitta could have made common cause with Anna. However, Anna had her own agenda. In any case, Melitta had insulted her in print, and Anna had complained to Jones about it. Freud and Anna were deeply grateful to the British. At the same time the German and Austrian analysts were bringing different ideas to the British Society, and Anna was to establish a separate camp in Hampstead, North London.

The disagreements in the British Society did not centre only on theory. It was felt that some analysts were rude to members of the public. Then there was the issue of analysts hanging on to offices for years. Four analysts – Melitta, Barbara Low, and Adrian and Karin Stephen – suggested a series of extraordinary business meetings to discuss some of the issues involved at the time. For once Melitta allied herself with a good cause, but unfortunately she tried to use these meetings to prosecute her war on Klein and her colleagues. The fact that these discussions took place during Second World War only added to the further drama to the meetings as from time to time bombs fell on London and members had to take shelter in the basement. By good fortune for us the meetings were recorded word for word by a stenographer specially employed for this purpose. During the extraordinary business meeting of 11 March 1942, both Melitta and Glover spoke against the Kleinians. Melitta excelled herself:

> *The Kleinians shelter behind ambiguity and vagueness . . . they lack the most elementary scientific discipline. In a manner somewhat reminiscent of Dr Goebbels (the Nazi propaganda minister), they try to impress us by repeating time after time the same slogans.*
>
> (King and Steiner, 1991)

Unfortunately Melitta undermined herself by telling the meeting that she had been diagnosed as a paranoiac by a senior member of the British Society who had tried to persuade her husband to take her out of the country "because I had dared to protest against certain intrigues and organised attacks".

Melitta then gave a list of (non Kleinians) whom she thought had been attacked or ill-treated by the Kleinians:

> *When Drs Bowlby and Middlemore brought original contributions, they were unfairly attacked . . . Mr Strachey has been patronised, disparaging remarks were systematically spread about Dr Brierley and Miss Sharpe.*

Reading Melitta's diatribe one is left with the impression that she may have indeed suffered from symptoms of paranoia, particularly as some of the analysts she mentions queued up to complain that they *had not in fact* been ill-treated.

Until now the British analysts had been horrified spectators, but finally it was too much. Sylvia Payne, who would shortly become president of the Society, finally 'read out the riot act':

> *At the last meeting accusations of what in law could be called malpractice were made against Mrs Klein . . . the charges were grave and in my opinion*

> *such charges cannot be made without the liability of libel actions being incurred.*
>
> (King and Steiner, 1991)

This successfully curbed Melitta's attacks. There were further meetings to discuss scientific differences, but Melitta hardly attended. There was nothing in them for her if she was prevented from attacking her mother.

Why was Melitta so hostile to Klein? Klein's biographer, Phyllis Grosskurth, accuses Klein of analysing Melitta and Hans, as if this was the source of their difficulties. This accusation has been shown to be false by Claudia Frank a psychoanalyst who has made a detailed study of Klein's clinical notes (Frank, 2009). Even if Klein *had* analysed Melitta and Hans, it does not prove anything. We know that Klein *did* analyse Erich, that he and his wife remained on good terms with her, and that Klein was devoted to her grandchildren.

The clinical preoccupations of Klein and Melitta allow us to construct the following hypothesis: although Klein loved her children, she was often physically and emotionally absent. Melitta was initially the 'star' of the children: well-behaved and very clever. In return, Melitta probably idealised her mother. A supportive father could have helped Melitta find a more helpful position in relation to her mother, but Arthur Klein was himself often away and there were tensions between him and Klein. We know from Klein's later work that idealisation covers up envy. Over time Melitta's idealisation of her mother seems to have broken down, as there was plenty in Klein's life to envy: her clinical brilliance, her creativity, her devoted colleagues and friends.

As for her daughter, when Melitta first came to England she went into analysis with Ella Sharpe. This seems to have helped Melitta put some distance between herself and her mother without falling out with her. Sharpe seems to have been the equivalent of a helpful father. Melitta was able to write her 1933 paper on the analysis of a three-year-old while using some of Klein's ideas and some of her own. It was good enough to win a prize.

Unfortunately Melitta then turned to Glover, who had initially admired Klein, but had turned against her. Instead of helping Melitta separate from her mother, he promoted an angry preoccupation. He seems to have exploited Melitta's hatred for his own ends. Furthermore it is an indication of Glover's character that when Sylvia Payne became president of the British Society, and not him, he left the Society in a fit of anger. Like Melitta he had alienated his colleagues by his aggressive behaviour.

Eventually Melitta also left the British Society, as well as her husband, and in 1945 moved to New York. There she continued, now *in Glover's footsteps*, by working with juvenile delinquents. As time went on she became increasingly disillusioned with psychoanalysis. However, she stayed on friendly terms with Walter Schmideberg.

This is not absolutely the end of the story. Klein died in 1960, and Melitta came back to England in 1961, and rejoined the British Society. What was she hoping for? To take her mother's place, to feel in some ways closer to her? Whatever it was, she did not seem to have found it, and left a year later.

Klein's will left to Melitta

> my gold flexible bracelet which was given to me by her paternal grandmother, the single stone diamond ring given to me by my late husband, my gold necklace with garnets and the brooch that goes with the said necklace, both of which I received as a present on my 75th birthday and I have no other bequest to my said daughter because she is otherwise well provided for and by her technical qualifications able to provide for herself.
>
> (King and Steiner, 1991)

Klein gave Melitta the family jewels as an expression of her love for her daughter. As usual, she expected her to look after herself.

Notes

1 The Berlin Psychoanalytic Institute (later the Göring Institute) was founded in 1920.
2 Anna Freud, 'Introduction to the Technique of Child Analysis' (1927).

References

Frank, C. (2009). *Melanie Klein in Berlin: Her First Psychoanalyses of Children*. London: Routledge.

Freud, A. (1927). *The Psychoanalytical Treatment of Children*. New York: International Universities Press.

Grosskurth, P. (1986). *Melanie Klein: Her World and Her Work*. New York: Alfred A. Knopf.

King, P. & Steiner, R. (Eds.) (1991). *The Freud-Klein Controversies, 1941–45*. London: Routledge.

Klein, M. (1932). *The Psychoanalysis of Children*. London: Hogarth Press/Institute of Psychoanalysis.

Klein, M. (1935). A Contribution to the Psychogenesis of Manic Depressive States. In: Klein, M. (Ed.), *Love, Guilt and Reparation* (pp. 262–289). London: Hogarth Press, 1981.

Riviere, J. (1932). Jealousy as a Mechanism of Defence. *The International Journal of Psychoanalysis, 13*: 414–424.

Sayers, J. & Forrester, J. (2013). The Autobiography of Melanie Klein. *Psychoanalysis and History, 15(2)*: 127–163.

Schmideberg, M. (1934). The Play-Analysis of a Three-Year-Old Girl. *The International Journal of Psychoanalysis, 15*: 245–264.

Schmideberg, M. (1935a). The Psycho-Analysis of Asocial Children and Adolescents. *The International Journal of Psychoanalysis, 16*: 22–48.

Schmideberg, M. (1935b). Reassurance as a Means of Analytic Technique. *The International Journal of Psychoanalysis, 16*: 307–324.

Schmideberg, M. (1936). A Note on Suicide. *The International Journal of Psychoanalysis, 17*: 1–5.

Schmideberg, M. (1938). After the Analysis. *Psychoanalytic Quarterly, 7*: 122–142.

Sharpe, E. F. (1927). Symposium on Child Analysis at the British Society in 1927. *International Journal of Psycho-Analysis, 8*.

Chapter 7

A tragic inheritance

The irresolvable conflict for children of perpetrators[1]

Coline Covington

The chapter that follows barely requires comment more than the author's own introductory words below. On reading her paper, the darkness of the shadow struck by the object during the harrowing years of the Holocaust is painfully clear. Analyst Coline Covington opens rhetorically with the following:

> *How do you live with the knowledge that your father ordered the deaths of thousands of innocent people? Children of parents who have committed or been involved in atrocities have to live with the guilt of their parents' deeds, even when guilt is acknowledged by the parents. Because of their family history, these children often become 'lightning conductors' for social guilt, tainted with the mark of evil. Drawing on clinical material and interviews with children of Nazi SS officers, this chapter examines the personal psychological repercussions and conflicts that children of perpetrators face in their lives. These conflicts live on not only within the children who have inherited their parents' crimes but within the larger society in the form of memory, denial and guilt. The psychological dilemma for children of perpetrators provides a prism through which we can better understand the impact of past atrocities on the collective.*

> For I the Lord thy God (am) a jealous God, visiting the iniquity of the fathers unto the children unto the third and fourth (generation) of them that hate me.
>
> Deuteronomy 5:9

Introduction

In her reflections on the aftermath of the German Reich, Eva Hoffman describes the experience of children of survivors of the *Shoah* (the Holocaust). She writes:

> what we children received, with great directness, were the emotional sequelae of our elders' experiences, the acid-etched traces of what they had endured. This perhaps, is always the way in which one generation's legacy is actually

> passed on to the next – through the imprint of personal and historical experiences as these are traced on individual psyches and sensibilities. But . . . the traces left on the survivors' psyches were not so much thoughts or images as scars and wounds. The legacy they passed on was not a processed, mastered past, but the splintered signs of acute suffering, of grief and loss.
>
> (Hoffman, p. 34)

Efraim Sicher refers to the invisible scars of the next generation, "the scar without the wound", as the marks of trauma, experienced not in real time but in a timeless psychic reality, affecting identity and the sense of self in relation to the world (Sicher, p. 27). Hoffman clearly states, "For me, in the beginning was the war, and the Holocaust was the ontological basis of my universe" (Hoffman, p. 278). The trauma of the parents, both individually and in this case as a group, resides in the unconscious of their children, silently shaping their internal world and their actions in the external world.

There is now an extensive literature on the transgenerational effects of trauma, and of Holocaust survivors in particular.[2] Starting in the late 1980s, a body of literature and film emerged giving recognition to the children of Nazi perpetrators and highlighting their own difficulties in coming to terms with the past of their parents.[3] Comparisons between the two groups are inevitable but also fraught with conceptual and experiential contradictions and problems. I will touch on some of these similarities and differences later in this chapter. However, there is a principal distinction between these groups, articulated by Dan Bar-On in *The Indescribable and the Undiscussable* (Bar-On, 1999). Bar-On distinguishes between a trauma that is too painful to talk about and a history that cannot be talked about, that has been "effaced from normalized discourse" (McGlothlin, p. 6 footnote). Hoffman argues that the latter cannot be classed as a trauma, with the implication of victimisation, but as a tragedy. She explains, "For tragedy, of course, involves a conflict – agon – between opposing principles and agents. Trauma is produced by persecution of subjects to whom all agency and principle have been denied" (Hoffman, p. 41). Perpetrators, on the other hand, have acted out a tragic conflict that then casts a shadow over their offspring and generations to come. The discovery that one's parents have committed evil acts throws up fundamental conflicts that affect the child's identity, sense of morality, and worldview.

In this chapter, I will present clinical material from work with a young woman whose father had been a leading military figure in a bloody civil war and had ultimately been indicted for torture. Her material touches on many aspects of the experience of children of Nazi perpetrators. While the relationship of each child with his/her parent necessarily varies, taken together these stories form a composite that sheds light on children of perpetrators in other similar situations (e.g. of the genocides in Cambodia, Rwanda, Kosovo, Syria and so on). It is important to clarify that these are perpetrators who have been involved in what would qualify as *evil acts that have been sanctioned by a higher authority*. I am defining evil in this context as an act intended to dehumanise another group of people who are distinctly targeted and categorised by race, religion, political affiliation, or place, to the point of extermination.

While there are numerous examples of children of criminally violent parents who also struggle with the contamination and shame this incurs on the family,[4] this is an intrinsically different experience to that of a parent who has perpetrated atrocities that are sanctioned by society. I also make the distinction between children of parents who have participated in extreme violence in armed conflict that is sanctioned and is not deemed evil. In these cases, while the parent's experiences may have been traumatic, the parent is generally perceived as a hero or fighting for a heroic cause, not as a demon who is corrupted by evil.

Case study: living in the cracks

Ana contacted me on the advice of her doctor because of recurring severe headaches that she had experienced over the last two years since her recent marriage. She also mentioned that she had nightmares of being attacked that made her feel very anxious.

Ana appeared for our first meeting exactly on time, immediately removed her shoes and left them by the front door, and hung up her coat on the hook I indicated. She was a very attractive woman, conservatively well dressed, and smiled at me as if she was inviting me to speak. This left a strange sensation in me of not just a reversal of roles but of being kept out by her, despite her seeming warmth. There was a brief silence and she then told me that at the age of 15 she and her mother, her younger brother and her baby sister had emigrated from their country of origin in the aftermath of terrible civil war. She told me in great detail about their harrowing escape, catching lifts from trucks, hiding in goods train carriages, and walking along deserted mountain paths with nothing to eat and no shelter. She smiled and said she had kept a diary of this time and was going to write a book about it someday.

Although her story was remarkable and she could express how very frightening is was at times, I was struck by the fact that it didn't seem to be the problem. Not knowing what to say, I asked her whether she thought there was some link between her headaches and her nightmares and this traumatic period in her life. Ana looked at me and said,

> No, I don't think there is a link because that's over now. It was a terrible time but it was also full of the excitement of a new life and freedom from what had happened in our country. My headaches only started when I got married and this is what I can't understand. I love my husband and he is very kind and loving to me. He is everything I could wish for, but I'm afraid I will somehow ruin everything.

Ana had eagerly agreed to see me three times a week and voluntarily asked if she could lie on my couch, not facing me. During the first few weeks, she dutifully arrived on time, lay on the couch and embellished her stories about her family's great escape, as if hoping we would find some clue from them to alleviate her headaches. She also picked her way through her feelings towards her husband, but there again it was clear she loved him and they had a good marriage. Then silence. I was beginning to feel a mixture of despair and doubt as to whether in fact Ana's headaches were analysable and I had made a mistake in taking her on as a patient.

In the following session, as Ana was recounting another episode in her escape saga, she remembered a dream from the previous night. In her dream she was seeing a doctor or perhaps it was a friend, she wasn't sure, who was going to give her some medicine for her headaches. Ana was wearing long white delicate kid gloves and the doctor asked her to remove them. She removed her right-hand glove but then hesitated with her left hand. The doctor insisted it was necessary to remove both and Ana reluctantly took off the glove from her left hand, revealing that her left hand had become disfigured as the muscles had atrophied. Ana was shocked to see what had happened but, more than this, she felt deeply ashamed to show the doctor something so grotesque in her.

I asked Ana what she thought of the dream and, after a moment, she replied that her father was left-handed and the family had always teased him about this. It made her wonder whether she was in some way like him.

Ana's response made me realise that she had never mentioned her father and that I too had blanked him out, as if he had not existed. I said, "I'm aware that in all your stories about the escape, you haven't mentioned your father once. Was he alive and, if so, where was he?"

Ana remained still for some time and simply said, "He stayed behind".

"Stayed behind?" I asked.

For the first time, Ana became irritated and answered sharply, "Yes! He stayed behind. Didn't you hear me?"

There was a long silence and Ana then relented,

> I'm sorry to be so rude. My father stayed behind because he was in prison. He's still in prison. . . . He's well known at home and after the war he was tried for torturing prisoners. He was found guilty. It's all out now, everyone knows. We couldn't stay after that. As soon as he was found guilty we started getting death threats. Everyone knew we were his family and in their eyes we were all to blame. He wrecked our lives there.

Ana's disclosure turned out to be the missing piece of the puzzle that enabled her to tell me about the events that had torn her family apart.

Like many of children of Nazi perpetrators, Ana had described a very happy childhood and loving parents. Her father put his family first, providing well for them, ensuring they had the best of everything, and, although he was strict with the children, he was also gentle and loving. One example Ana gave of her father's kindness was when he caught her as a young child prodding a bird with a broken wing. She remembered him lecturing her about how cruel it was to torture animals and feeling ashamed and exposed before him. She commented, "This is not the same man who was found guilty of torture – how could he be the same?"

Ana was her father's favourite and had felt particularly close to him as a child, playing games and making up stories that were special between them. She remembered during the war an occasion when her mother had interrupted her from asking her father to play, explaining he was tired and needed to rest. Ana had felt irritated with her mother, whom she normally got along well with, and linked this to her irritation with me for asking her about where her father was. She said,

> I think it was the first time I became at all aware that there was something wrong. It wasn't that my father was tired, he looked ill, like he was breaking apart and I didn't know what was going on. I was irritated that there was something I didn't know about and it was clear then that my parents knew. My parents never talked about what was going on outside our family and I had grown up thinking this was normal. My mother still doesn't. Of course, I knew that terrible things were happening in the war and my father was brave, but this was a different feeling. My father prided himself on being in control at all times – and this time he was cracking. It wasn't exactly a sadness that was the problem, it was something else indefinable. I remember when I was upset and cried when I was little and he didn't comfort me but he would say in a gentle voice, "You mustn't cry. It's important to be brave and strong and then you won't feel sad anymore." So I knew what it was like to be strong and not to be sad. I knew the war was going badly and we were losing and wondered if my father felt he had failed. It was so important for him to do his best and to do what was right.

Over the next few sessions, Ana told me about her father's trial, or what she knew of it, and described some of the allegations that had been made against her father. He was a high-ranking officer and had not only instigated the torture of prisoners but had also authorised localised mass killings. The evidence was clear that he had both given orders and had been directly involved in these events. His defence was consistently that he was doing his duty for his country, that the torture was required to obtain information and that the killings were for self-protection, particularly when his military unit was threatened with reprisals.

Ana admitted that, putting herself inside his mind, she could understand it all made sense. But when she looked at it from her perspective, she was horrified not only at what her father had done and had been capable of doing but of what she felt was a total betrayal of her. She suddenly complained of a headache coming on and started crying. She sobbed,

> This is so hard to live with. He is the father I have loved so much, who made me feel so loved, and he is now the father whom I hate for what he has done. How can I have any respect for him? Yet I still love him. This is why my head is splitting. I can't keep these two fathers together. And I don't know where this puts me.

An integral part of our childhood psychic development is the painful realisation of hating the object of our love. However, for Ana, as for other children of perpetrators, the problem is not simply that of holding these opposites together. The problem is how to think about a father who has acted like a loving parent in one world and a monster in another. Ana was articulating how hard this is to live with – and to recognise – and what it means about her as a person and whether she could trust what she saw of herself in the mirror, as her view of her father and his reflection of her had cracked. At the same time she desperately wanted to protect the father of her childhood and deny he was responsible for the crimes he had committed.

In the sessions following Ana's insight about her splitting headaches, she became noticeably paranoid in her behaviour towards me, accusing me of being critical of her, not believing her, and of pretending to be concerned about her. In the transference I alternated between being a father whom she could no longer trust and being her critical superego that castigated her for her hatred and sense of betrayal of her father. Ana began to see what she was projecting on to me and at the end of a session in which she had been especially rejecting of anything I said, she exclaimed,

> I don't want to be like this! But I'm also angry with you because I don't want to have to understand! I have to make someone – whether it's you or myself – an enemy. I don't know how else to manage what I know. I fluctuate from not wanting to believe any of it – that my father was really only my father and never did any of the horrible things he did – and from attacking myself for being so stupid not to have seen this before and wanting to kill him and everything about my past. I want to believe I've been duped all along – but then I remember other things. . . . I can't find a place for what has happened inside me. I am left with this crap, this horrible hand in my dream that I can't get rid of. And I can't get rid of feeling I am to blame, I'm guilty!

Ana was trying to grasp the world that had been kept secret from her and to square this with her own experience. She spent hours venting her fury against her father, continually questioning how he could have done these things. Her anger and disbelief eventually gave way to trying to think about how her father had been able to justify what he was doing – how he could remain the same person. She saw his obsession with duty and doing his best as something which had resulted paradoxically in two very different outcomes. He was the dutiful father and the dutiful military leader – but what was admirable behaviour in one context did not necessarily apply to another. Seeing how driven her father had been to perform well, Ana then remembered the time when she thought he was breaking apart. As if speaking to him, she said,

> I think that was the moment when you couldn't go on any longer, when you saw that all your efforts to do well, to be a good soldier, to be brave, to be loyal, all of it had failed and that was your tragedy and it's mine now. You

> believed what you were doing was for the right and then you were let down, it all crumbled and everyone could see the cracks. And now it's the cracks that I have to live in. You've covered them over and go on trying to convince yourself – but you can't be with me in my world any longer.

In finding some explanatory thread to keep her father's identity together, Ana was able to incorporate a fuller and more complex picture of him, and eventually of herself. She was not so naïve as to think that her father's fault line had been his propensity to follow orders, but this was the beginning of her understanding of how he could be the "same" person and how elusive the boundary between these seemingly different persons can be.

Ana's headaches stopped. She had reached some form of reconciliation with her father, accepting her love for him but at the same time knowing she could not be in contact with him because to do so would be to perpetuate the deceit between them. Like Schlink's narrator, Ana also realised that "there was nothing to say".

She was nevertheless left with the question as to why her headaches had started soon after her marriage, especially as there seemed to be no significant problems in her marital life. Her persecutory dreams continued periodically and also signalled that she had her own internal demons to deal with. The penny dropped one afternoon when Ana heard herself talking about trying to be a dutiful wife. She turned round to face me as if wanting to confirm that I was there with her but, most importantly, that I was separate from her. She lay back again and said,

> That's it! You remember when I said I was worried I might do something to ruin my marriage? I have this dutiful streak in me just like my father – this flaw that can ruin everything if I'm not careful and if I let it rule me. I think all along I've known I have this and I've also sensed some danger inside me but I haven't been able to see what it was. I think it's what makes me feel so frightened in my dreams. I can also see that if I had been in my father's position, it is possible I could have behaved as he did. I hope I wouldn't have. But I can see how close this is inside me.

I commented that there might be another problem in trying so hard to be the dutiful wife as it might mean leaving things unspoken with her husband and jeopardising their intimacy, as her father had done with his family. Her splitting headaches had contained the lacuna of what could not be spoken about, of a discrepancy she could not make sense of and yet could not suppress altogether.

Ana replied,

> It's true, I'm always watching myself, censoring what I say, as if some awful secret will come out. I put up a wall with my husband – and within myself.

Ana's awareness of her own proclivity to step over the boundary and enter into a perverse, dehumanising world did not resolve the pain and betrayal she felt from her father and the rupture this had made in her life, but it did help her to bear the contamination her father had brought on the family and to become her own agent who could make different choices. It also enabled her to dismantle an internal wall she had constructed to keep what was so horrifying apart – in a hidden place inside her.

A background of silence

In listening to and reading accounts of the children of Nazi perpetrators, the most striking feature that stands out in their experience of family life is the silence surrounding what was going on in the outside world and, specifically, their fathers' involvement in these events that were unspeakable within the privacy of the family.[5] This was reflected in Ana's initial silence about her father and what I later realised was my unconscious collusion with this. Outside the confines of my consulting room, there was another reality that could not be spoken or thought about without serious breach of the world Ana had tried to preserve for herself and those close to her.

In some families there was a clear process of splitting whereby internal family life was idealised and revered and the external world presented a struggle to contain and combat what was impure and life threatening. Rudolf Hoess's daughter, Ingebirgitt, describes this split graphically in her memories of "my beautiful Auschwitz childhood" (Hall, 2015), living in ease in a house adjoining the perimeter of the concentration camp her father had designed and built. What happened on the other side of the garden wall was not known or spoken about. Despite the fact that the servants were often prisoners from the camp, the family maintained a wall of silence that was critical in maintaining the existence of these two seemingly antithetical worlds. Just as the garden wall physically demarcated a world of love from a world of hate, so did the silence.

While in retrospect we may want to interpret the silence experienced during the war as a form of denial or dissociation, it is important to acknowledge that for many families, such as Ana's, there was no conscious awareness of violations taking place. The belief system that enables atrocities to take place rests on adherence to duty and duty to a higher authority that is perceived to be safeguarding and promoting the interests of the group. In order to exist within this environment, especially when active engagement is required, the belief system needs to be upheld. Silence then serves to protect the group not only from the horrors of war but it suppresses questioning of the prevalent belief system. When atrocities do come to light at the end of a war, the ensuing shame and guilt are so intense that the need for silence then becomes acute – but it is a silence of a different order. This was palpably evident within Ana's own family after leaving their homeland and a father imprisoned for war crimes.

Post-war silence within families could also be tinged with coldness and emotional distance. Hoffman describes children of perpetrators "growing up in homes where a heavy atmosphere of secrecy reigned; of parents perceived as chilly and distant; of subjects that were seen as untouchable, and of gradual or sudden realisations that something had been recently and deeply rotten in the state in which the children were growing up" (Hoffman, p. 120). For a child, the presence of a secret held by the parents has profound emotional consequences, to the point where the child is unsure what to believe and what not to believe within the family history. There is also an inevitable sense of exclusion that casts a shadow over the child's sense of himself, conferring unconscious guilt as to whether the child himself has been the cause of something so terrible it cannot be spoken about. A borderline patient of mine, who grew up in a family involved with the French resistance, described a childhood of mysterious references to relatives who had disappeared and the fear it instilled in her and her siblings that this could either happen to them or that they would discover the truth and be murdered themselves. What she came to realise in the course of her analysis was that the threat of murder was her anxiety that unravelling the family history would destroy not only the fiction that the family had lived by but her own make-believe version of her parents and siblings.

The silent shrouding the past is painfully portrayed in Bernard Schlink's story about a son trying to make contact with his ageing father. Schlink writes:

> Why did his questions pressure his father? Because he didn't want to turn his insides out, particularly in front of his son? Because his insides, where the doors and windows had never been opened, were all shrivelled and dead, and he didn't know what his son wanted of him? Because he's grown up before psychoanalysis and psychotherapy had made revelations a daily occurrence and he had no language to communicate his inner feelings? Because whatever he'd done and whatever happened to him, from his two marriages to his professional obligations before and after 1945, he saw in it such a continuity that it was in fact the same and there was nothing to say about it? . . . Wordless intimacy had been too much to hope for.
>
> (Schlink, 2012, p. 187)

Schlink's narrator struggles to understand his father's silence and in the end wonders whether it reveals what he describes as a "continuity", as if the silence itself maintains a connection between past and present that would be betrayed or broken by speech. There is then "nothing to say". This passage evokes what Hoffman refers to as a kind of 'endorsed amnesia' during the post-war years in Germany, in which the subject of the Holocaust was virtually censored (Hoffman, p. 120). She goes on to observe that when the post-war generation discovered the truth, it came as a shock and led to explosions within families and within German society, as if waking up *into* a nightmare. While Hoffman suggests that there was some form of mass repression, Schlink's question about "continuity" reveals the essential importance of maintaining an identity and set of beliefs underlying one's identity that continues over time, despite ruptures in one's experience of the world and oneself.

Repudiation, idealisation and acceptance

My brief account of Ana's analysis illustrates only some of the features and conflicts experienced by children of perpetrators. Ana is also perhaps an exception because she sought an analysis to help her come to terms with her past. Overall, children of perpetrators seem to fall into three categories in terms of their relationships with their fathers; these categories can be broadly classed as idealisation, repudiation and acceptance. Philippe Sands's film, *My Nazi Legacy*, vividly portrays the opposing relationships between two sons and their respective high-ranking Nazi fathers, Hans Frank, governor of occupied Poland and Otto von Wächter, governor of Galicia in Ukraine. Niklas Frank bitterly repudiates his father, Hans Frank, in contrast to Horst von Wächter, who idealises his father, Otto von Wächter, refusing to accept the crimes he committed. But the distinctive difference between these men is that Niklas had a cold, unloving father whereas Horst viewed his father as "a good man, a liberal who did his best. . . . Others would have been worse" (Sands, p. 246). For Niklas, the decisive moment in his relationship with his father is when, at the age of seven, he visits him in prison at the time of the Nuremberg trials. Niklas remembers,

> I didn't say goodbye. The whole thing lasted not more than six or seven minutes. There were no tears. I was really sad. Sad that he lied to me. Sad that he didn't tell me the truth about what might happen to him. Sad about what would happen to us.
>
> (Sands, p. 364)

This final estrangement and deceit contributed to Niklas's decision to repudiate his father, a repudiation made easy as it was consistent with his experience of his father.

For Horst, however, his loyalty to his father is a stumbling block that prevents him from repudiating his father and leaves him with a conflict. In Horst's attempt to preserve the good in his father, he transforms the narrative of his father from perpetrator to victim. He admits,

> I cannot say I love my father. I love my grandfather. . . . I have a responsibility for my father in some way, to see what really happened, to tell the truth, and to do what I can do for him . . . I have to find some positive aspect . . . I know that the whole system was criminal and that he was part of it, but I don't think he was a criminal. He didn't act like a criminal. . . . There was no chance to leave the system . . . he was completely in the system.
>
> (Sands, pp. 250–251)

As Sands observes, Horst was "on a mission of rehabilitation" (Sands, p. 246). The problem with Horst's "rehabilitation" is that it is predicated on his father's innocence. What Horst cannot accept is that his father may have been a 'good' man *and* he committed evil acts. This is the fundamental paradox that evil poses, particularly when evil acts occur en masse; that all evil deeds are committed by humans who also, by and large, have loving relationships.

Idealisation effectively collapses the conflicting reality of the past but is at the cost of denying reality. Both positions are markedly different from my example of Ana, who did not hate her father but who also did not try to excuse or justify what he had done. This was perhaps what helped her ultimately to separate from him psychically.

The most outspoken child of a Nazi perpetrator has been Niklas Frank, who published an excoriating account of his father, *Der Vater*, in 1987. As Hitler's personal lawyer, Hans Frank rose to power and became chief jurist in occupied Poland from 1939 to 1941, where he was known for his reign of terror over the civilian population, establishing Jewish ghettos and responsible for the mass murder of Jews. Niklas describes his father as narcissistic, distant and at times cruel. His parents' relationship was fraught, both greedy for power and wealth. Niklas's memories of his childhood include being driven with his mother in the family's chauffeured car while his mother raided the Jewish shops for discounted luxury goods. His childhood comes across as lonely, harsh and frightening. He describes his father as a 'weak' man. Referring to his father's change of plea to guilty during the Nuremberg trial, Niklas commented, "His true character emerged with that second statement" (Sands, p. 362). The fact that his father was accused and ultimately hung, following the Nuremberg verdict, for crimes against humanity seems to underscore Niklas' pre-existing hatred of his father. He did not have to reconcile contradictory realities; he had one father whose behaviour was relatively consistent at home and at work. Niklas repudiation of his father could be complete. As he said about his father in a television interview,

> Having your neck broken spared me from having a screwed-up life. How you would have poisoned me with your brainwashing, just like they did to the silent majority of my generation – those not lucky enough to have had their father hanged.
>
> (Hitler's Children, 2012)

Another tortured scion of the Nazi legacy is Rainer Hoess, grandson of Rudolf Hoess and nephew to Ingebirgitt. The stigma of his grandfather's crimes has taken on an ontological meaning in his life. He asks, "Why am I alive? To carry this guilt, this burden, to try to come to terms with it? I think that must be the only reason I exist" (Hitler's Children, 2012). And yet when the grandson Hoess describes memories of his own father, we can begin to see some of the foundations for his bitterness. He explains,

> There was no warmth between my father and us. Never. He told us what to do and we obeyed. He set the rules and we obeyed. My father never let us show weakness, show emotion. He hated that to death. Whenever we cried,

> we were beaten even more, just for crying, not for what we had done. . . . He remained a zealot of the Third Reich.
>
> (Hitler's Children, 2012)

Rainer Hoess's burden of guilt seems to be proportionate to his hatred of his father and, ultimately, of his grandfather's deeds.

Others, who did not have such hostile relationships with their fathers, nevertheless chose to go into hiding and to distance themselves from their pasts. Ingebirgitt Hoess never used her father's name, even on her mother's gravestone, for fear of reprisals, explaining, "There are crazy people out there. They might burn my house down or shoot somebody" (Harding, 2013). Ingebirgitt Hoess also finds it hard to believe the full horror of her father's crimes, asking, "How can there be so many survivors if so many had been killed?"(Harding, 2013) Bettina Goering, Hermann Goering's grandniece, emigrated from Germany to New Mexico to start a new life. Both she and her brother had themselves sterilised to ensure that their family line would be killed off, curiously and perhaps unconsciously, repeating the Nazi drive for racial sterilisation of the Jews as a way of cleansing the Aryan population of contaminating elements. Even though she was born after the war, Bettina Goering claims, "I feel responsible for the Holocaust . . . because of my family, who had an active part in it" (Hitler's Children, 2012).

Gudrun Himmler, daughter of Heinrich Himmler, architect of the Final Solution, also went into hiding, marrying and assuming her husband's name and keeping her family identity secret. Like Ingebirgitt Hoess, Gudrun Himmler may have gone into hiding out of fear of reprisal. She continues to assert her father's innocence of genocide. Her efforts to care for her father's former associates along with her active participation in the NPD (Nationalistiche Partei Deutschlands), the right-wing German Nationalist Party, suggest that she has remained loyal to ideology of the Reich (see Lebert & Lebert, p. 13).

While Gudrun Himmler kept her connections to the past alive but secret, other Nazi children demonstrated their loyalty to their fathers by immersing themselves in their fathers' history in an attempt to defend and vindicate their crimes. Wolf-Rudiger Hess, son of Rudolf Hess, spent most of his life arguing for an investigation of his father's death, claiming the British Secret Service had murdered him in order to prevent his parole and the disclosure of embarrassing information about the British Secret Service. Hess's argument was incontrovertibly refuted in 2007 (six years after Hess's death) by the publication of documents that clearly demonstrated British support for Rudolf Hess's parole. Before his death, Wolf-Rudiger, stressed, "I never had any time. I spent all my free time on my father" (Lebert & Lebert, p. 76). Hess's compulsion to defend his father suggests that his own narcissistic identification was at stake. Niklas Frank observes, "There are two ways to survive for a child of a war criminal – to defend him until the end like my older brothers or to confront with his actions and to admit, 'Yes, our father was a criminal'" (Hitler's Children, 2012). Confronting the truth is inevitably more difficult because of it narcissistic implications. The Leberts argue that the Nazi children who failed to disavow their fathers also claim to have benefitted from their father's legacy. They comment,

> There seems to be a connection there: a child that so passionately deifies its father draws from his pretended significance and one-time lustre a considerable part of its own sense of itself – and is simultaneously incapable of owning up that its family history is, in truth, a serious psychological handicap.
>
> (Lebert & Lebert, p. 213)

The Leberts explain the need amongst some Nazi children to deny their tainted family history as a defence against their own narcissistic injury. For many Nazi children, such as Ingebirgitt Hoess, it is important to remember that their childhood was lived in the reflected glory of their fathers, many of whom were highly admired and revered amongst their peers. They were Hitler's blessed children. With the failure of the Reich and, worse still, with the arrests and imprisonment of their fathers, these children experienced a sudden and devastating loss of grace. Ingebirgitt Hoess describes the British search for her father at the end of the war,

> I remember when they came to our house to ask questions. I was sitting on the table with my sister. I was about 13 years old. The British soldiers were screaming: "Where is your father? Where is your father?" over and over again. I got a very bad headache. I went outside and cried under a tree. I made myself calm down. I made myself stop crying, and my headache went away.
>
> (Harding, 2013)

As another daughter of an SS officer succinctly put it, "I was a nobody now" (Children of the Third Reich).

Katrin Himmler, Heinrich Himmler's great-niece, like Niklas Frank, has chosen to publicly acknowledge her family connections and history as a way of coming to terms with her past. In her documentary, "Family members of Heinrich Himmler", Katrin states,

> In our family, it was useful to have this evil personified in Heinrich Himmler, the culmination of all evil. All the others could easily fade into his shadow. This had an impact on the family, and still does for some, so that for a long time no one examined what the other family members had done. Heinrich eased the burden for the rest of us.

In another interview, Katrin admits to feeling sick when she discovered her grandmother had been a Nazi (Hitler's Children, 2012).

Katrin has perhaps been able to explore her past so openly because, unlike many other Nazi families, the history of her family was spoken about. She recalls,

> My father told us about the family constellation very early on, he spoke openly about the fact that Heinrich Himmler was his uncle, his god-father even, and that he had committed terrible crimes. As a young child it was clear to me how difficult this was. How emotionally difficult this was for him and therefore for us, to be related to this mass murderer. I remember it as an emotional burden. When we were children, my sister and I thought it was good that only girls were in our family, so that the name of Himmler would eventually die out. We wanted the name to disappear or be erased.

Katrin makes it clear that she wanted her name to 'disappear' out of shame. In contrast to Bettina Goering, Katrin asserts, "I was never afraid that in my genes there is 'the bad blood from Heinrich Himmler'. I think that if I believed that, then I would be upholding the Nazi theories that everything is genetically determined" (Hitler's Children, 2012).[6] In acknowledging what for so many German families could not be spoken about, Katrin seems to have accepted her history and the collective guilt of her family and society, without being crippled by it.

My patient, Ana, began to accept her own tie to her father's crimes when she became aware of her disfigured left hand in her dream. Seeing this grotesque part of herself allowed her to realise that, while she was like her father, she could be different from him. Katrin comments, "There came a point when I felt I could live with this name. But I wanted my son to have the chance to start again, to have this different name. That's different than giving up a name that is part of your life" ("Family members of Heinrich Himmler").

Transgenerational guilt

For the children of perpetrators who deny their father's crimes, there is no consequent guilt to contend with. Just as the crime is disavowed so is the guilt attached to it. This is not the case for those children who acknowledge their father's crimes, like Niklas Frank, Rainer Hoess, and Katrin Himmler, who are faced with the burden of guilt by association. As Niklas Frank asserts, "Yes, I feel responsible for my father's actions and I'm ashamed for this".

Shame and guilt are interwoven. There is the contamination attached to the proximity of evil that imbues shame. Primo Levi describes this in the faces of the Russian soldiers as they liberated Auschwitz and witnessed the atrocities that had taken place:

> They did not greet us, nor smile; they seemed oppressed, not only by pity but also by a confused restraint which sealed their mouths, and kept their eyes fastened on the funereal scene. It was the same shame which we knew

> so well, which submerged us after the selections, and every time we had to witness or undergo an outrage: the shame that the Germans never knew, the shame which the just man experiences when confronted by a crime committed by another, and he feels remorse because of its existence, because of its having been irrevocably introduced into the world of existing things, and because his will has proven non-existent or feeble and was incapable of putting up a good defence.
>
> (Levi, p. 54)

Levi starkly points out that it was the victims and the observers who experienced shame, not the Germans. This highlights the fact that there was no place in the system of the camps, or indeed within the administration responsible for devising and implementing the Final Solution, for shame or guilt as this would signify a deep flaw at the heart of the Reich's ideology. The totalist belief system ascribed to by most Nazi officers was consistent within its own particular closed world. This, more than anything else, explains why so many of the Nazi war criminals did not plead guilty when brought to trial. Although Hans Frank changed his plea at the end of his trial, Niklas scoffed at his father's confession of guilt, assuming this was a kind of safeguard or deal his father was making with God to save face. However, this initial failure to acknowledge guilt on the part of those who had committed the crimes was the principal cause of the damage suffered by the next generation in Germany. Unacknowledged guilt was passed on to the children, left to atone for the deeds passed on to them from their fathers and to untangle the remnants of a perverse belief system that had corrupted everyone's lives.[7]

The guilt experienced by the children of perpetrators is not only the consequence of being left to deal with the sins of their fathers. For those children who loved their parents were also left with another form of guilt – that of loving someone who is tainted by evil. In his novel, *The Reader*, Schlink writes about a young German boy's coming of age love affair with an older woman, Hanna, who suddenly, and inexplicably, disappears at a time when he was beginning to have his own, separate life from her. It is only years later, as a student attending a war trial, that the narrator discovers to his horror that the woman he loved is there in front of him, standing trial for her acts as an SS officer in a concentration camp. It becomes clear in the course of Hanna's trial that she fails to defend herself because, he realises, defending herself would mean revealing her illiteracy. It was more important to her to keep this a secret than to deny charges that she had issued written orders for the killings of prisoners.

The narrator understands,

> She accepted that she would be called to account, and simply did not wish to endure further exposure. She was not pursuing her own interests, but fighting for her own truth, her own justice.
>
> (Schlink, 1997, pp. 132–133)

The narrator then has to confront his guilt for a series of betrayals; his betrayal in pushing Hanna away when he was young and beginning to be interested in other things in his life, his betrayal in deciding not to reveal to the court that she was illiterate, a fact that would have spared her a life sentence, and, finally, his guilt in "having loved a criminal" (Schlink, 1997, p. 133). The poignancy of the story lies in the symbol of illiteracy. Although at the time of the Third Reich Germany had the highest literacy rate in Europe, illiteracy signifies the ignorance that allowed ordinary people to become swept up in committing atrocities. Another interpretation of Hanna's illiteracy is that it represents the Third Reich's "moral illiteracy" (Wroe, 2002), something even more shaming, and hence to be kept hidden, than the acts to which this gave rise.[8]

Hoffman addresses the dilemma expressed by Schlink of "loving a criminal" and the predicament of being in what she refers to as a "no-win position". Hoffman writes,

> for to remain fixed in hatred and fear of one's parents, one's first objects of love, is to risk emotional stultification, or even death. But to give in to impulses of attachment and affection, when they are directed towards parents who have committed horrific crimes, and who have done so not out of passion but from conviction and belief – to accept this is surely to give up a part of one's own moral being.
>
> (Hoffman, p. 122)

However, what Schlink's narrator shows us is quite the reverse. He has not given up his own moral being in continuing to love this woman, he has in fact confirmed his moral being through his own awareness of his betrayals and his guilt. Hoffman seems to be confusing accepting the reality of evil with condoning it while the two are very different. Not to accept is to perpetuate a psychological splitting and denial that gives credence to the idea that evil can be located outside us, if not eradicated altogether.

Restorative guilt and false guilt

Children of perpetrators carry not only carry their own family histories but also the history of their communities. By virtue of their close association to evil, children of perpetrators are at the forefront in being forced to find a way of living with extreme moral contradictions that many of us do not have to confront in our everyday lives. In their study of the children of Nazi leaders, the Leberts question whether they have "become a kind of lightning conductor for German history?" (Lebert & Lebert, p. 76). Certainly they have played an important role as receptacles and scapegoats for collective guilt. However, this is also a role that, at least potentially, carries social influence and transformation. The guilt experienced by the children for the crimes of their fathers, especially in light of the denial expressed by so many perpetrators, can also be understood as a means of restoring a sense of moral order. The commission of an atrocity, or an act that intends to dehumanise a person, forces us to recognise that something outside the bounds of our perceived social norms has occurred. Our immediate sense of social and moral order is turned upside down and fundamentally threatened. The world that we can count on and, in most instances, trust no longer exists. This creates a state of anomie, taken from the Greek 'anomia' meaning lawlessness. On a social and collective level, the emotion of guilt affirms that harm has been done, that someone is responsible, that there is concern for the injured person, and that something destructive has happened that may not necessarily be possible to repair but needs to be acknowledged and mourned. By feeling guilty, these tenets of both a social and moral order are restored and re-confirmed. The shame and guilt experienced by children of perpetrators both enables and is the process by which they can restore a sense of moral order and integrity within their families and for the future. This is similarly so on a collective level.

Our guilt not only protects us from the threat of anomie, it also serves as a reminder of the past and keeps our ability to observe and judge alive. The act of remembering in itself performs a cathartic function as it validates our experienced reality and enables us to separate past from present. Kertesz, in writing about the Holocaust, stresses the necessity to remember and to have a history in order to go on being a person. However painful the memory is, it brings with it the knowledge that we are responsible towards ourselves and others. Kertesz exclaims,

> 'No!' something bellows, howls, within me, I don't wish to remember, . . . remembering is knowing, we live in order to remember what we know, because we cannot forget what we know, . . . we are not able, to forget, that is the way we are created . . . the reason why we know and remember is in order that somebody should feel shame on our account . . . *in any case you're always partly to blame.*
>
> (Kertesz, pp. 26–27)

Kertesz conversely warns us that without memory, there is no one to blame. This is the plight of children who deny the crimes their fathers have committed and, in doing so, deny a part of themselves, their own self agency. In this respect, guilt helps to protect us from dissociating from our past and from ourselves. Guilt preserves our humanity.

While it is evident that guilt serves a variety of important functions, it can also be used in a malignant or false way, becoming a kind of politically correct smokescreen that actually hides other ills. The young narrator in Schlink's novel describes his peers' blanket condemnation of their parents simply because they had been of the generation of the Third Reich. Despite the fact that his father had lost his job as a philosophy professor on political grounds, the son condemned both his parents 'to shame'. The narrator admits, "We all condemned our parents to shame, even if the only charge we could bring was that after 1945 they had tolerated the perpetrators in their midst" (Schlink, 1997, p. 90). But the narrator's shame, or guilt, in this regard is conveyed as a reaction conforming to the zeitgeist of his time. He notes the feigned interest expressed by his fellow students in the horrors of the Holocaust,

> When I think about it now, I think that our eagerness to assimilate the horrors and our desire to make everyone else aware of them was in fact repulsive. The more horrible the events about which we read and heard, the more certain we became of our responsibility to enlighten and accuse. Even when the facts took our breath away, we held them up triumphantly. Look at this!
>
> (Schlink, 1997, p. 91)

The students are filled with the self-righteousness of the converted; their eagerness to acknowledge guilt belies their disavowal of it.

During the trial of his lover, Schlink's narrator comments on the "general numbness" that seemed to take hold of perpetrators, victims, judges, members of the court and others attending. "When I likened perpetrators, victims, the dead, the living, survivors, and their descendants to each other, I didn't feel good about it and I still don't" (Schlink, 1997, p. 101). Kertesz's phrase, we are all "partly to blame", does not mean that we can all be likened to one another and in this way erase the horror and the significance of the distinctions between us.

A number of children of perpetrators have been recorded as saying that they wish their own lives could be taken in expiation of the deaths caused by their fathers. They are expressing not only a wish to absolve themselves of their own associated guilt but also a primitive notion of social justice – an eye for an eye – in the hope that one death would cancel out the other. But underlying the idea that they deserve such retribution, is the wish to be recognised as a victim too. The difference between perpetrator and victim can then be ignored and the child of the perpetrator can become an honourable victim rather than a person dirtied by his father's past. It is a form of narcissistic masochism that washes clean the sadism that is perceived as dangerous and taboo.

Hoffman distinguishes this kind of extreme guilt as a form of "pseudo-identification with Jewish victims". In describing a patient, the daughter of SS parents, Hoffman writes,

> She felt she was like them; she wanted to know Jews and feel close to them. This, too, is a theme that surfaces in German second-generation literature, and it is a delicate and troubling one. Sympathy for the victim and a reparative urge are the decent responses in genocide's wake. But the desire to impersonate or appropriate the identity of the other in order to disburden oneself of one's own carries with it the risk of inauthenticity and the seeds of bad faith . . . in stories like this . . . we can find clues as to the roots of that wider identification with the victim that has been such a prominent feature of postwar German politics.
>
> (Hoffman, p. 123)

These are examples of how guilt can be misread and perverted into bad faith, motivated by and disguising narcissistic needs. Like the students in Schlink's novel, it is the triumph of the self-righteous that negates genuine guilt.

The irresolvable conflict of evil

A son of a Nazi perpetrator reads his father's last words to his mother before being hanged,

> "I swear I never ordered or committed a crime." The son remarks in disgust, ". . . how many lies? . . . Of course he's lying, or he can't see what he did as a crime . . . because he sees himself as just a tool – that's particularly awful for me. I've read his statement of defence. In it, he describes the Gestapo as a normal administrative body with normal tasks. That was even more shocking for me because it was such a stupid argument. He seems to have had such a naïve attitude to this system. I was really shocked. I would almost have preferred a cleverer father. It's shaming".
>
> (Children of the Third Reich)

And how unbearable to have had a father who was so blind to what was going on and his part in it. But the son also assumes that if his father had been 'cleverer', he would have been different. Unfortunately, this is far from the case. The problem of the Reich was that what wasn't 'normal' could not simply be attributed to the stupidity, sadism or madness of its administrators – there is plenty of evidence to show that the SS cannot simply be classified as monsters and madmen. And the son's reaction to his father's professed innocence goes deeper than shame and loss of respect, there is also his disbelief that points to something that is unthinkable about what his father did. And by virtue of the fact that it was his *father*, what does this mean about him?

The legacy that these children, along with my patient, Ana, have inherited is precisely this struggle to make sense of how such evil could have happened without attributing it to a single cause and therefore something we can process mentally that is in some way familiar. The experience of evil is that it is *unthinkable*, it is not only beyond the bounds of our everyday existence, it is antithetical to the world we know, it is a world that is *ahuman*.[9] Because evil destroys our social norms it is by its very nature hard to integrate in our thinking and in our experience of life. This is true for all of us, but especially so for people who have been touched by evil – victims and the families of perpetrators. Trust in a seemingly predictable and consistent reality is shattered and, even more importantly, trust in those we are closest to and most dependent on is thrown into doubt. Niklas Frank, speaking to a German audience, warns,

> I don't trust any of you. Who knows? If the economy turns bad again, you might get those ideas again, to follow a strong leader, restrict ethnic minorities,

> maybe even imprison them. You don't have to call it "concentration camps". Here and there you have a little murder, a little killing. It might help purify the bloodline. Besides, it will create more jobs for the real Germans.
>
> (Hitler's Children)

How close our realpolitik is coming to this now.

What is most disturbing for children of perpetrators and what they are acutely aware of because of their close links to evil, is that the kernel of evil does not reside in others, it resides in all of us. We are all born with the mark of Cain. Niklas Frank conveys the anguish of his identification with his father when he says, "I'm sure I've hated (him) so very much because I kept finding him in myself" (Lebert & Lebert, p. 16). Ana's dream image of her atrophied left hand also signified her identification with a father who had kept hidden a lifeless and life-destroying part of himself. Both Niklas and Ana could only hate this aspect of themselves and yet it was their hatred that allowed them to acknowledge and incorporate the presence of evil within themselves.

The experience and proximity of evil is contaminating and disorienting; it is also alienating. The children of perpetrators share with victims the knowledge of a ruptured world, a loss of innocence that can never be regained. There is an initial shock that numbs the capacity for memory or piecing together the two strange realities of past and present. Modiano describes this state of mind in post-war France,

> I told myself that nobody remembers anything any more. . . . And yet from time to time, beneath this thick layer of amnesia, you can certainly sense something, an echo, distant, muted, but of what, precisely, it is impossible to say. Like finding yourself on the edge of a magnetic field, with no pendulum to pick up the radiation.
>
> (Modiano, pp. 124–125)

Those who try to resolve the contradictions left in the wake of evil by expelling or masking the truth continue to live in a twilight world without a centre. Paradoxically, it is the act of remembering and what this entails that centres us and allows us to create a different future.

Notes

1 An abridged version of this paper first appeared in the *British Journal of Psychotherapy*, February 2018, vol. 34, no. 1.

2 See Fromm, M. G., ed. (2012). *Lost in Transmission: Studies of Trauma across Generations*. London: Karnac. Fonagy, P. "The transgenerational transmission of Holocaust trauma." Chapter 20 in *Terrorism and War: Unconscious Dynamics of Political Violence*. Eds. Covington, C., Williams, P., Arundale, J., and Knox, J., London: Karnac. Volkan, V. (2006). *Killing in the Name of Identity*. Charlottesville, VA: Pitchstone.

3 See Sichrovsky, P. (1988). *Born Guilty: Children of Nazi Families*. New York: Basic Books. Bar-On, D. (1989). *Legacy of Silence: Encounters with Children of the Third Reich*. Cambridge, MA: Harvard University Press. See also "Children of the Third Reich," film produced by Catrine Clay, BBC2, 10 November 1993.
4 Studies of families of violent offenders demonstrate that they often experience associative shame, ostracism and victimisation. See Condry, R. (2007). *Families Shamed: The Consequences of Crime for Relatives of Serious Offenders*. London: Routledge.
5 Nazi perpetrators were most commonly men, but women were also actively involved in committing atrocities, either as Nazi officers or as adjutants to their Nazi husbands. See Lower, W. (2013). *Hitler's Furies: German Women in the Nazi Killing Fields*. London: Chatto & Windus.
6 The thrust of Hitler's vision of the Reich and the new German supremacy was to re-create the purity of the Aryan race.
7 In commenting on the conflicting belief systems evident in post-war Germany, Hoffman writes: "the public climate in which the younger German grew up was diametrically opposed to the belief system of their parents. Indeed, Peter Sichrovsky interestingly suggests that the contradictions between what he calls a 'fascistic family structure' and the postwar democratic ethos both increased the tensions between the generations and ultimately enabled the young to rebel against the parents and break the bonds that tied them to the past" (Hoffman, p. 124).
8 The German title of Schlink's book, *The Reader is Der Vorleser* (1995) and reinforces this interpretation. The preposition *vor* (German for 'in front' or 'before') unfortunately gets lost in the English translation and with it the suggestion that the reader would read *in front* of the child, be a role model and thus place *before* the child a set of moral values, which the child then internalises. In Hanna's childhood this was missing and would only be replaced later by Michael, the Vorleser.
9 For an account on the nature of evil and its effects on us, see Covington, C. (2016). "Do we need a theory of evil?" In *Everyday Evils: A Psychoanalytic View of Evil and Morality*. London: Routledge.

References

Bar-On, D. (1999). *The Indescribable and the Undiscussable: Reconstructing Human Discourse after Trauma*. Budapest: Central European University Press.

"Children of the Third Reich." Produced by Catrine Clay for BBC2, first shown on 10 November 1993.

Hall, A. (1 June 2015). "'My beautiful Auschwitz childhood': Daughter of camp commandant Rudolph Hoess describes life growing up next to a concentration camp-and how she has hidden her identity for decades." London. *MailOnline*.

Harding, T. (7 September 2013). "Hiding in N. Virginia, a daughter of Auschwitz." *Washington Post*.

Himmler, K. (19 June 2012). "Family members of Heinrich Himmler." Documentary film available on www.docsonline.tv.

"Hitler's Children." Produced by Chanoch Zeevi, first shown on Israeli Channel 2 on 1st May 2011, BBC2 in 2012.

Hoffman, E. (2004). *After Such Knowledge*. London: Vintage.

Kertesz, I. (2004). *Kaddish for an Unborn Child*. London: Random House.

Lebert, S. & Lebert, N. (2000). *My Father's Keeper: Children of Nazi Leaders: An Intimate History of Damage and Denial*. London: Little, Brown.

Levi, P. (1989). *The Drowned and the Saved*. London: Abacus.

McGlothlin, E. (2006). *Second-Generation Holocaust Literature: Legacies of Survival and Perpetration*. London: Camden House.
Modiano, P. (2014). *The Search Warrant*. London: Harvill Secker.
Sands, P. (2016). *East West Street*. London: Weidenfeld & Nicolson.
Schlink, B. (1997). *The Reader*. London: Phoenix.
Schlink, B. (2012). "Johann Sebastian Bach on Ruegen." In *Summer Lies*. London: Phoenix.
Sicher, E. ed. (1998). *Breaking Crystal: Writing and Memory after Auschwitz*. Urbana: University of Illinois Press.
Wroe, N. (9 February 2002). "Reader's guide to a moral maze." *The Guardian*.

Chapter 8

Making my way out of the shadow into the sun

A painful confrontation with my past

Martin Miller[1]

With disturbing complexity, the chapter that follows offers an unusual and distinctly personal view of events 'in the shadow' both during the war years and, for our next author, events that continued to dictate his personal life for so many years thereafter. Allow me to begin and for the author to elaborate:

> *Swiss psychotherapist Martin Miller's parents survived the Second World War in Warsaw. Their relationship was anything but simple. His Jewish mother survived thanks in large measure to a relationship with a Polish man – a blackmailer who worked for the Gestapo.*

After the war, they stayed together, moved to Switzerland and married. Martin was born in 1950. Of his life with his parents he writes, "I was born into a family traumatised by war and was ultimately treated as the persecuted Jew during the war".

It was only after his mother's death that Martin could articulate and make public his experiences: "This was finally the time when I felt empowered to write a biography of my mother", he says. In the chapter that follows, Miller reflects on his own past and the career that he was eventually able to develop for himself as a psychotherapist. In this light, he considers how parents can split their own wartime experiences, and he reflects on a transgenerational inheritance borne of these experiences.

So many people are barely conscious of their own background – their history, their past. Some, of course, know many *facts* about it, and can refer to experiences to the last detail, but upon listening to them, one immediately has the sense that they are completely split off – as though talking about someone else. What is missing is any connection to feelings experienced.

Then there are those who either refer to their history incorrectly or so poorly, appearing to make a point of only allowing their story to be seen in a shining, bright and beautiful light. All was good, they purport, whilst not allowing for any critical comment. They defend their family's history like a lion: embellishing and glorifying it. Unconsciously, however, they recount experiences that have occurred in their family which make you shudder. These experiences are then completely and, I would suggest, defensively split off from the personal meaning they hold. Indeed it is rare that I come across situations where someone recounts their story realistically, factually and with sensitivity.

On the other hand, I feel personally and, as a psychotherapist, professionally privileged when I have experienced what can happen to people when offered the opportunity to gain access to their own history. As a psychotherapist, my principle aim through the course of a therapy is to allow every patient's biography to become a differentiated, coherent and, above all, honest narrative for him or her. A personal narrative is, after all, one's biographical story reflecting one's consciousness and which when gained through therapy, can remain at one's side as a protection of sorts in the present and which, at all times, helps one to connect the here and now with the past.

Today, I am pleased to feel that I have developed this narrative for myself, because this consciousness has effectively pulled me out not only of bad moods but of bad and indeed trying situations (i.e. those I judge as detrimental to myself). Another advantage of this knowledge is that never again will I feel helpless in my daily dealings with others. Whilst I still face difficulties, I am now able to resolve emotional conflicts equipped with a greater sense of independence. Today, when faced with emotional difficulties, I am better able to help myself, as a good mother would do, and it is *this* form of autonomy that constitutes for me its decisive aspect.

This paper highlights for me a special situation. My mother was a world-renowned psychologist, *expert*, author and researcher in child development. At the age of 30 I began work in the same profession as hers, with the result being that existing conflicts intensified – and at a staggering rate.

I should add here that from birth, my relationship to my mother was a disturbed one. The conflict we had – or to use Balint's terminology, the *basic fault* – was very closely linked to her experiences as a Jew who had survived the war in Warsaw. Apart from the problematic issue of being the son of a famous mother, needing to fight to find his place in the limelight of fame, or rather, its *shadow*, I was affected by the consequences of my mother's and my father's unresolved war experiences. In this chapter I will not deal in any depth with the issue of transgenerational inheritance, but rather focus on the issue of how it is even possible to develop one's own individuality whilst being thrust into the shadow of one's famous parent.

When addressing this topic it has occurred to me that very few children born into such constellations have managed to find themselves a position of independence and autonomy within society. Two alternatives seem to present themselves: either one is and remains a small attachment and exists as sort of an appendix to one's famous parent – an ardent admirer, perhaps worshipper of their celebrity and, in a narcissistic manner, tries, like a bee, to feed off the admiration bestowed on the parent. Or one rebels. You too gain fame, but you do so by creating scandal and, in this way grabbing the attention you feel you need.

In my case, after fighting a gruesome battle, I did manage to develop my own identity. Only after the death of my mother, however, have I dared to emerge from *under cover*. All previous efforts to become noticed for my own sake – unrelated to her – had felt futile. Any hope of success had somehow needed to be abandoned, or so I imagined.

Still today wherever I go and introduce myself, I am invariably greeted with the words: "Oh, you are the son of the famous Alice Miller". Immediately I am diminished. As a person I am insignificant and uninteresting, transformed in their minds as merely the practical *medium* for the interlocutor to gain further knowledge about the famous Alice Miller. Similarly, whenever I give a talk, the organiser finds it extremely important to have the poster announce that the event will feature the son of the famous Alice Miller. He then can rest easy as there will be a sufficient number of attendees. This is my reality and I have to learn to live with it – any attempt to overturn this socio-psychological pattern is futile. Of course a positive aspect of such experiences, I might add, is that I usually am successful in drawing a distinct separation between myself and my mother and, by the evening's end, everyone in the lecture hall has become aware that I am my own person who *also* has a contribution to make.

Allow me now to cover two stories which complement one another – both relating to my shadow.

I will start with my biography: I was born under what can only be called the gruesome shadow of the Second World War. Though it was shortly *after* the war, to me it felt like I actually grew up *in* the war, without ever knowing what it was about. I never had the opportunity to really get to know my parents. For them I was a foreign being – remaining a constant symbol of their war experiences. It is for this reason that I will explore the brutal world of war into which I was born and how I succeeded in liberating myself from this war-like shadow.

In the second half of this chapter I will cover my experiences as a psychotherapist. Here is where I found myself caught up in a critical conflict with my mother – both her present and a past with which she could not come to terms, but which was reactivated in later years.

In my conclusion, I state from experience that for a child it is highly dangerous if one's parents have been fundamentally unable come to terms with their own past. Even if they have travelled an arduous path in life, they are likely to have projected their unresolved and awful experiences unconsciously onto their children. My own parents seemed, almost without thought, to have done exactly that. Throw in an unresolved war situation and you can thank the dear Lord if you survive such hell!

My parents cast over me their brutal shadow of war

I was born into a marriage that was under emotional strain from the start. In 1947 my parents moved from Poland to Switzerland for study. There, respectively, they read psychology and sociology at the University of Basel before settling in Switzerland and marrying.

My mother came from an orthodox Jewish family living in Piotrokov, a small town south of Lodz, and survived the Holocaust in Warsaw hiding underground. Her grandfather, owned a hardware store, was considered one of the well-to-do inhabitants, and an acknowledged religious scholar. Her father, though pious, was not financially successful, and not well respected by his daughter – my mother Alice. Though she suffered greatly under her own mother's authoritative (and *authoritarian* – often violent) upbringing, she managed to insist on being permitted to attend the Polish school rather than the Jewish one. Alice's relatives describe her as a very difficult child, who would always withdraw with her books – overall, making a very arrogant, albeit brilliant impression on others whom she loved to outwit.

When the war broke out in 1939 and the Germans attacked and occupied Poland, the first ghetto was built in Piotrokov. Together with a large part of her family, my mother moved to the ghetto. Though only 16 years old, she knew to make contact with the ghetto's underground movement and through it obtained a false passport identifying her not as a Jew but as a Polish citizen. From then on she was no longer Alysha Englard, but became known as Alice Rostovska. After acquiring false papers for both her sister and her mother (thereby rescuing them), she escaped the ghetto. Sadly she needed to leave her father behind in the ghetto because, as an orthodox Jew who spoke only Yiddish, he would never have survived outside of the ghetto. Indeed, sick and abandoned, he died there.

Alice hid her mother and sister in a convent. Her mother, however, deeply resenting being forced into assuming the Catholic faith for reasons of shelter, objected. As a favour to her, Alice herself felt forced to find a flat in the Arian part of Warsaw. Such a step would have meant suicide for Jews, as being caught outside the ghetto spelt certain death. My mother, however, decided to take that risk, saw an advertisement for a flat rental and responded to it. She was extremely unfortunate. She had fallen straight into the clutches of a Polish informant working for the Gestapo who was behind this advertisement which was a death trap.

The following story is something I am only able to reconstruct based on research and different stories told to me, but in view of what I experienced later on whilst living with my parents, much points to the fact that my father was the same man who blackmailed my mother during the war. I will explain this later.

My mother never spoke to me about her wartime experiences. Mostly she recounted episodes that were 'defamiliarised' to such an extent that the listener, in any event, could not understand what had actually taken place. I, as her son, never questioned her, as I felt instinctively that she would not tolerate any further questions.

But there was the one time when she let down her guard. It was on this rare occasion that my mother, albeit only in vague terms, spoke about her wartime experiences and suddenly revealed to me a secret that took me by total surprise. Unfortunately, however, in the midst of our heated conversation, I didn't dare ask any questions. 'Incidentally', she had said, the man who threatened to inform on us in the name of the Gestapo had the same name as your father. His name was Andreas Miller.

Only many years later, whilst writing the biography of my mother, the magnitude of what my mother had actually revealed started to dawn on me: So it was my own father who had been the Nazi criminal, the same man who had forced my mother to surrender to him in return for his not betraying her, her mother and her sister to the Gestapo – the same man whom she would not be rid of after the war.

It was a coincidence, but Andreas fell in love with Alice the Jewess. At the same time my father continued persecuting the innocent. As he, of course, needed to earn a living, he did so by continuing to place advertisements for flat rentals in an attempt to attract those desperate to hide in the Aryan sector. He would then deliver their names to the Gestapo. To survive, my mother was forced to cooperate with him and his crimes – crimes that both my father and mother, undiscovered during their lifetimes, would take to their graves. Alice became the classic victim of the Stockholm syndrome.

After the Warsaw Uprising, my mother together with her sister fled to the Russian side. There stood Stalin's Russian Army, who then betrayed the Polish people to the Germans. My mother worked in a military hospital at the time and I can only imagine that what she must have seen at the time would have left deep scars – traumatising and damaging to her.

When the war ended she returned, together with her sister and mother, to Piotrokov. But no one they had known was there. All Jews had been killed. A few members of her family survived – now dispersed around the world. Most though had been killed in the Treblinka extermination camp or in the ghetto.

She then decided with her sister to move to Lodz and study there. At first she thought she was rid of the fraudster who had blackmailed her throughout the war, but soon Andreas found out where my mother was studying, travelled to Lodz and embarked there on his own studies.

As for me, I was born in 1950 and my parents immediately gave me away to an acquaintance of theirs. Deposited with these people who were strangers to me, I was said to have never stopped screaming and throwing tantrums. Then, my story has it (as confirmed in later years by my mother), on a chance visit, my mother's aunt, a refugee at the time living in Zurich, appalled by my treatment, spontaneously decided to take me away to her own home and family – without asking my mother's permission. There for the first six months of my life, I thrived.

As for my mother, she had declared then, and confirmed in later years, that I would disturb her whilst she was writing her thesis. I would be in her way when, as a child, I would make my needs known.

Based on what I know today, my mother had been concealing something critical from me. Newly married, she was indeed writing her thesis, along with my father. But as for my father, a convinced Nazi, how must it have been to have a Jewish son? As my mother had never mentioned to me that I was unwanted by her, I am convinced today that it was my father who forced her to give me away. It seems though that at some point my mother could no longer bear being separated from her child and proceeded to remove me (I understand, brutally) from my caregivers.

Throughout my life my early separation from my mother had deeply traumatised me, and to this day I have never been able to come to terms with it. From then on, my mother and I were never able to build a warm and loving relationship. The separation of the first few months could never be compensated. All future conflicts that I had with my mother were marked by this early separation. I am convinced today that my father had hoped that I would die as a result of the neglect to which the *acquaintance* had subjected me.

But this did not happen. Instead, in later years, he would let me experience – with a vengeance – the fact that I did not do him the favour of disappearing as a Jew. I was brutally beaten, persecuted, humiliated and literally tormented at every turn. Sadly, I never defended myself, but then again, I was always alone, nobody had ever helped me stand up to this sadistic and violent father – not then and not later on.

I was thus born into a family traumatised by war, and became myself engulfed in its *dark shadow*. During my own early life my parents' relationship to one another remained as cruel as it had been during the war and thus I became the victim of a transgenerational inheritance. Throughout my life my father, still a staunch anti-Semite and Nazi, continued to bully me relentlessly. I had turned into the persecuted Jew of the family. He would regularly beat me, but never once did my mother come to my defence. It seemed she had remained consumed with the same fear she experienced during the war. When, against his will, I stayed alive, my father immediately re-established the same constellation as he had with my mother during the war.

Years later I would often ask my mother how she would explain to herself this contradiction of not defending me against the beatings of my father yet her being able to present herself to the world as the heroic advocate for battered children. My mother never responded directly but instead, with deep reproach, would only blame me for accusing her of something she had never committed.

In my family I have suffered practically the same range of humiliations and persecutions from which the Jewish people had suffered during the war. I do not identify myself as a Jew in the common sense of the term. Jewish holidays mean nothing to me. However, what I do know only too well is the feeling of suffering the same pain and persecution that the Jewish people had experienced, and it is this that has become an important part of my Jewish identity today.

Under such circumstances I found it impossible to freely develop my potential. I became the victim of horrible projections. Not only did I have to live the life of a Jew in war-torn Poland, but I had to continue living in its polluted shadow.

Later on, in my work as a psychotherapist, I realised how some parents can split off their experiences of war and transfer them – project their experiences as victims onto their children. Having forced a false identity onto the child, they may then try their utmost to undermine any attempt by the child to free him/herself from this enforced identity. The child is confronted with sinister parental fears and anxieties because the parent justifiably is afraid to have to re-experience/live out that part of themselves that they had split off

In many respects, the psychological humiliations I endured from my father were worse than the physical abuse to which I was subjected. At school, when I encountered difficulties, even with homework, he would seize the opportunity to demean me. Always finding a reason to justify his behaviour, he would beat me over the head daily while screaming that I was pure filth and would turn out to be nothing but a failure in life. Should I want to spend time on my own, my father would immediately disturb my privacy, yelling at me to devote myself to school and to stop being such a slug. Nothing would help, not even when I had already completed my homework. At table he control me at all times: dictating *how* and, above all, *what* I was to eat.

I had a sister with Down syndrome. Both parents used her against me like a weapon. Often, when I was about to say something, my sister would interrupt me. If I objected to this, my father would immediately interject: "but you are normal and she is mentally delayed". Unfortunately, I was to develop a profound hatred of my sister but kept such feelings to myself. Today, I know that this hatred had little to do with my sister but mostly to do with my tormenting parents. It is, however, typical that one bears one's hatred towards the weakest.

Even in this respect my father proved to be the perfect Nazi. He manipulated me against my sister to such an extent that I became entirely convinced that mentally delayed people are worth nothing – not worthy of life. He succeeded not only in making me the persecuted Jew but somehow turning me into a racist Nazi. As for my mother, she would always reproach me for rejecting my sister and for considering her as worthless life. Today I understand the relationships, but in those days I didn't.

At the time, my parents would also systematically exclude me from any of the gatherings of the academic elite that would take place at our home, clearly signalling that they wanted absolutely nothing to do with me – that I was of no value to them whatsoever. For years I simply thought that, through me, my parents lived out the migration problems they experienced in Switzerland. Later, after I had found out about my parents' past, I realised that this was almost beside the point. Rather the point seemed to be that I should be turned into the persecuted Jew in wartime Warsaw, whilst also made a foreigner within my own family.

My mother took great pains to avoid acquainting me with Jewish culture. It was as though her husband was going to betray her to the Nazis and deport her to Treblinka. My mother would never lose that fear.

The slow and painful escape from the shadow of the war

Whether consciously or not, I had also learnt something from my mother, particularly how to hide and survive. Whilst I never spoke with my parents about their behaviour, never stood up to them, inwardly I distanced myself from them as far as I felt possible. I lived a life of my own, never showing anybody what I *looked like inside*. I began meeting all of my needs, all on my own. I became so adept at it, that, despite their severe monitoring, my parents practically never found me out.

At the age of 17 an educational opportunity opened up for me and I was able to move into a Catholic boarding school. I was ecstatic at being finally able to escape this hell. The school was governed by strict orders and regulations and many of my schoolmates complained about its repressive environment. But here is what I once wrote to my mother:

> Dear Mummy, I feel like I am in paradise here. Never before in my life have I felt so free. I am relieved to no longer live at home. That had been a dreadful prison for me.

My mother was utterly shocked when she received this letter. Whilst claiming she could no longer understand the world, she had, consciously or not, selected the boarding school that had saved me from my Nazi father – just as she had saved her sister and mother by finding for them a Catholic convent during the war. My father, of course, managed to meet up with me once a week in order to check whether I actually did my schoolwork. For me, these encounters were sheer hell.

I narrowly passed my A-level exams – perhaps my teenage expression of freedom from any authority whatsoever. When I then expressed the desire to go to university to read psychology and sociology – the same subjects as my parents had studied – I encountered their strong resistance, with my father working himself up into his typical fit of rage. As in the past, raising his fist, he was all set to beat me as he had always done, when suddenly he realised that I was no longer a little child, but was standing eye to eye with him. When I too raised my fists, in total shock, he stammered: "Do you seriously want to hit your poor father?" I answered: "If you hit me, then I will hit you back". Ever since this incident, he never beat me again.

But there were other ways he could and would completely wear me down. Having the apparent temerity to ask for his financial help for my university studies filled him with fury as he screamed,

> What has got into you to expect something like this from me. You are the biggest fool I know. How on earth did you come up with the absurd idea to actually ask me to finance the studies of such an asshole, such a total loser like you? You only barely passed your A-levels and now, look at yourself, becoming so arrogant as to want me to pay for your studies?

His verbal and violent orgy left me feeling totally numb and incapable of standing up for my rights. Later in life I would blame myself as, according the law, I had an absolute right to request from my parents that they support me during my studies. When, shortly after this incident, I spoke to my mother about what had happened, she too let me down. Though in the past she had often ranted to me about my father, now she cooperated with him just as she had done during the war. "You must understand your father", she said, "as he was so upset when you nearly failed your A-levels. And anyway, I completely agree with him on this matter. Studying will overwhelm you and if you were to begin studying now, it would not end well".

I decided to train as a primary school teacher and after training had become completely independent of my parents – earning my own money. Instinctively I realised two things: if my parents remained in contact with me, it would be dangerous for me. Further, that I would never be able to rely on them.

Unfortunately I was unable to follow through completely. Though I became a teacher, I did not at all enjoy this work. Meanwhile my desire to work as a psychologist never went away. I had my independence, made my own money and, to some extent had fled the shadow of my parents. But I was extremely dissatisfied with my situation in life, above all with my professional life. Again I felt the *ignorant, persecuted Jew* – the identity that my parents had forced on me. My personal development had been so hindered that I felt a complete outsider in the school where I worked, falling out with most of my colleagues, unable to integrate. Yet I enjoyed a wonderful relationship with the children and in that respect had no problems with authority.

During those years as a teacher I increasingly realised that within me lay a dormant gift: that of being a psychologist. My desire to realise my professional dream grew steadily but I still did not yet know how to transform this passion into a reality.

The courage to embark on one's own professional career and meet one's own needs: I completely step out of the shadow, but the price I was to pay for my escape from the parental prison was immeasurable

My parents created remarkable careers for themselves. My father became professor at the University of St. Gallen and chairman of the Swiss Commission of Higher Education. He thus became the most important person in the organisation governing all Swiss universities.

My mother, Alice Miller, underwent training as a psychoanalyst and became a member of the renowned Zurich Psychoanalytical Society. For 25 years she worked as an independent psychoanalyst. In 1979 she published her first book, *The Drama of the Gifted Child.* Against all expectations this book became a gigantic global success. My mother became famous throughout the world – a star.

It was in America that her career really took off. She left her profession as a psychoanalyst and became an author. From then on she called herself a researcher in childhood and would campaign for the rights of children, vehemently attacking parents for their brutal parenting techniques. In all those years my mother was a courageous, aggressive fighter for her ideas. Nobody would have guessed that she was still beset by anxieties.

My mother's transformation became for me a huge issue. During those years when my father would so torment and persecute me, my mother never once protected me. Throughout her career as a childhood researcher she behaved as if she had always been committed to the cause of persecuted children. For me, her shadow was growing increasingly darker. All readers envied me for having such a great mother, but in truth the book-Alice-Miller was totally different to the real-life-person. As always, I protected my mother whilst remaining silent in the face of this lie.

I was already 30 years old when my mother embarked on her global career. Perhaps like many who become famous the world over, she too seemed to change personality – and to such an extent that after the transformation I could barely recognise her To follow one's own path alongside such people is infinitely difficult and if one dares take the in spite of it all, life can mete you out a horrible punishment. Today I fully understand those people who live in the shadow of their famous parents and can appreciate if they don't dare disentangle themselves from them.

At the age of 30 I decided to become a psychotherapist myself and thought that my mother's fame would help me in my own work to become also a psychotherapist. Initially, my mother promised that she would support me. By 1979, I started my own psychotherapy practice, at the same time enrolling in the University of Zurich's psychology faculty. Though I never asked my parents for permission, of course, upon hearing of my intentions, my mother reacted seriously insulted. Reproachfully she said: "Why would you want to study when all they do there is convey total nonsense to you. Anything you need to know, you can just come to me". These remarks frightened me to the core: it was the first time I noticed that my mother, by then already famous, had extreme difficulties with me wanting to carve my own future in the same profession that she had. Simultaneously I was confronted by her enormous appetite for power.

Within this short period of time her perception of reality had become completely distorted. As the famous Alice Miller she owned the monopoly of knowledge, and the rest were idiots. It suddenly felt as if I was standing in front of my father, who had the same tendency to put on airs, who had nothing but contempt for everyone else and who, instead, praised his own self to the sky.

No longer was my mother the most important person to whom I would turn. From the start I recognised the treacherously dangerous umbrella my mother was holding over me, and so as fast as I possibly could, I tried to escape. Unfortunately this escape took me a full 30 years, as I was all alone having to deal with it.

One can hardly imagine how, even as a grown-up, one can feel totally helpless and at the mercy of such insignificant, and outwardly weak people whose behaviour belie their inner steeliness. Below, I will describe this situation in more detail. For now, I will leave it at this: at the time, unlike me who had nothing, my mother was extremely influential and her clutch over the power of the media felt so strong that she could easily have been able to blackmail me – and this indeed is what she later did.

I thus found myself in a precarious position of having to decide – at first unconsciously, later with increasing awareness, that in front of me were two possibilities: I could stand under her umbrella and be looked after, serving my mother like a slave and remaining in bondage – a lucrative life, no doubt and perhaps one offering a degree of power. Her desire, it felt, was to seduce me into willingly placing myself under this deceptively protective umbrella.

Alternatively, my own openly expressed desire to be autonomous from my mother would have been a declaration of war. Reflecting on my past history helped me remain steadfast in my wish and finally feel able to determine and forge my own path. Steadily, my relationship to my mother deteriorated and her eyes looked at me with growing mistrust, deep insecurity, and increased paranoia. I was familiar with this gaze ever since my childhood: seeing it whenever my father would hit me at the table or humiliate and torment me. She just sat there and remained silent.

Independent, free, I embarked on a psychotherapeutic training with Professor Bastiaans from Leiden – a move that was already to damage further any good professional relationship I might have with my mother.

Why Professor Bastiaans? The background though simple, felt significant to me: being the star that she was, my mother was invited to a psychotherapy conference in Lindau. I accepted her invitation to accompany her, going along admittedly as a small appendage. At this conference participants literally fought for the opportunity to exchange a few words with Alice Miller. I felt completely lost – instinctively recognising the unpleasant feelings arising in me. Automatically I separated myself from my mother and set out to discover the conference for myself. Gradually, still unconsciously, I made the first steps towards moving out of my mother's dangerous black shadow. Spontaneously I decided to attend a seminar given by Jan Bastiaans on how people tend to react in situations of stress – aggression or escape: basically, fight or flight.

He also dealt with trauma. I was totally fascinated by the man and after his talk introduced myself to him – using, of course, my advantage of being the son of the famous Alice Miller. Agreeing a date to meet with him in Holland already made me feel a bit more free and independent.

As always I did not tell my mother anything about this encounter – it was to remain my secret. After all, had I not been taught by the *master of deception* herself? Secretly I was emerging from the shadow and, without necessarily conscious intent went about taking control for my *personal prison escape*. First though, just like my mother had done, I went into hiding, *joining the underground* so to speak, and assuming, unofficially, a new identity. I played being ignorant, but was, in truth, secretly beginning to develop my own new identity as a psychotherapist. Unfortunately this game of hide and seek lasted until after my mother's death. The price I had to pay to survive was to practice for decades as *an underground therapist*.

Not once did I allow myself to show publicly who I really was. For years I renounced on a career, never feeling permitted to show openly my aptitude, dare

I say gift, as a therapist. I could not, however, stay totally in hiding forever: the few times when I revealed myself to my mother had led to serious confrontations with her. This escalated to such an extent that my mother, consumed by hatred, appeared bent on killing me.

At the convention she never once showed any intention of seriously engaging with me as much as ask what I was actually up to all day. She seemed drunk on the narcissistic nourishment on which she fed herself throughout the convention.

Surreptitiously I commenced my training with Bastiaans and learnt a great deal. It was the mechanism of projection that made a particular impression on me – in a sense, staked its claim. Projections are after all separations from the repressed parts of oneself. In my case (as in the case of many others) I sensed myself to be, as previously noted, a victim of my parents' projections. For my father and, in part, also for my mother I had become the object of their projections, for example, as the persecuted Jew in wartime Warsaw. My parents were for me completely unaware of their projections, as indeed so many of us are. I experienced them as believing that I was somehow a filthy Jew; and, feeling no guilt whatsoever, my father could thus treat me as a Nazi would have done. For him the war was still on.

This is what happens to victims of war or to people exposed during their childhood to severe trauma or parental oppression. If never having reflected on their projective behaviour, then it is their nearest, albeit not necessarily dearest, who, above all, will become potential victims of these dangerous projections; and dangerous they are, as these split off psychological parts are invariably hugely destructive.

Once I started working as a psychotherapist, the relationship between my mother and me underwent a profound change. At the beginning, I suddenly became her best and most intimate friend. I helped her with the writing of her first book, I listened to her when she embarked on her second book, and came up with good ideas for her to use. You cannot imagine my relief at now being accepted by my mother. I truly felt liberated and was looking forward to a future when I would finally be able to develop and live my life as my own self. I had witnessed, of course, how my mother's ideas had come about and thus was firmly convinced that now I too would able to benefit from these ideas.

Soon I realised, however, that this assumption was ill founded. I had blundered into a trap, felt literally held hostage and, to this very day, haven't quite recovered from its consequences.

At the very back of my mind, I knew that my mother had a hate-filled relationship to her sister. Whilst only some fragmented bits of the story were ever communicated to me by my mother, these should have been sufficient for me to realise that my mother was a psychological bombshell marching through life ready to explode at any moment.

In the first throws of euphoria whilst training to become a psychotherapist, I failed to notice this. To the contrary, I was elated that my mother was actually interested in my work as a therapist. She had asked questions with curiosity, leaving me feeling that the famous expert was actually engaged with my work.

It is only today that I know that, in order to survive, my mother had perfected the art of completely reinventing herself in her dealings with others, including myself, as she had done during the war. Hard as I tried, I just couldn't believe at the time the incredible energy she would mobilise to put a stop to my development. As she was losing control over me, it seemed she had had to find ways and means to destroy me.

Finally it struck me that the rage I knew my mother to have harboured against my aunt (her sister whom she had saved during the war) was now being turned against me – whether consciously or not. (As it happens, I look very similar to this aunt.) This sister was known in the family to be creative, easy going and, like my mother, highly intelligent. Yet she was always presented to me as the very opposite: stupid, uneducated. It was only later that I learnt that my aunt who lived in Mexico had become a pre-eminent professor expert in the history of the Native Indians and the Inca, and had published several books.

Hitherto keeping this under wraps, my mother was now faced with the reality that her son was also creative and was perhaps even becoming a competition to her in her own field – *her empire*. Whilst my mother was writing her books I had been listening to her intently and, within a short time, had found it easy to translate her theory into practice.

In my euphoric state, I, of course, told my mother about my experiences of working as a therapist. I spoke freely, without giving it further thought. My mother listened to me intently and, yes, I have to admit that never before had she shown so much interest in me as then. I suspected nothing. Nothing at all. After all those years of neglect, I was finally getting to enjoy the attention and the interest of the famous Alice Miller. Did not thousands of people listen to her? Now suddenly I had become, in her arena, a fascinating person. Unfortunately this was to be short-lived. Suddenly the wind turned: my mother was to reveal her true self.

Having listened to me attentively, she proceeded to steal my ideas for her third book. Ironically, it was called 'Thou Shalt Not Be Aware'. At first I always believed that my mother would, of course, be proud of me for having so adeptly translated her theory into practice, but I know today that I was brutally robbed of my intellectual property.

Meanwhile, in Berne my mother had gotten to know a primary therapist called Konrad Stettbacher. One day in 1983 I received a letter from him informing me that my mother had secured with him a coveted place for me to enter into 'primary' therapy with him and that I should not let give up this opportunity but, instead, should immediately transfer into his account SFR 12,000 (at the time some GBP 9,677). The waiting time for this therapy was set by Mr Stettbacher at three years.

Reading this letter, I felt as though I was being hit over the head. When I confronted my mother, accusing her of committing a dreadful psychological attack, she exploded, with a fury I had never experienced before, saying it was time I accepted something from her, seeing that as a mother she had been unable to care adequately for me when I was a small child.

Clearly I was no longer an infant and there is no way to make up for childhood losses to an independent 30-year-old. As always though, I failed to stand up to her, but sensed that this attack had forever destroyed my relationship with her. Using all her persuasive skills my mother tried to persuade me to start a therapy with Stettbacher. Finally Stettbacher phoned me wanting to convince me of this therapy. When I then started questioning Stettbacher about his therapeutic experience and knowledge, I realised that this man didn't have a clue. I declined to enter therapy with him, informed my mother – a decision which precipitated a further violent explosion whose verdict it was that I would present a serious danger to my clients seeing that I had no understanding of therapy. In my mother's words, she deeply regretted having enabled me to embark on this profession and was now officially in battle against me as a therapist. With her subsequent threat to expose me as a charlatan, I clearly knew where the enemy was hiding and was starkly aware that I was all on my own with my career as a therapist.

There was another side to this experience, however, and one that carried with it a significant advantage: I was forced to develop my own methodology as a therapist – but sadly, only in hiding. Given my mother's celebrated status, coupled with her threats, it felt safest for me to keep a low profile, lest I risk my life by revealing my own identity. Unable to prove openly my own capabilities, was I in the same position as my mother's during the war? Has the deadly shadow of the war again fallen over me?

For several years I had no contact with my mother and lived my own separate life. It sounds easier than it was. I got married, bought a house and enjoyed life. Though I never saw my mother, her *emotional presence*, so to speak, was never far away. During this period I experienced first-hand how emotional introjects have an impact on one's day-to-day adult life – how they become intertwined in one's daily life. My father, who had persecuted and tormented me so severely for decades, also did not disappear. I often had the feeling that both parents continued to see their sole mission in life to make my life as difficult as possible. They would do this by meting out on me whatever aggression and hatred was within them. This is where, despite their hatred for one another, they harmonised beautifully.

Whilst I constantly felt persecuted, I came to realise later that once such introjects come vividly to the fore, one can experience a feeling of being split. I was indeed being confronted with an inner life that had taken hold of me. The result was that within me a painful drama and complete chaos reigned supreme.

On the surface I displayed a Martin who was a fine therapist and one who enjoyed the pleasurable aspects of life. Unfortunately beneath the surface my marriage was falling apart. My wife and I simply didn't fit as a couple anymore, and we got divorced. As soon as my mother heard that I was divorced she harassed me to start therapy with Mr Stettbacher. I was totally devastated by my divorce, but she turned to me coldly, saying:

> You now realise that the only reason you are divorced is because you didn't listen to my advice and go into therapy with Mr Stettbacher. I just hope that now you are prepared to go into this therapy for your own sake.

Shamelessly she exploited my weakness; and in my distress I finally agreed to enter into his therapy.

As I did not want to go to Mr Stettbacher himself, he offered me the name of one of his students in Munich. I thus went into primal therapy with Eva, one of Stettbacher's students. As it turned out, several months later I found out that this therapist had taped the sessions and immediately sent the tapes off to Mr Stettbacher. He in turn sent these tapes to my mother; and this was how she could control my entire therapy. Subsequently, and throughout many months I was literally inundated by faxes from my therapist, my mother and Stettbacher. At every opportunity they let me know that I had no idea what I was doing being a therapist, that I was a wicked charlatan and that I should at long last obey them and adhere to the strict therapy methods developed by Stettbacher.

It all became too much for me. Thank God I finally had the idea to investigate with whom I was actually dealing. In the end it took no time for me to find out that Stettbacher had never studied psychology, but that he was a conman. His actual profession was selling lamps.[2] He had clearly been very adept at worming his way into my mother's life. My suspicion, however, is that she herself had selected him for me as the instrument to ply her dirty trade.

I immediately confronted my mother, who was then living in France, with what I had found out about this criminal. Then, just as she had always done during the war, she straightaway adjusted to the situation and colluded *with me*. She had done the same with my Nazi father: working her charm with him to survive.

Suddenly Stettbacher was an evil man and I the poor victim. I calmed down instantly: my mother had brilliantly managed to loosen the noose around her neck. I now finally understood when people say that mafia bosses are both serious criminals and highly intelligent at the same time. I had to reflect over a long period time to clarify for myself whether I was being paranoid about my mother and her behaviour towards me. But I always ended up concluding that this petite lady who was so brilliantly intelligent really and truly had wanted to kill me.

My mother was a pure master of deception. She manipulated me into an impenetrable mesh of lies and there was nothing I could do to defend myself against this. This went on for decades. After her death, I overcame my fear and started writing her biography. Soon I began to realise that I was actually also writing my own biography and I was horrified to see what was coming to the surface. At first I thought that after the book was published, I would finally find peace. Instead I had opened a Pandora's box.

Today, I have finally reached the point where I no longer have to face and grapple with any secrets. Both of my parents can consider themselves lucky to be dead as it would have been sheer torture for them to be confronted by their son with the truth: with their horrendous war crimes against those who were innocent, and against me, their son whom they wanted to destroy. Helpless and naïve, we had put our faith in my parents but were cruelly betrayed. Today, I myself no longer need to hide anything.

Sadly, I also no longer have the opportunity to show them what I know, but fortunately I have the opportunity to publish my knowledge everywhere and at any time. Today I realise that over the years I have developed an entirely new method to practice psychotherapy and I have been very successful at it. Until now, I have never dared show myself. To have now found the courage to write a book on my own method of practice – a result of rigorously analysing my own biography with the finest toothed comb.

With the help of this paper and future publications it is my wish to assist others who have also suffered and suffered deeply throughout their childhood. So many people have been forced to stagnate under an umbrella that holds back not only rain or sun but life itself. If I succeed in offering them some small support so that they may free themselves and escape the grip that is suffocating them, then I can honestly say that my pain to break out from my own imprisonment was truly worthwhile.

Notes

1 Essay translated from the German by Eva Szpiro-Burke.
2 The Swiss authorities withdrew Konrad Stettbacher's permit to practice in 1995 due to lack of proof of qualifications. He died in 2016 at age 86.

In socio-political life

Chapter 9

Closed doors

Sylvia Paskin – with Coda by Sara Collins

Leaf through the daily papers, switch on the news: are we the readers and listeners not bombarded daily by images and stories of figures in power – figures who cast shadows to behold and about whom we might naturally wonder, envy or perhaps even disdain? What has been the fate of some of these figures – including those from the not-so-distant past? Our next author, Sylvia Paskin, went to look for herself in what may appear to many as the far-flung reaches of an ancient empire, and opened the door to a remarkable story of power, politics and fear.

On completing her work below, Sylvia sought input from the analyst Sara Collins, and it is with Sara's psychoanalytic perspective that she concludes this chapter.

The scene set by T. S. Eliot with the opening words of his 1963 poem *The Journey of the Magi*: "A cold coming we had of it", could well have been written for Leon Trotsky. Other experiences of exile for Trotsky had been in Russia itself – in Siberia, in Alma-Ata on the border with China, but this was to be Trotsky's first taste of external exile. Others would follow, journeys to France and Norway, finally Mexico – but he was destined never to return to his homeland. It would prove to be a 'long journey'.

The father

It was indeed a very cold winter when on 12 February 1929, having travelled 22 days on a train west from Kazakjstan to Odessa, Trotsky, his wife Natalia and son Lyova Sedov (taking his mother's maiden name) took the steamer *Ilyich* to Istanbul. The ship had no cargo and no other passengers save these three. In front of the ship an ice-breaker was needed for the 60 nautical miles that were required to reach their Turkish destination.

This was not a journey of choice – Trotsky was being deported. How did Trotsky, a brilliant political analyst and theoretician, one of the foremost creators of the Russian Revolution, a charismatic and spellbinding orator, the organiser and commander of the Red Army come to find himself in this situation? After all he had many, many supporters and was a revered figure amongst the workers, peasants and soldiers. Trotsky had travelled the length and breadth of civil war Russia in his armoured train stopping only to make forceful speeches, received and acted upon by adoring crowds of supporters.

In 1924, after several strokes, Lenin, an ally of Trotsky had died, and this opened the door to Stalin's ambition.[1] He chipped inexorably away at others he felt were dissident or rivals – some were driven to suicide, some were imprisoned, others murdered. Stalin was ready to do battle with Trotsky since he too had a wide following and a clear claim to leadership. This had to be undermined and, if necessary, destroyed.

Apart from their rivalry, Stalin and Trotsky had fundamental differences on the future of the Revolution. Stalin was in favour of running the country under the aegis of merciless bureaucracy, employing a ruthless authoritarianism. Stalin also wanted the Revolution to stay within the country's borders.

Trotsky, on the other hand, had a grander, more expansive vision. He believed in 'Permanent Revolution' – broadly speaking, that a country's continuing revolutionary progress was dependent on the continuing revolutionary process occurring in other countries. In a word, Trotsky believed in the internationalism of socialism.

Their enmity increased: an Opposition party was formed under Trotsky, but Stalin wanted socialism in one country, and he prevailed. Trotsky could not manage the Bolsheviks and when party congresses had to choose between Stalin's approach and Trotsky's, they chose Stalin's.

Trotsky thought the Russia of 'icons and cockroaches' too backward. He wanted to provoke revolution in Germany but his policy failed. This left him in a very vulnerable position. Stalin wanted him out of the country. He had his way.

Stalin was on good terms with the Turkish government. The two countries had emerged at roughly the same era – the time of the First World War. Both countries had embarked on a policy of modernisation wanting to turn peasants into literate citizens. The old Arabic script in Turkey had been Latinised and the same happened in Russia with the Cyrillic script.

At this point Stalin did not feel confident enough to have Trotsky assassinated. He came to an accommodation with Turkey's leader, Ataturk: the Turks would give an assurance of safety for Trotsky and in return Trotsky was banned from publishing anything in Turkey itself.

Trotsky felt himself to be in Turkey under duress, and in a letter to Ataturk, wrote the following:

> Dear Sir, I have the honour to inform you that I have arrived at the Turkish frontier not of my choice, and I will cross this frontier only by submitting to force.

He did not want to stay in Istanbul – he did not speak the language. He was concerned about being isolated. He was put in a wing of the Soviet embassy, and initially received with courtesy. But he was under constant surveillance by Stalin's agents and his GPU – the Russian Secret Police. His wife and son could walk freely in the city but Trotsky himself was, to all intents and purposes, a prisoner: if he left the embassy, he would be flanked by guards.

Trotsky did everything possible to get visas to Germany, to France, even to England – but to no avail. He named the last chapter of his autobiography 'Planet without a Visa', as that was indeed how he experienced his situation. Istanbul too was full of White Russians then only able to get lowly posts as doormen and waiters; and any one of them would have been pleased to assassinate him if given the opportunity. It is possible that Stalin had already thought of this and was hoping it would happen.

But the stay at the Soviet embassy was an embarrassment and the Trotsky family were moved to a nearby hotel. It was too dangerous for them to stay long-term in Istanbul, so other living quarters needed to be found. Natalia and Lyova looked at several places and finally found one.

Off the coast of Istanbul lie nine islands: the Princes' Islands, the largest of which is known in Turkish as Büyükada: a "red-cliffed island set in deep blue". The American poet and political activist, Max Eastman,[2] who was a subsequent visitor to the island, wrote of it that it "crouches in the sea like a pre-historical animal drinking". It had a large Greek population at that time and they called it Prinkipo. It was an hour and half by ferry from Istanbul. It felt safer than the city.

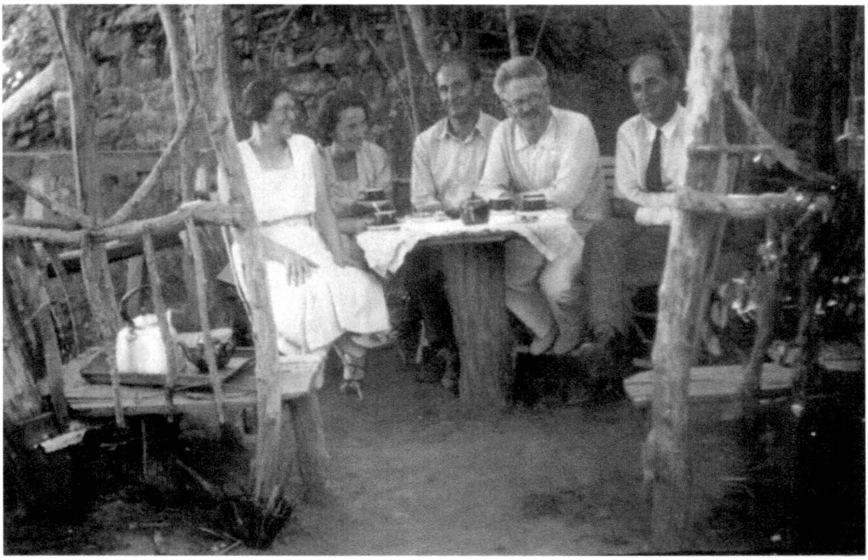

Figure 9.1 [Collection Trockij, Lev Davidovič], International Institute of Social History (Amsterdam). In Prinkipo (Büyükada island, Turkey). From left to right: Zina Trockij, Jeanne Molinier (?), Roman Well (ps. of Ruvin Sobolevicius), Trockij and Adolf Senin (ps. of Abraham Sobolevicius).

Ironically Büyükada was already famous as an island of exile: historically the enemies of the Sultans-rebels, rivals of the royal blood, usurpers were imprisoned there and sometimes blinded.

Traditionally however, Büyükada provided ornate residences for wealthy visitors wishing to escape the stifling heat of an Istanbul summer and, in that respect, it was also a 'fantasy' island. It had massive wood-framed houses, with ornately decorated plaster ceilings and sumptuous gardens. There were no cars – all transport was by gaily decorated horse-drawn *phaetons*.

Donkeys, however, pulled the more mundane carts for milk, fruit and vegetables, as it was here, in a rented villa, at Hamlaci Sokak 4, that Trotsky, his family and entourage set up home.

The villa had belonged to a bankrupt: Izzet Pasha. He had been Sultan Abdulhamid's head of security. Surrounded by a garden – on the edge of the sea, the villa was spacious but also dilapidated – providing only the very basic accommodation. Writing about the state of the house Eastman, who had once been a comrade but subsequently fell out with Trotsky specifically noted its "lack of comfort and beauty". Comparing it to a bare barrack, he wrote "a man and woman must be almost dead aesthetically to live in such an abode" . . . "for a few dollars they might have made of it a charming home".[3]

But domestic aesthetics were not Trotsky's first consideration. This exile afforded him time to think and, more importantly, to write. If Stalin thought he had isolated and silenced Trotsky, he was to be proved wrong. Trotsky now had a freedom far greater than he had in Russia. He could express himself exactly as he wished and more importantly from his point of view, communicate with the wider world. He took over most of the first floor as an office, creating an enormous desk out of bricks and planks. Within months of being there Trotsky had completed the first draft of his autobiography, *My Life*, and started his massive three-volume *History of the Russian Revolution*. He had also created a *Bulletin of the Opposition* which his son Lyova edited.

Trotsky was offered book contracts and publishing deals from Germany and America. He edited essays, wrote for major newspapers worldwide eager to publish his thoughts on the world situation. Apart from the recognition which he relished, and his need to promulgate his theories, Trotsky desperately needed the income generated by this work as, on leaving Russia, Stalin had allowed him only 1,500 dollars. Now in exile he was not alone and needed to support not only himself and his family but a whole entourage of international supporters and admirers including the French writer Alfred Rosmer, the Belgian mathematician Jean van Heijenoort and German Otto Schüssler. There were also other young disciples, a secretary, bodyguards/gardeners and a cook.

A constant stream of books and journals arrived for Trotsky on the island until a huge library was amassed in the attic of the villa. There were many visitors from abroad. Stalin must have been angered by Trotsky's global profile – he would have liked to have him killed. For now though, he was to be held. Some years later, when the last stage of Trotsky's permanent exile was reached – in Mexico – this would change.

The life of exile on Büyükada, however, afforded Trotsky a time of industry and order. In his *Farewell to Prinkipo* he writes, in retrospect, that it had been:

> a fine place to work with a pen, particularly during autumn and winter when the island becomes completely deserted and woodcocks appear in the park.

Amusingly he adds:

> Graphologists demand that I forward my handwriting to have my character analysed. Astrologists request to be told the day and hour of my birth to draw my horoscope. Autograph collectors wheedle for my signature to add to those of two American presidents, three heavyweight champions, Albert Einstein, Colonel Lindbergh and of course Charlie Chaplin.

Trotsky's household was strictly regulated, with assiduous attention paid to security. There were Turkish guards at the gate while the young disciples kept a 24-hour watch. Trotsky and the others all carried guns – in one incident a visiting doctor was nearly shot by Trotsky when he reached into a back pocket for a stethoscope. Trotsky felt under constant threat.

Trotsky worked hard with Lyova, the eldest son of his second marriage to Natalia Sedova. He was his father's confidante, secretary and factotum. However when Lyova had wished to return to Russia – probably to see his brother, Sergei (who hadn't been interested in their father's political aims) Trotsky interfered, writing to him that it would be "a big mistake in every respect . . . a big blow". Lyova stayed in Berlin.[4]

The daughter, Zina

Into this dynamic but tense environment, two new visitors arrived in January 1931: Zina, now 30 years old, and her five-year-old son, Seva. (In Trotsky's early life he had married another young revolutionary, Alexandra Lvovna. They married on a prison transit train carrying them to Siberia. This was Trotsky's first exile. Here they set up home and in the space of two years two daughters had been born: in 1901 Zinaida [Zina], and in 1902 Nina.)

But Trotsky could not stay confined for long. He wrote in *My Life*:

> The necessity of creating a centralised party was engaging many revolutionaries. . . . My handwritten essays, newspaper articles looked small and provincial to me. . . . I had to escape exile.

Trotsky knew this would be very difficult for Alexandra Lvovna.

> But she met this objection with the two words: "You must" . . . She was the first to broach the idea of my escape when we realised the great new tasks.

She believed he was destined for greatness, and for a time, he was.

Winston Churchill, who was no admirer of Trotsky, wrote of this incident in his essay *Great Contemporaries*:

> He found a wife who shared the Communist faith. She worked and plotted by his side. She shared his first exile to Siberia in the days of the Czar. She bore him children. She aided his escape. He deserted her.

Churchill called Trotsky a "bundle of rags and sacking" in the first version of this essay, then "a skin of malice" and finally "the Ogre of Europe". His daughter Zina thought this last description of her father to be amusing, and inscribed a photo to him with those words written on it.

A singular event then occurred – one which would have lasting and tragic consequences. In order to keep the soldiers from pursuing and arresting Trotsky, his wife Alexandra said he was suffering from an infectious disease and sleeping. The door was constantly kept closed.

This story was also told to Zina, but one day, with the innocent curiosity of a two-year-old, perhaps wanting to show her father a doll that a soldier had made for her, she opened the door and went into the room. She did not find her father underneath the covers but rags and bones which were meant to simulate her father's sleeping form. This would have been shocking and traumatic for the little girl. She must have felt abandoned and betrayed.

Trotsky hardly saw Alexandra again, though they maintained contact throughout their lives. Alexandra never remarried. Finding life as a single parent difficult, Alexandra sent Zina away to be brought up by Trotsky's sister Yelizaveta but she continued to raise Nina. Zina in effect 'lost' both parents.

A year later Trotsky met Natalia Sedova in Paris, divorced Alexandra and married Natalia. Zina and her sister Nina barely saw their father again either, but they did attend some of his political meetings and were then rewarded with a look and a smile. . . . Zina did, however, see him once when she was seven and he was living in Vienna,[5] attending political meetings in the Café Central.

In the wake of the Russian Revolution, Trotsky's daughters grew up in impoverished circumstances, though Trotsky did send money. They attempted to create their own families. Nina married Man Nevelson and had a son and daughter. Sadly Nina contracted tuberculosis, received little or no medical attention, and died in 1928. Zina had nursed her to the end.

As for herself, Zina first married Zakhar Moglin with whom she had a daughter. Later Zina divorced and married Platon Volkov with whom she had a son, Seva.

Both Zina and Nina had a high regard for their celebrated father and became politically active. By 16 years of age Zina was editor of the newspaper of the Petrograd Komsomol (the All-Union Leninist Young Communist League). She taught in a local school before fighting in the ranks of the Opposition with her husband, Platon Volkov. Intelligent and clearly politically engaged, Zina had a passionate, intense but highly strung nature. She had been arrested twice.

Of all of Trotsky's four children, Zina bore the most resemblance to her father physically, with dark sharp features, similar, piercing eyes and facial expressions. She had also contracted tuberculosis.

After Nina's death, Zina felt bereft. Her life lacked purpose. She wanted more than anything to spend time with her father, to get to know him. She wanted to be with him on Büyükada. Most of all she wanted to ally herself to his political life, to be of use to him.

It was very difficult at the time to get the necessary visa to leave Russia – Stalin granted it, eventually, on medical grounds but on one cynical condition: that she leave her little daughter behind as a hostage. At first the meeting between father and daughter on Büyükada was tender – they both wept over Nina. She had been too ill to wave him goodbye when he left Russia.

The household in Büyükada had a strict and regulated regime – Sara Weber, an American born, Russian-speaking secretary wrote in her memoir how she came to work for Trotsky. She had been told by "a leading member of the American 'Left Opposition' who had just returned from a visit":

> LDT is now facing a real tragedy, he is losing his Russian secretary and needs to find someone suitable in Constantinople which swarms with old-time Russian white-guardists' and with GPU agents, is practically impossible.

Sara took the job.

'LD' (as Sara Weber called Trotsky) never sat down but dictated walking to and fro:

> LD spoke without any use of notes, at an even speed, sentences following smoothly one after the other . . . at the sound of the bell LD would stop dictating, at times in mid-sentence.

After lunch and a brief rest, Trotsky would dictate again,

> "Watching him dictate", Sara wrote,[6] "I had an almost *physical* sense of his thought processes; the thinking was so intense it seemed I could *feel* it. His thoughts were transformed into words, sentences, paragraphs as if read from some inner memory tape".

Sara also commented on the deep and tender relationship between Trotsky and Natalia: apparently he would always butter her bread at breakfast.

As for Zina, she came armed with huge expectations. She needed to give focus and meaning to her life. Photos of her on Büyükada show her to be a vulnerable figure – a slight slouch to the shoulders and an intent gaze often towards her father rather than to the camera. Zina was also suffering from a lung condition – she had a pneumothorax. But over and above what she needed for this condition, she needed love and affection, wanting as she did to make up for lost time, a lost father, wanting to embrace him and his work.

Trotsky, however, had neither the time nor the inclination to nurture this – he was totally absorbed in his literary output, as was Zina's half-brother, Lyova. In a short space of time, Trotsky had given over the responsibility for Zina's wellbeing to Natalia, her stepmother. For her part, Natalia tried to be helpful to Zina, taking her to doctors' appointments, engaging her in conversation. But Zina, unsurprisingly, did not interpret this as kindness – quite the opposite: she experienced Natalia's actions as deliberate attempts to get in the way of her relationship with her father.

Trotsky was obdurate and oblivious to his daughter's emotional fragility. He refused to work with Zina – shutting himself away in his study behind a closed door. She was forbidden to interrupt him.

Hoping to gain attention, Zina wrote an article which Trotsky promptly rejected. He could not let her in on secret codes or addresses. He thought that if she were to be put under pressure she would divulge the information on her return to Russia. To add insult to the injury she experienced of being passed over and rejected, it must have been obvious to Zina how passionately attached her father was to Natalia and indeed to their son. Naturally Zina was loyal to her mother and could not accept Natalia as a substitute. When Zina would be critical of her to Trotsky, he would respond very angrily by shouting her down. Zina was clearly also very jealous of her half-brother Lyova with whom her father worked so intimately.

An additional aspect of Trotsky's life stood in the way of Zina's spending time with her father: an 'obsession' she experienced her father as having, namely fishing. Indeed Trotsky was a passionate fisherman – going out often twice a day with a local Greek fisherman, Charolambos and fishing for mullet, bonito and lobster. Natalia accompanied him on some of these trips but never Zina.

Zina already suffered from depression. Her childhood and adult life had been very difficult. She became needy and demanding – frustrated that her father would not give her what she wanted, namely, the love and attention she had never had from him and which she craved. But the more she asked for it, the more withdrawn, cold and distant Trotsky became. Their relationship seemed to mirror the Greek tragedy, Antigone, with Trotsky in the role of Creon, a believer in moral precepts, the rule of political law. Indeed Trotsky believed in *reason*, structure and logic. Zina by contrast was far more labile and unpredictable. Zina unnerved her father with what he considered were her *unreasonable* demands. Her inner life was not forged – or at least for her father, certainly not forged *enough* – in iron.

On 1 March 1931, a few months after her arrival, there was a flash fire – a water heater in the loft had caught fire. Trotsky's precious library suffered. For a time it was Zina who was blamed – giving some indication of what people thought of her mental stability. It later transpired it had been an error on the part of the cook.

As Zina's behaviour became more distressed, Trotsky increasingly felt her to be a disruptive burden and distraction in the house.

Meanwhile Trotsky's son, Lyova had returned to Berlin, having befriended and begun a relationship with Jeanne Molinier, the wife of the banker and Trotsky supporter Raymond Molinier. This had created a difficult situation as Raymond continued to visit Büyükada, providing considerable financial help to Lyova's father. (For his part, Trotsky had decided Lyova and Jeanne should go to Berlin to carry on the political struggle there.)

Trotsky felt that Zina would also benefit from being in Berlin, as he hoped Lyova and Jeanne could keep an eye on her. At the same time he wrote to his friend in Berlin, the German journalist and Marxist writer, Franz Pfemfert for a reference for Zina, and was given the name of a highly reputable psychoanalyst, the Adlerian, Arthur Kronfeld. (Unusually for a Marxist, Trotsky was interested in psychoanalysis and admired Freud.) Kronfeld was Jewish and spoke Russian fluently. Trotsky felt Zina would benefit from seeing him, but Zina felt very resentful, suspecting that the true reason for her father's insistence was her departure. When she left Büyükada, Trotsky said to her "You are an astonishing person. I have never met anyone in my life like you". Zina told Lyova it was said "with a severe expression".

Trotsky and Natalia thought Zina should go alone to Berlin to recover and they would look after Zina's son, Seva. In the event, Zina went to Berlin in the autumn of 1931. But this action did not in any way provide her with the respite she so needed.

Though Zina would see Lyova and Jeanne in Berlin occasionally, she felt very lonely there. Her acute jealousy prevented her from making any real relationship with Lyova. In fact she indicated that seeing him gave her a "nervous breakdown". As for her physical health, Zina was operated on in Berlin to make good on a lung operation she had had in Istanbul. Financially, though her father would send her money, she could barely survive. She tried to involve herself in local communist politics.

As for psychoanalytic treatment, Zina attended some sessions but said that she hated dwelling "in the filth of her unconscious". She also found out that the private letters she sent to her father (to which he rarely replied) were sent by him to her analyst. Zina regarded this, quite rightly, as a serious breach of trust. Trotsky maintained he was merely being helpful.

With the rise of the Nazis, the presence of 'Brownshirts' on the street, Berlin was without doubt a frightening city in which to live, not least for the lonely and deeply troubled Zina. She would write again and again to her father seeking affection but again and again he would fail her. Indeed he hardly wrote to his daughter because he found her letters to him so fractious. When she became frustrated by his lack of response she wrote in an even more accusatory fashion which would distance and anger him even more. Nor could he forgive her for her criticisms of Natalia which he brought up time and again in letters to Lyova.

Lyova himself was in fact fond of Zina and many times wrote on her behalf to their father begging him to write to Zina. "She is desperate" were the words repeated in his letters to his father and his mother – at one point, accentuating the desperation, writing:

> Zina is terribly oppressed, depressed, she looks utterly destroyed. I pity her Daddy, very, very much.

But what Trotsky wanted from his son was not that, but rather to further the cause.

(Meanwhile Lyova, himself was often cold and hungry. Whilst his father would send him an allowance, he spent most of it pursing political activities on his father's behalf. Otherwise he would be studying.[7] As for Jeanne, whilst living with Lyova in Berlin, from time to time she would travel to Paris to visit her husband Raymond who, wanting a reconciliation, had begged her to return – even threatening suicide. Jeanne stayed with Lyova.)

Trotsky became more and more infuriated and threatened Zina that if she did not change her attitude towards him he would break off all relations with her. She missed her husband and son. Then, apart from her lack of a relationship with her father, in February 1932 the Soviet government revoked her citizenship along with that of Trotsky and all his relatives. As a result Zina could never go back to Russia to see her husband, son or mother. She was stateless.

An added complication was that Zina may well have been pregnant, though no one knows by whom. By December 1932, however, she appeared to rally, her physical health having improved. It was thought that if her son should join her in Berlin that would help them both. Indeed on 14 December Seva arrived in Berlin. But another hammer blow occurred a week later when the chief of police ordered Zina to leave. Russia was impossible, Büyükada another impossible destination, and now Zina had to leave Germany.

Zina took Seva to a neighbour. On the morning of 5 January she telephoned Lyova, begging him to come and see her, but he could not come immediately. He and Jeanne and Franz Pfemfert reached her boarding house in Karlshort (then a poor area of Berlin) at 2 p.m. By then Zina was already dead. She had turned on all the gas taps in the kitchen and, exerting huge physical effort, had pushed all the furniture against the bedroom door. She lay down in bed and covered herself up – a chilling reminder of how she once thought she would find her father. Papers and notes were strewn about the room. In one she begged Jeanne to look after Seva. "He is sweet", she wrote. In another note she wrote,

> I feel the approach of my terrible disease. In this condition I do not trust myself, not even with the handling of my child *in no circumstances* should he come here. He is very sensitive and nervous . . . he is with Frau K.

Seva was not told for a year that his mother had died – rather that she was in hospital with an infectious disease.

Zina's 'faint smile' was noted in a letter to Trotsky sent by Pfemfert on 20 January. Clearly it was interpreted as a sign of release. And a relief to those who mourned her. Zina's bag and all her money had been stolen. She was cremated. Her place of burial unknown.

As for her papers, most were seized by the police on their arrival, others were kept by Jeanne and Lyova. Later, however, after Lyova's death (most probably a murder), all these papers were stolen from the couple's Parisian apartment by the French police.[8] Zina's faint smile in death was noted – and red roses were put in her coffin.

Lyova sent the following telegram to his father:

> Zina has taken her own life. Alexandra Lvovna and Platon must be informed. I have not said anything to them. Stop. Seva does not know anything about Zina's death. He is with us.

On receipt of the telegram, Trotsky and Natalia retreated into their bedroom for several days, only appearing to ask for tea. When Trotsky came out of the room it was noted that two deep wrinkles had formed on either side of his nose and ran down both sides of his mouth, and his hair had turned white.

But Trotsky accepted no responsibility for the part he played in his daughter's demise. A few days after her death he penned an open letter to Stalin blaming him for driving Zina to her death:

> On the twentieth of February you published a decree by which not only my wife, my son and I, but also my daughter, was deprived of Soviet citizenship – "a wretched and stupid act of vengeance".

As for his grandson, Trotsky added:

> he was hardly near his mother for a week when General Schliecher's police in collusion with Stalinist agents decided to expel my daughter from Berlin.

Trotsky also mentioned Nina who had written to her father when she was dying:

> The letter was held up by you for seventy days so that my answer did not find her alive.

Trotsky even blamed Lyova for Zina's suicide. In response Lyova called the letter "monstrous", writing that his father was not taking any of his own behaviour towards Zina into account; moreover, sounding as though everyone was to blame but Trotsky himself.

Trotsky also wrote to his first wife Alexandra who had by now lost two daughters. In response Alexandra wrote to him, "I will go mad myself if I do not learn everything". She wrote subsequently, "much is explained by your character, by the difficulty you have in expressing your feelings".

On 15 July 1933 – a few months after Zina's suicide and two days before he left Büyükada for France, Trotsky, having secured a long-awaited visa, wrote his farewell to the island which had been his home for four years, and "in praise of this intricate and primordial art which has not changed for thousands of years" (i.e. fishing).

> Now "oddly I feel as if my feet had got somewhat rooted in the soil of Prinkipo." . . . 'The house is already empty. The wooden cases are already downstairs; young hands are driving in the nails.,. the floor of the old and dilapidated villa was painted with such queer paint in the spring that even now, four months later, tables, chairs and our feet keep sticking to it'.

Whilst the essay touches on his residence in Büyükada, he reserves most of it to extolling the virtues of fishing with the young illiterate fisherman Charolambos who "could read [it] like an artist the beautiful book of Marmara". They spoke to each other in gestures and a few Turkish, Greek and Russian monosyllables.

In 1940 Trotsky was in his last place of exile – the 'Blue House' in Mexico City owned by the painter, Frida Kahlo. He lived there with Natalia and his grandson Seva. Jeanne wanted to bring him up but Trotsky fought a bitter but successful court battle and won custody of his grandson. By this time all four of Trotsky's children were dead – Nina and Zina, recovering from an appendix operation in a Paris clinic, was most likely poisoned by the GPU. His younger son Sergei, an engineer, was arrested and probably shot in 1938.

Trotsky's first wife also disappeared, her granddaughter imprisoned but later freed. Nina's son and daughter disappeared and died young, Lyova, his wife and son as well. A tragic harvest of people. People say revolutions eat their children, but here in Trotsky's case, they were simply devoured. Financially, whatever money they may have had seemed to have been lost during the revolution.

As for Natalia, she lived another 15 years – writing her own memoirs with Victor Serge titled *The Life and Death of Leon Trotsky*. Stalwart and dedicated to the end, she had never left Trotsky's side – supporting him through every precarious and tumultuous aspect of his life.

The house of exile on Büyükada now lies in ruins. Its roof has fallen in, walls have crumbled, the garden is completely overgrown. The iron gate still stands ajar at the bottom of the garden looking out onto the pier from which Trotsky set sail on his many beloved fishing expeditions. The lobster pool is still there. The kitchen area is strewn with broken green tiles and the yellow painted doors are hanging off their hinges. Some doors still have a few blue and clear stained glass panels intact. It was never a beautiful house but viewing it now it has a certain grandeur as a ruin. Birdsong proliferates amongst the lavish green of the garden but, as with other ruins, there is little to give evidence of the human activity both rich and tragic that once filled it.

In the last chapter of his autobiography, *My Life* – a chapter titled 'Planet without a Visa' – Trotsky writes:

> Since my exile. I have more than once read musings in the newspapers on the subject of the "tragedy" that has befallen me. I know no *personal* tragedy.

This autobiography was published in 1930. In the same chapter he quotes a line from Proudhon which he admires: "Destiny – I laugh at it".

I wish to acknowledge the help given to me by the Editor, Jonathan Burke in the writing of this article. His lucid questions, comments and insights were invaluable to me.

SP

Coda: some psychoanalytical insights into the complex and troubled relationship between Trotsky and his daughter Zina

by Sara Collins

Given that these are political public figures, rather than patients on the couch, these comments are speculative.

Central to Zina's life would have been the trauma she experienced at two years of age. Her father simply disappeared: Trotsky was there and then he was not. Zina must have struggled with this abrupt and secretive desertion of the man who was her father, surrounded as it was by subterfuge and actual lies. His escape had to be manoeuvred and Zina had to be fooled. She probably felt abandoned and perplexed in equal measures as to what had happened. We cannot know but she must have found it difficult to come to terms with his mysterious departure. It is unclear to us, and it must have been baffling to his daughter, why he left his young family behind – and why he did not take them with him. Possibly the daughters were too young – Zina's younger sister Nina was only four months old. But what is certain is that they never joined him and he never returned. His departure was just as final as it was abrupt.

It is not clear what the nature of the relationship between Trotsky and his first wife was or what Zina heard from her mother about their marriage. There was a strange dichotomy in the fact that on the one hand for Zina, her father was revered, famous and powerful, but he was also in constant fear for his life. He was constantly on the move, running away from political opponents. There was no safety or anchor for him anywhere. Even in exile, he was constantly guarded and virtually a prisoner.

But one thing is clear from this early incident and it was a constant in his life: Trotsky always put his political ambitions first – the pursuit of his ideology was paramount and it transcended all personal attachments. For Trotsky people were either assets, and thus near him, or they were not, which greatly impacted on Zina's relationship with him. In his absence, Zina must have developed an elaborate matrix of fantasies about him, and longed to be with him one day, to fulfil those fantasies. No doubt the death of her beloved sister Nina from tuberculosis led Zina finally to seek her father out, so much so that she took her son with her to Turkey, even though she had to agree to leave her daughter behind in Russia. Zina never saw her again.

Alexandra, Zina's mother, was a conspicuous absence in Zina's life: Zina was brought up by her aunt, Trotsky's sister Yelizaveta, after her parents' divorce, while her sister Nina stayed with the mother. This might explain why Zina did not seek her mother out at crucial times in her life. The woman who brought her up was closely linked with Trotsky. In leaving one child behind, while seeking to re-unite with her father, Zina was following a family pattern of sacrifice and abandonment intertwined with the pursuit of political ideals. On the other hand, Zina held an unrealistic vision of what a reunion with her father might be. His absence from her life seemed to create a passionate yearning in her, and when she couldn't be with him physically, she joined his ideology, and became politically involved in what he believed in. As fantasies about absent figures often are, she probably felt that seeing him again, being reunited, would change her life for the better. However once Zina arrived on Büyükada, where her father was exiled, an intense Oedipal situation arose. There was a triangle – Trotsky, his second wife Natalia (Zina's stepmother) and Zina herself. Being reunited with him, hoping to gain his approval and inclusion in his political life did not transpire. Fierce competition for his attention got in the way. Trotsky now loved another woman and he made it clear to Zina that Natalia was paramount in his affection.

Trotsky and Natalia did not handle the situation well. Trotsky's main attachment was to his ideology, to those who served it, and indeed to his own standing. He held himself in high regard. To make matters worse, the place Zina craved, to be included in her father's life – to be a political collaborator, confidante and disciple – was taken. Indeed it was already taken by her half-brother Lyova who had become Trotsky's right-hand man. The situation for Zina on Büyükada personally and politically was very fraught.

On Büyükada, Trotsky led a small restricted life after having a very large one. To intensify matters still more, Zina sensed another Oedipal conflict being played out. Trotsky had wanted to be the 'Alpha male' of the revolution but Stalin had taken this from him and supplanted him. Trotsky had lost his place and once in exile he was reliant on the uncertain favours of foreign governments. His potency was being challenged. For a man with a strong predisposition to narcissism, this must have been intolerable. Trotsky wanted the Revolution to be played out on the world stage and he, Trotsky, would lead it. Even in his semi-humorous comments on the autograph hunters he puts himself alongside American presidents and world heavyweights. However, his own diminished circumstances must have affected his state of mind and his capacity to pay attention to his daughter's neediness of him.

Zina's mental state on Büyükada gradually deteriorated. The more emotional, and in Trotsky's eyes, needy she became, the more Trotsky distanced himself and the more implacable he became. He showed Zina he had contempt for her emotionality. It stood in the way of his work, his writing, his need to still be a recognised force in the wider world. It is also possible that the chaos and confusion she expressed reflected the turmoil of her father's inner world. So much easier for Trotsky to unconsciously make Zina the container of his unwanted anxieties and projections, the crazy one. Tragically for her, it seems she readily accepted these projections and enacted them.

We know Trotsky spent several years in Vienna. One of his friends and comrades, Adolf Joffe, introduced him to psychoanalysis and took him to meetings at the Vienna Psychoanalytic Association, where he was receptive to psychoanalytic ideas. Joffe received treatment from Alfred Adler. He took Trotsky to some of Adler's lectures. It is said that Trotsky and Adler played chess together. When Trotsky decided Zina should go to Berlin and receive treatment, he carefully chose Arthur Kronfeld, an Adlerian.

And although Trotsky thought he was being helpful in this regard, in encouraging the psychoanalysis, he forwarded the letters Zina sent him to her analyst Kronfeld. He showed no regard for Zina's right to privacy. This understandably distressed Zina, and must have felt like another betrayal. It could have seemed as if the two men were in league with one another against her.

Zina committed suicide. After her suicide Trotsky and Natalia went into a five-day purdah. It was said he emerged with white hair and even deeper wrinkles. One wonders whether these were signs that he felt remorse and guilt for her death. In any case he quickly sought to blame others – his own son and Stalin. He never blamed himself. But once Zina was no longer alive, Trotsky fought for custody of his grandson. Perhaps this was an attempt at reparation, for had he not had any feelings for Zina's fate, he could have avoided the responsibility. Maybe there was an unconscious feeling of self-blame and perhaps he wished to keep something of her alive within him, by raising her son.

These events were enacted during a time of great political upheaval in Russia. On the one hand, there was the Revolution with all its ideas for massive social reform. 'Great' men rose to power. They gathered together, plotted, planned and fulminated wanting to create a better world for the masses. Counter to this, people lived in a state of constant dread and persecution. For many Russians, the reality of the Revolution was exile to Siberia, suicide, mysterious deaths and disappearances. These were treacherous waters to navigate and many floundered, including the daughter of one of its central figures.

Three years after reuniting with her father, Zina was dead. It is as if this meeting led to her demise and ultimate act of self-destruction. Zina's meeting with her father destroyed her final hopes and fantasies about him. Her internal life and objects were shattered. He was not a hard act to follow, he was an impossible one to follow, and more so to live with.

Notes

1 Stalin was born Joseph Vissarionovich Dzhugashvili. The word 'Stalin' means 'man of steel.'

2 Max Eastman was Trotsky's unofficial literary agent. They fell out over money for an article he had written for *Liberty* magazine in America. He made notes on his visit to Trotsky but only wrote them up in the 1940s.

3 On his visit to Trotsky in Büyükada, he wrote "after twelve days in Trotsky's home, my mood has changed to such an extent that I could hardly write them down . . . I feel 'injured' by his total indifference to my opinions, my interests, my existence as an

individual . . . He lives instinctively in a world where other persons (except in the mass, or as classes) do not count . . . He lacked the gift of mutuality".

4 Lyova Sedov studied mathematics and physics at the *Technische Hochschule* in Berlin with a view to gaining an engineering degree.

5 Vienna features in the family history at least once before when, in 1912, Trotsky's father travelled there with Zina for a short visit and for the grandfather to receive medical help. It seems that Zina had seen her father fewer than a handful of times, before Büyükada.

6 Sara Weber wrote in the journal *Modern Occasions*, Spring 1972, an article titled 'Recollections of Trotsky'.

7 Lyova studied mathematics and physics at the *Technische Hochschule* in Berlin with a view to earning an engineering degree.

8 This is what Jeanne Molinier told Jean van Heijenoort, as recorded in his memoir, 'With Trotsky in Exile: From Principe to Coyoácan'.

References

Churchill, Winston S. (1938) *Great Contemporaries*. London: Thornton Butterworth.

Heijenoort, Van Jean (1978) *With Trotsky in Exile: From Prinkipo to Coyoacán*. Cambridge, MA: Harvard University Press.

Trotsky, Leon (1933) *Farewell to Prinkipo, Writings of Leon Trotsky 1932–1933*. Atlanta, GA: Pathfinder Press.

Trotsky, Leon (2007) *My Life: An Attempt at Autobiography*. New York: Dover Value Editions.

Weber, Sara (Spring 1972) *Recollections of Trotsky*. Cambridge, MA: Modern Occasions.

Chapter 10

Kafka

'Parental superiority' as the act that feels hard to follow

Steven Mendoza

Though the contribution that follows might well have found itself solely under the rubric of 'Literature', it felt best to follow the instinct of our author who writes:

> *In the chapter that follows, Franz Kafka is treated less as a literary figure and more as a protester against a system in which history can see Nazism to be incipient. This is seen to be relevant today as increasing instability and anxiety favour fascism and impede democracy. From his extensive letter to his father Kafka is seen as the victim of negative attributions. Like so many of us he seems to have identified too easily with what can be seen as his father's projections. The letter can be read to indicate not so much an oppressive bullying father as one who could not recognise his son's considerable abilities and achievements. This might have been a function of his own negative identification as a self-made Jew in an anti-Semitic society. Although Kafka is commonly seen as a psychological author he himself seems to have seen his work as exclusively social, political and satirical. We can recognise the strength of inner persecutory functions in his personality but he seems more to belong to the literature of Orwell and Swift than of Dostoyevsky and Eliot.*

I had always thought of Kafka as the fearful champion of all of us who are oppressed by the bureaucracy, the family, the right to life murderers,[1] the politicians whose unfulfillable promises command the votes of the stupid. As an undergraduate I read in compulsive horror Kafka's short story *The Penal Colony* and wondered why he would wish to impose such suffering even if only in fantasy. I was repelled that he might indulge the wish to write so. I did not go on to read those classics of victimhood – *The Metamorphosis* and *The Trial*. I did see Orson Welles's film of *The Trial* and it commanded all of the alienation, cruelty, rigidity, perversity, arbitrariness of the bureaucracy, the totalitarian state, the persecutory state of mind. But the book itself has the collusive naiveté of its protagonist Josef K, with his inappropriate formality, his helpless bondage to social mores, his fatal compliance. This was disturbing in a way quite different from *The Penal Colony*. In the book he dies, as the book prescribes, like a dog, stabbed in a ditch.

Quickly in the book we discover that the officers who confine him to his lodging wear clothes that look like uniform but are not. They establish that he is under arrest but not by the police. They reassure him of the limited comfort of the greater discretion and lesser disgrace of an arrest like his, compared with being arrested by the police. But he still faces a judiciary and an advocacy that is exploitive, impervious, arbitrary, perverse, omnipotent. Since he is arrested, this must be a criminal proceeding not a civil one. Since he is not arrested by the police, it seems to me that the legal system he faces cannot be the legal system of the state because its officers *are* the police. Perhaps the persecutors here are society itself and its mores and their sentence is the self-imposed one Kafka wrote of in *The Judgement*.

Writing for his 'The Kafka Project', the Italian literary researcher and poet Mauro Nervi[2] tells us that 'Kafka obtained the degree of Doctor of Law on June 18, 1906 and performed an obligatory year of unpaid service as law clerk for the civil and criminal courts'. Perhaps this experience is part of the external origin of his rendering of judicial settings and processes. Josef K may be up against a secret state system like the state's secret police, the OGPU of Lenin, the notorious Stasi of the German Democratic Republic or the Special Branch of the United Kingdom which anticipates so much terrorism. But I think Kafka is finding in the process he describes a more general sense of the elusive and yet pervasive powers that oppress and control us. As I write this, President Trump extends his rule of the inversion of reality, the defiance of law and the attempts to suppress freedom of speech to which dictatorship aspires. As I write of Kafka, we the educated liberals of self-professed humanity, recoil from Trump in the resentment, anger, fear and disgust which I think Kafka seeks to inspire and certainly does in me.

Fascinating is the flogging of the arresting officers in response to K's complaint. Here is a system which applies even to its own its arbitrary cruelty. I think such cruelty is possible only for those in whom the capacity for identification is defective. I think this lack of basic humanity is necessary to the establishment of pseudo-moral, oppressive, tyrannical systems such as those that can and do proliferate in these difficult times.

But we can go beyond the secret state and even the alien intrusive system such as we may see in science fiction (Dick, 1968). Many critics see in Kafka's system not only a social institution but a persecutory state of mind pervaded by anxiety, guilt and fear. I have seen no suggestion in literary criticism that Kafka (K!) himself thought he was uttering an allegory not only of the evils of oppressive society but of his own neurosis.

His extensive letter (Kafka, 1953) to his father acknowledges his own weakness and vulnerability whilst also addressing his fear of his father as a function of his contempt and withholding of affection and affirmation. His father, Hermann Kafka (1852–1931), was described by Kafka himself as

> a true Kafka in strength, health, appetite, loudness of voice, eloquence, self-satisfaction, worldly dominance, endurance, presence of mind, knowledge of human nature.[3]

But the letter seeks not only to explain his fear but to justify it. As for himself, he acknowledges only his own sensitivity. He treats it not as function of his disturbance but the fault of the father of a sensitive child. I recall a writer, I think of him as John Banville, saying: 'It's his father I'm sorry for'. No search has regained this material but I might say for myself that it is the father I am sorry for. Certainly Banville does posit Kafka's exaggeration of his father's stature as we shall see later.

Actually the father comes across to me in the letter as a materialistic, domineering man of little refinement, sensitivity, philosophy, love or wisdom. We might recognise such ostensibly well-meaning Jewish fathers today, materialistic, loud, ignorant, domineering and it is customary to be contemptuous of them. A hard-working, able, tenacious man of poor origin in an uncharitable state, Hermann Kafka, by his own efforts and those of his employees, gives his family the comfort and opportunity of a gentle upbringing. He complains in the letter of there being no gratitude for this, no acknowledgement, no love and no reciprocity. Franz seems to justify this omission by his father's contempt and lack of feeling for him.

There is no account of Hermann pretending ingenuine affection!

Although Kafka complains of his father's treatment, there does not seem to be any record of him being physically violent and this in an age when the child spared the rod was a child spoiled, when children were birched till they bled, when the martinet was not a stickler for discipline. It seems that Hermann had a mean mouth but a merciful hand. Perhaps he was not that bad. In the letter to his father, what Kafka does report is:

> There is only one episode in the early years of which I have a direct memory. You may remember it, too. One night I kept on whimpering for water, not, I am certain, because I was thirsty, but probably partly to be annoying, partly to amuse myself. After several vigorous threats had failed to have any effect, you took me out of bed, carried me out onto the pavlatche[4] and left me there alone for a while in my nightshirt, outside the shut door. I am not going to say that this was wrong – perhaps there was really no other way of getting peace and quiet that night – but I mention it as typical of your methods of bringing up a child and their effect on me. I dare say I was quite obedient afterward at that period, but it did me inner harm. What was for me a matter of course, that senseless asking for water, and then the extraordinary terror of being carried outside were two things that I, my nature being what it was, could never properly connect with each other. Even years afterward I suffered from the tormenting fancy that the huge man, my father, the ultimate authority, would come almost for no reason at all and take me out of bed in the night and carry me out onto the pavlatche, and that consequently I meant absolutely nothing as far as he was concerned.

A child who practiced such provocation might not have been a child in fear of abuse. So we understand that Kafka was not a conventionally abused child but one whose self-esteem suffered the attrition of negative attributions. There is no need to diminish the seriousness of this because it was not worse, but this passage is reminiscent of one in Donald Winnicott's paper *Hate in the Countertransference*:

> Did I hit him? The answer is no, I never hit. But I should have had to have done so if I had not known all about my hate and if I had not let him know about it too. At crises I would take him by bodily strength, and without anger or blame, and put him outside the front door, whatever the weather or the time of day or night. There was a special bell he could ring, and he knew that if he rang it he would be readmitted and no word said about the past. He used this bell as soon as he had recovered from his maniacal attack.
>
> The important thing is that each time, just as I put him outside the door, I told him something; I said that what had happened had made me hate him. This was easy because it was so true.
>
> I think these words were important from the point of view of his progress, but they were mainly important in enabling me to tolerate the situation without letting out, without losing my temper and every now and again murdering him.

Clearly Hermann had none of the analytic finesse prescribed here as essential but his action can be seen as insuring against violence just as Winnicott's was. It does not seem to me so terrible to put the whingeing little brat out!

As a social worker I encountered parents who were the very opposite of those who beat their children. They could not bear their anger with their children and they could not bear their children to see their hate of them. In some families I had the feeling that a child who cannot make his parents angry is a child who can only feel impotent, a child who can only amplify his provocations for lack of finding any limit. As a young man I would criticise and even rebuke my elders for lack of any sense of myself as a person whose expressions had any power to affect a grown-up at all.

Painfully cognisant as he was of his son's inadequacies, it seems that Kafka's father had no realisation of his son's success, his doctorate of law, his application, success and advancement in a learnt profession and in corporate office, his persisting literary pre-eminence. The failure of appreciation seems to have been mutual. I think of the virtue of a man of Hermann's type as the virtues of a hard-working peasant, characterised by honesty, loyalty to family, a fundamental adherence to religious doctrine, and a respect for materialism uncompromised by idealism.

But the man who advances himself and, by hard work, gives his children advancement not available to himself, seeks to see them exceed him; and many such say so unambiguously.

Kafka professes himself a frightened weakling and it seems that his father also made this attribution, and probably rightly so. But Kafka's lack of his father's phallic masculinity seems to have blinded both father and son to the son's literary and professional potency.

Still I wonder if Hermann possessed the peasant virtue of seeking the child's advancement as just described. I fear he had only the sense of the child's inferiority. If as a Jew in a society contemptuous of Jews, and as a man of little formal learning he could not bear his own destructive feelings of inferiority, he might have evacuated them by projections his son could not but identify with.

Kafka had from his father so much that he *did not* want that it may have been difficult for him to appreciate what he had that he *did* want and that he needed. The Buddhadharma[5] I was taught began with the contention that our parents are very kind.

The first example of their kindness I was given was that after our birth they allowed us to go on living. I understood this to mean that we do not acknowledge the real extent of their kindness. From Melanie Klein I have learnt to think of gratitude as an emotion that arises spontaneously when we feel that we have been given something good:

> it is enjoyment and the gratitude to which it gives rise that mitigate destructive impulses, envy, and greed.
>
> (Klein, p. 186)

and

> The more often gratification at the breast is experienced and fully accepted, the more often enjoyment and gratitude, and accordingly the wish to return pleasure, are felt.
>
> (Klein, p. 188)

Kafka's father, in the son's letter to him, reiterates how much he has to be grateful for, but the letter makes it clear that the son has no sense of the giving nor of the getting of the good. We have just seen Klein prescribe that gratification at the breast must be experienced and fully accepted.

Klein lays emphasis in her book on how envy can destroy the capacity for enjoyment and prevent the consequent gratitude. In Kafka I think not so much of his envy of his father. Instead, from his letter I sense his anger, hatred and self-pity. In much the same way as Klein attributes to envy, I think Kafka's reactions to his father, as expressed in his letter, might well have had that very effect of subverting the experience of gratitude, and the consequent acceptance and enjoyment it might have brought.

I can sympathise with the entire family but *Kafka's analyst* must see his patient as needing to bring good faith to his construction of reality. He needs to judge for himself instead of complying with attributions. To do this he might need first to find a more realistic sense of his actual potency. He does not apperceive his own potency and I can attribute this failure to his father's negative attributions.

In *The Politics of the Family*, R. D. Laing gives a social psychological and psychodynamic account of the significance of attributions in the family in the development of identity. The book was written at the time when Laing believed that the pathological family praxis was the cause of schizophrenia. His work in this period has something of the outrage with which Kafka can have us identify protectively, some of which I have tried to convey. But, wrong as Laing has proved to be about the aetiology of schizophrenia, the iniquities of small mindedness in the family remain. We do identify so easily with attributions within and beyond the family. Indeed, psychoanalysis may be defined as the work of discovering, through deepening introspection, the reality of who we are in contradiction of the host of attributions, including our own, which have prevailed over actual experience.

Ron Britton's work on the ego hostile superego impressed upon me the importance of what we do within the self to consolidate attributions such as those of Kafka's father. Freud represented the superego as a composite of the conscious and the unconscious, of the internal and external, of parent and self, such as we find in the Christian conscience. I have heard Britton assert that 'Only the ego is fit to occupy the seat of judgement'. Thus does he dismiss the imprecations of the conscience as pseudo-moral and actually destructive in intent. The ego has to take the seat of judgement and, in good faith, assess our moral responsibility and the truth.

The patient may actually have done wrong, and may feel guilt – not as paranoid apprehension (as in Klein's paranoid schizoid position) but as one in the depressive position. On such an occasion the analyst is concerned with the strength of the ego to bear depressive phenomena. Otherwise he addresses himself to the vulnerability of the ego to the hostile superego's imprecations.

Barry Proner (1986) approaches this as envy of the self. On this basis, we can think of the superego as a narcissistic principle demanding, in a persecutory way, that the self be self-sufficient, omnipotent, omniscient – an object depending only upon itself. As such, it envies the capacity of the ego for love of and gratitude to the object. This ego, able as it is to bear dependency, finds in it the promise of receiving from a loving *unenvious* parent all the parent's own power along with the promise of being able to develop more of his own. Sadly Kafka's father could not see in his son the power he himself had engendered. Even more sadly, Kafka himself could not feel he was in possession of his own power.

In chapter 28 of Learning from Experience, subtitled '-K', the analyst Wilfred Bion is trenchant in his condemnation of the superego in what he says he can only describe as 'withoutness'. In his chapter he describes how the concept of 'container-contained' is inverted into 'minus container-contained' and then functions to deplete thinking of real meaning and substitute it by hypocritical moral superiority. In *The Syzygy* Jung gives a similar account of this function characterised as the negative animus, a woman's assumption of phony stern masculine rectitude and a man's identification with his mother's negative animus. In Bion, as in Laing, as indeed in Kafka, I hear notes of contempt of hypocrisy, notes of protest and indignation.

How often does religious doctrine degenerate to hypocritical pseudo-morality. *The Inquisition* finds the Murano in his persisting Jewish observance to be a heretic. It hands him over to 'the secular arm', the laity, to be burned as though absolving itself of the breach of the commandment prohibiting killing. In this alone we hear echoes of Bion's 'withoutness'. The Taliban chastely veil women and abuse young boys. Daesh veils its women and sells girls into sexual slavery. Christians are so jealous of the sanctity of life that they murder doctors to protect the unborn child. All further are expressions of Bion's 'withoutness'.

My thesis is that Kafka's father, as a Jewish man of common origin in an anti-Semitic society was himself possessed by the spirits (Grotstein, 1979) of the ego hostile internal objects enacting that very 'withoutness'. Later we will consider the derivation of such hostility to the ego from the inner and outer worlds, and the vicious circle of amplification between the two that Wilhelm Reich suggests. We have no clinical account of Kafka's father but we can attribute narcissistic rivalry to his being distracted from his son's achievements by what he may have considered to be his son's unmanliness. Indeed Bettelheim has shown us how the Oedipus Complex began not with Oedipus' rivalry but with his father's fear of rivalry. Had he not sought to murder his child he might never have been murdered *by* him! Kafka's artistic achievements, his learning and social status commanded greater approbation than his father's. Hermann, in the spirit of King Laius, might have seen this as his castration instead of conferred gratification. This would imply that Hermann was possessed, as I have suggested, by such intrusive ego hostile attributions of inadequacy as we hear Kafka profess of himself.

Ironically the origin of the inadequacy his father despised may have been Hermann's projections of his own sense of inadequacy, and his son's identification with them. We have learnt of projective identification that the infant projects and the mother identifies. When this communication is reversed, then the child may not be able to modify projections as the developed breast can.

Work in the consulting room may show how many of us need to analyse our own such identifications and the extent to which we might replace the ego hostile superego with the ego itself, on the seat of judgement. It is often difficult for us in repudiation of imprecations of wickedness and inadequacy to believe ourselves in good faith. The ideal peasant is immune to the need to make such projections because he has no sense of adequacy or otherwise. There is only duty, hard work and the avoidance of the disapproval of others. He believes in the virtue of hard work and hard cash. He has no thought for his own virtue, positive or negative.

Had Kafka's father this freedom from self-regard, he may not have made such projections. As for the son, his own emotional development seems to have taken place before his ego felt strong enough to supplant his superego. Indeed this is the work that is required of many of us in analysis, both as analyst and as patient. Where popular psychology values positive self-regard, I suggest psychoanalysis posits freedom from the regard of self. I posit the regard of self as the pernicious navel gazing attributed to psychoanalysis by the ignorant.

Instead of finding ourselves good enough, we learn *to be* ourselves. In the Dharma we are taught the emptiness of the self of inherent existence: that the self as a thing in itself is veiled from our cognisance, that the self we perceive is a perception capable of only limited realisation.

The first violin of the Takács Quartet attests to the ecstasy, literally the displacement from the self, of the realisation of emptiness:

> To perform, say, the slow movement of a late Beethoven quartet is to attain a blissful state, liberated from the confines of individual personalities.[6]

I have known patients who, like me, would continually return 'home' determined that this time they would say the right things. Inevitably the family would wrong-foot them. It was not a matter of what was said but of who said it. We see this painfully dramatised in Xavier Dolan's film, *It's Only the End of the World.* So inadequate do his family feel that they can experience his attempt to restore communication only as a further put-down. He never gets the chance to tell them that he is dying.

In my own clinical experience, a young man of a perniciously critical military father needed only to register his own validity to find the work for which he had qualified and to proceed with his own life. Hitherto even his Lotus kit car would not endorse his masculinity. Effective as was my brief treatment, it hardly qualifies as analysis and might at most be considered re-fathering, a corrective emotional experience, God forbid!

As a social worker I remember a teenage girl whose mother would say in repeated and emphatic patois: 'She think she a big woman. But she just a little girl'. Actually she was a young woman of voluptuous secondary sexual development and strong, genial, reticent character. As I lectured her, in the name of casework, on the importance of self-belief, she remonstrated with me: 'I feel the spirit'. I felt like a charismatic preacher of her mother's church. Perhaps that was the best work for this case.

I recall once hearing my own cousin, the poet and teacher of poets, Myra Schneider say: 'My teens ended and, lost in the world, I failed my parents' expectations'. Her father was an important scientist, her mother a fervent Latinist. As with Kafka, it was not that her achievements did not equal theirs but that they could not recognise her potential. As a young woman she had not yet equalled the achievements of their maturity. In their incomprehension of her need to develop, their own maturity is questionable, as was Hermann's.

In show business an act is hard to follow when it is of a quality and an appeal that will be hard for the following act to exceed. Hermann Kafka's act was hard to follow not because his achievements defied emulation but because of his dissatisfaction with and contempt for his son. This made it hard for Kafka junior to act at all and certainly to feel that his act was good enough.

Jasper Conran is a designer in many modes, a multi-millionaire, an hotelier, an Officer of the Most Excellent Order of the British Empire and a snapper-up of unconsidered stately homes. As the son of Sir Terence Conran and of the soi-disant superwoman Shirley Conran he had the double challenge to follow parents who both confronted him with achievements hard to equal and projected into him attributions of inadequacy hard to disavow. London's Evening Standard reported his predicament thus:

> 'Being a design tycoon? It doesn't impress mum and dad,' says Jasper Conran. The designer recently opened his first hotel, L'Hôtel Marrakech in Morocco.
>
> He launched his first collection aged 19, became a multi-millionaire design magnate, won fans including Princess Diana and now owns stunning homes in Dorset and Greece.
>
> Yet Jasper Conran admits that even these achievements are often not enough to impress his 'extraordinary' parents, Habitat founder Sir Terence and bestselling author Shirley.
>
> In an interview with the Standard, the 57-year-old revealed that he often turns to his siblings for moral support as his high-achieving mother and father 'like to remind you, even into their late eighties, of how very successful they are'.
>
> Conran told how he rings up brothers Sebastian and Tom or sister Sophie to vent his frustration, saying: 'Oh my God, can you believe it?'
>
> The second son of Sir Terence and Shirley added: 'It's not easy to be the child of two very successful people, because you wonder how you're going to come out from under their yoke.' He called them 'omnipresent' and 'two very interesting, fascinating, extraordinary parents who are who they are'.
>
> He famously resigned from Conran Holdings last year – the day after Sir Terence gave an interview to the Standard suggesting his son lacked experience.
>
> Jasper was also reportedly estranged from his mother – author of bonkbuster Lace and self-help book Superwoman – for more than a decade until a reconciliation at his wedding to Irish artist Oisin Byrne in 2015.
>
> Charlotte Edwardes, Jonathan Prynn
> *Evening Standard*, Wednesday, 25 January 2017

I note that it took but a day for him to resign a post of stewardship of his father's estate after his father's disavowal of his competence. Franz Kafka had no such integration of ego able to posit his achievements in the face of his father's contempt. Conran could leave his father to manage his own shop. Franz Kafka was not even required to manage his father's shop but he had not the ego strength to repudiate destructive imputations of his manhood.

It may be that Conran as a homosexual and Kafka as a Jew had to contend not only with an Oedipal onslaught but also with society's projection of its uncleanness. Whether you are a *dirty queer* or a *dirty Yid* you have to disavow the imprecations if you are to have an act at all, never mind one to follow that of the father. And so many patients show their analysts that you do not even have to be a member of a scapegoated minority to find it difficult to defy attributions of inadequacy. Kafka, of course, had the option of being both. John Banville suggests 'repressed homosexual yearnings' and disgust with women:

> Friedländer follows the Kafka scholar Mark Anderson in thinking it 'highly improbable that Kafka ever considered the possibility of homosexual relations'. Nor does he for a moment seek to suggest that the 'imagined sexual possibilities' Kafka may have entertained are a key to unlock the enigmas at the heart of the Kafka canon. All the same, once this particular genie is out of the bottle there is no forcing it back inside. Repressed homosexual yearnings certainly would account for some of the more striking of Kafka's darker preoccupations, including the disgust toward women that he so frequently displays, his fascination with torture and evisceration, and most of all, perhaps, his lifelong obsession with his father, or better say, with the Father – the eternal masculine. For surely poor old Hermann Kafka, small-time businessman and purveyor of fancy goods, could not have fitted into the shoes, indeed, the nine-league boots, that Kafka fashioned for him in the story he considered his first real artistic success, 'The Judgment', in which a father condemns a son to drown himself.
>
> *A Different Kafka*, John Banville
> *New York Review of Books*, 24 October 2013

Readers may identify disgust with women in some of his writing but Kafka did have a series of sexual liaisons with women and did intend to marry, only to withdraw. In his letter to his father he writes of marriage as if it were the domain of the father and the indication in this of the classical Oedipus complex seems clear. This aspect of Kafka's implicit dynamics is explored by Meg Harris Williams in her paper *The Oedipal Wound in Two Stories by Kafka: The Metamorphosis and A Country Doctor*.

I think it possible that it was not so much that Kafka had real homosexual yearnings as that he had only the normal homosexual responses that are a function of a man's bisexuality. With the contempt of his masculinity borne by both himself and his father he might have felt these normal apprehensions as signs of his epicene failure of masculinity. It seems to me that many men confuse a homosexual orientation with the failure of masculinity. Actually some homosexual men are phallic and dominant in ways typical of the stereotype of the male chauvinist pig. It is not so much that the drive to penetration and ejaculation is pathological. The pathology may be in the lack of the genital impulse of love, cherishing, protection and procreation. The phallic drives us toward love, as Donne says:

> Whoever loves, if he do not propose
> The right true end of love, he's one that goes

To sea for nothing but to make him sick.

'Elegy XIX: To His Mistress Going to Bed'

I have so far thought about Kafka and his work in terms of the individual and the family. But it seems to me that Kafka himself saw his work not as an exploration of his own difficulties, real as he acknowledges them to be, and not as an indictment of his father, iniquitous as, in his letter, he finds him to be. Rather it seems that Kafka's work may be seen by himself and his readers as an indictment of the family but, on a greater scale, of the family as the microcosm and, indeed, as Reich holds, germ, of the cultural, social, political system.

The difficulties arising from identification with parental projections, I have proposed, constitute a dynamic of what Reich might have called the authoritarian family. Kafka's books, like Reich's are concerned with the cultural, social and political implications and negative opportunities of this dynamic. Kafka is too vulnerable to identification with parental projections. We can see the bureaucratic system he depicts as one immune to feeling where he is too sensitive. The administrators of such a system direct it as though they were incapable of identifying with the victims of their ordinances. They require their officers to execute their policies as though they themselves were equally immune. Such a system justifies itself by principles like justice, morality, the common good, the superiority of the race, the ends that justify the means. These principles are invoked not in good faith but in accord with the 'withoutness' we heard Bion describe earlier.

Sociologists protest that societies, cultures and organisations cannot be described by the functions and organisations of individual psychodynamics. But the sociologist may see such systems as fostering the development and proliferation of such psychic organisations among individuals. The sociologist trying to understand the inception of such systems may think of them as engendered in the first place by individuals afflicted by such psychic organisations. Most simply these individuals may be characterised as in the paranoid schizoid position in which primitive defences, splitting, projection and denial, prevail over functions depending upon a psyche organised in the depressive position.

Wilhelm Reich's *The Mass Psychology of Fascism* was written at the same time as Klein was formulating such concepts. He sees social organisations emerging from psychological ones. He calls the family 'the germ cell of the authoritarian state'. Sadly Hermann's paternal style is all too authoritarian in just the spirit Reich intends:

> From the standpoint of social development, the family cannot be considered the basis of the authoritarian state, only as one of the most important institutions which support it. It is, however, its central reactionary germ cell, the most important place of reproduction of the reactionary and conservative individual. Being itself caused by the authoritarian system,

> the family becomes the most important institution for its conservation. In this connection, the findings of Morgan and of Engels are still entirely correct.
>
> *The Mass Psychology of Fascism*, ch. 5

Ian Thomson is even more specific. He finds in Kafka's society the precursor of Nazism:

> In 1982, the Italian writer and Nazi concentration camp survivor Primo Levi embarked on a translation of Franz Kafka's The Trial. At first he was enthusiastic, hoping to improve the German he had learnt so imperfectly at Auschwitz. Instead, Kafka involved him more terribly than he could have imagined. Levi found only bleakness in the hero Josef K, who is arrested and executed for a crime he probably did not commit. The more Levi became immersed in Kafka, the more he began to see his own life mirrored in that of 'St Franz of Prague', as he called the Czech writer.
>
> Kafka's three sisters had all perished in the Nazi gas chambers – victims of the grotesque bureaucracy foretold by their brother two decades earlier in The Trial. Kafka must have had a seer-like sensibility, Levi thought, to have looked so accurately into the future.
>
> *Financial Times*, 19 July 2013

The personality of a Hitler, a Saddam Hussein, or a Bashar al-Assad prepared to decimate his people and raze his cities, even a Donald Trump, is of perennial interest. Commanding the same interest is the personality of the fanatic, the suicide bomber, the would-be beheader of a drummer.[7] We have thought of the fanatic with his belief that the Godhead seeks and rewards the deaths of girls who want to go to school and the deaths of Christians who do not believe in transubstantiation, as possessed by powerful emotions of religious fervour. As we think of the feelinglessness of Kafka's society, I suggest we need to think of a manic state of psychotic conviction, of freedom from uncertainty, a state enjoying the certainty of rightness. Such a state can be distinguished from real emotions like love and guilt which depend upon the capacity to bear the uncertainty of the Kleinian depressive position. The arts have the power to endow us, at least in the temporary transport of catharsis, with the capacity for feeling. This I think is quite different from the manic state which we might characterise as motivational rather than emotional.

I write this in a political atmosphere which reminds us of the development of fascism in the economic crisis of the thirties of the last century. For Yeats it began even earlier in the First World War:

> Turning and turning in the widening gyre
> The falcon cannot hear the falconer;

Things fall apart; the centre cannot hold;
Mere anarchy is loosed upon the world,
The blood-dimmed tide is loosed, and everywhere
The ceremony of innocence is drowned;
The best lack all conviction, while the worst
Are full of passionate intensity.

Surely some revelation is at hand;
Surely the Second Coming is at hand.
The Second Coming! Hardly are those words out
When a vast image out of Spiritus Mundi
Troubles my sight: a waste of desert sand;
A shape with lion body and the head of a man,
A gaze blank and pitiless as the sun,
Is moving its slow thighs, while all about it
Wind shadows of the indignant desert birds.

The darkness drops again but now I know
That twenty centuries of stony sleep
Were vexed to nightmare by a rocking cradle,
And what rough beast, its hour come round at last,
Slouches towards Bethlehem to be born?

The Second Coming
William Butler Yeats (1865–1939)

I suggest that the 'passionate intensity' of the 'worst' be no more than the manic state I have suggested. As for we, 'the best', the thinking, chattering, classes who write and read this: I do not think it is so much that we lack conviction as that we have lost the belief in the efficacy of protest. When I was young we protested against nuclear weapons, American adventurism in Vietnam, the proscription of cannabis, homelessness. I am told that the young now are just as active as my coevals were in the unparalleled sixties.

I am afraid that historically the reforms of the middle of the twentieth century were the temporary aftermath of the Second World War . . . that the generation that gained weight under rationing, that witnessed the liberation of Belsen, that did not elect Churchill, have had their time and it has gone. I lack conviction! I am afraid that as terrorism got the IRA power sharing in Ulster so, finally, it may be only terrorism which can instigate reforms when democracy is kettled.[8] I do not mean by this that terrorism is a means justified by its ends. I mean that it is a historical fact borne of historical causes. I am afraid that the proletariat, what is left of it, can no longer depend upon the intelligentsia to lead the revolution. Too many purges have followed too many revolutions. I think the greatest value of Kafka's work is neither literary nor psychological but the evocation of political anger and it is in that spirit that I conclude this essay.

Author's personal addendum

In my own case, hard as my own father's act was to follow – he was an editor, director and writer of sponsored films – harder still was it to believe in my own potential and apply myself to its realisation in the darkness of my mother's apparent disappointment.

Kafka's father could see in his son no potential for an act to follow his triumph. My mother missed in me the promised Messiah. The act that is hard to follow may be not the act we must exceed but the ideal to which we cannot aspire.

Notes

1 Society for the Protection of Unborn Children (SPUC).
2 The Kafka Project is a non-profit literary research initiative. Mauro Nervi is an Italian researcher and poet in the Esperanto language.
3 Kafka, Franz. The Complete Stories (Translated by Willa and Edwin Miur, Tania and James Stern). New York: Schocken Books, 1983. www.kafka.org/biography.
4 'Pavlatche' is the Czech word for the long balcony in the inner courtyard of old houses in Prague.
5 Buddhadharma at its simplest is the teachings of Sakyamuni Buddha, the Buddha of our earthly history, the principles and practice which lead to enlightenment. Dharma is an elusive epistemological concept: at its simplest it is the way things are, the truth, what western philosophy might call 'that which is the case'. In the teaching on emptiness dharmas are mental phenomena, the only objects available to our apprehension. As mental phenomena they lack inherent existence as what Kant would call things in themselves. They are merely subjective. So dharma is the way things are and dharmas may be things as we construct them subjectively in our consciousness!
6 Edward Dusinberre in the *Guardian* 16.01.15 www.theguardian.com/books/2016/jan/15/takacs-quartet-beethoven.
7 British Army soldier, Fusilier Lee Rigby, 22 May 2013.
8 Kettling: the isolation of small groups of protesters for hours at a time to make demonstration impractical as a democratic expression.

References

Banville, J. *A Different Kafka* (24 October 2013) New York Review of Books (1949). *International Journal of Psycho-Analysis*, *30*:69–74.

Dick, P. K.(1968). *Do Androids Dream of Electric Sheep?* London: Panther Books, 1972.

Donne, J. (1654). *The Harmony of the Muses, 'Elegy XIX: To His Mistress Going to Bed', originally spelled 'To His Mistris Going to Bed'*, re-printed (2004) in Broadview Anthology of Seventeenth-Century Verse and Prose. Peterborough, Ontario: Broadview Press.

Grotstein, J. S. (1979). Demoniacal Possession, Splitting, and the Torment of Joy: A Psychoanalytic Inquiry into the Negative Therapeutic Reaction, Unanalyzability, and Psychotic States. *Contemporary Psychoanalysis*, *15*:407–445.

Harris Williams, M. The Oedipal Wound in Two Stories by Kafka: The Metamorphosis and a Country Doctor. *Psychodynamic Practice*, Published online: 24 March 2017. https://doi.org/10.1080/14753634.2017.1304828.

Jung, C. G. (1959). The Syzygy: Anima and Animus. In *Collected Works of C. G. Jung, Volume 9 (Part 2): Aion: Researches into the Phenomenology of the Self.* Edited by Gerhard Adler and R.F.C. Hull. Princeton, NJ: Princeton University Press.

Kafka, F. (1953). *Letter to the Father.* English translation by Ernst Kaiser and Eithne Wilkins; revised by Arthur S. Wensinger. Schocken Books.

Klein, M. (1975). Envy and Gratitude and Other Works 1946–1963: Edited by: M. Masud R. Khan. *The International Psycho-Analytical Library, 104*:1–346.

Nervi, M. 'The Kafka Project' (Revision: 2011/01/08) www.kafka.org/?biography.

Proner, B. D. (1986). Defences of the Self and Envy of Oneself. *Journal of Analytical Psychology, 31(3)*:275–279.

Reich, W. (1933). *The Mass Psychology of Fascism*, New Edition (13 February 1997). Souvenir Press Ltd (also new (1969) translation from the revised German manuscript, *Die Massenpsychologie des Faschismus* by Mary Boyd Higgins as Trustee of the Wilhelm Reich Infant Trust Fund).

Winnicott, D. W. *Hate in the Countertransference*, in Klein, M. (1975). Envy and Gratitude and Other Works 1946–1963: Edited by: M. Masud R. Khan. *The International Psycho-Analytical Library, 104*:1–346.

Yeats, W. B. (1919). *The Second Coming.* First printed in *The Dial* in November 1920, and afterwards included in his 1921 collection of verses.

In philosophy

Chapter 11

Attachment and doubt in the work of Stanley Cavell

Robbie Duschinsky and Serena Messina

"In his autobiography, Little Did I Know*", note our authors, "the Harvard philosopher Stanley Cavell traces the roots of his philosophical approach to his childhood, examining what he had to learn to make sense of his father's anger at the world and at him. He describes the huge shadow his father cast over his work, even as Cavell himself achieved success in an academic sphere 'quite beyond comprehension' for his uneducated father".*

This chapter will begin by considering Harvard philosopher Stanley Cavell's account of his relationship with his father, and what it was that he learnt about doubt and acknowledgement in making sense of his father's hate towards him. The section that follows will outline the main current of Cavell's philosophical work: his thinking about what is at stake in scepticism regarding the pain of others. The powerful implications of his reflections on this issue will then be demonstrated through attention to Cavell's work on Shakespeare, with particular attention to themes of attachment and doubt in *King Lear*.

He is as alone as I am

Cavell is known as a philosopher of the analytic tradition, a branch of philosophy that focuses largely on questions of how to achieve surety regarding truth or moral judgement. Yet his first love was music. As a teenager, Cavell played alto saxophone as the sole white member of a black jazz band in Sacramento, California (earning more money per week as a musician than his father's pawnshop, *Pitch of Philosophy*, p. 24). He used the name Stanley Cavell as a stage name, and aged 16, legally changed his surname from Goldstein. Later, he majored in music at the University of California, Berkeley, before beginning studies in composition at the Juilliard School of Music in New York. However, he found himself unable to work and was drawn instead to reading Freud and works of philosophy in the library. In his autobiography Cavell describes a powerful feeling he had during this time in his life – a feeling that he was falling apart. The experiences of his childhood, which had made him who he was, were now also undoing him. The turn from music to philosophy was made in the context of a period of receiving psychoanalytic psychotherapy, seeking recovery from great inner pain. The insights that Cavell found in psychotherapy led him to serious exploration as to whether he should train as a psychoanalyst, though ultimately he brought these insights to academic philosophy. This is important for understanding Cavell's unusual approach as a philosopher.

In *Little Did I Know* (pp. 457–458), Cavell would describe the political conditions in Austria and Germany in the years during the rise of National Socialism that fed his focus on analytic philosophy, transplanting it into Anglophone academia wherein he was continually in search of certainties and avoiding errors of thought. An influential exemplar of the analytic project is Bertrand Russell's theory of descriptions which evaluates statements using a logical procedure to demonstrate whether they reference the world correctly or in error. As a young man, Cavell entered this analytic philosophical tradition, despite the fact that it had little place – at least at the time – for considering the inevitabilities and logic of error and loss, and what we do after experiencing either or both. Yet he found, or made a space within this tradition, for his own philosophical thoughts. He came to see in ordinary language philosophy (Wittgenstein and Austin) and American transcendentalism (Emerson and Thoreau) good, supportive forebears of his own direction of reflection. Cavell gave particular attention to passages where these thinkers write about the inevitability of imperfection, of incompleteness, and he considered their reflections on the different ways we might respond to this inevitability.

In his autobiography, Cavell details the roots of his work as a philosopher in his experiences as a child. In particular, he gives central place to his father, an immigrant Jew from Eastern Europe enraged by the daily battles of living in a society that made him feel out of place and by a family that was unable to offer respite from this feeling. Cavell relates the moment that he recalls knowing for sure that his father hated him. It was 1933, during the Depression. After a failed business venture, the family had needed to downsize and so they moved to a new apartment. Cavell was six years old at the time of the move. He describes wandering around in the new apartment, trying to take an interest in the combination of familiar furniture and the unfamiliar space of the unlit living room. Cavell reports noticing a bowl and lifting off the lid to find it filled with small chocolate wafers, one of his favourite treats. Only then does he realise that his father is standing silently in the semi-darkness on the other side of the room:

> As I took one of the speckled wafers from the purple bowl, I said aimlessly, but somehow to break the silence with my father, "I didn't know we had these here." He lurched at me, wrenched the dome top and the wafer out of my hands, and said in a violent, growling whisper, "And you still don't know it!"
>
> (*Little Did I Know*, p. 19)

Cavell reports that this is his first memory of ever being alone in a room with his father. He describes the moment as one of certainty for him: utter conviction that his father wanted him dead. In considering this quality in the father–son relationship, Cavell reports that "from as early as I can recall, it seemed less that my hatred was caused by his famous temper than that my sense of distance from him or ignorance of him was the cause of his rage at me" (p. 19).

Just as his father's anger cast a large shadow over his development, even as a child Cavell sensed that in turn there was some shadow that he was casting over his father:

> When later in my bedroom at the back of the new apartment I found a time and place to release my state of numbness and to cry uncontrollably, I seemed to find I was crying for my father as much as for myself, crying over whatever it was that had left this man bereft and incoherent. He is as alone as I am . . . It is as if I knew then that I would one day find a way out of the devastation he could make of his island, and knew that such a day would never come for him. (Don't tell me no man is an island.) Not of course that I escaped it entirely, but I have made headway.
>
> (*Little Did I Know*, p. 20)

Cavell situates his work as a philosopher firmly in the context of what he learnt, what he *had* to learn, in trying to make sense of his father's anger and survive within a family utterly shaped by its presence.

Philosophers had made it seem like doubt about the reality of the world or other people was a problem that could be solved through finding the right method for finding certainties. However, the whole question seemed misconceived to Cavell. After growing up within a family environment coloured by his father's rages and despair, he was acutely aware not only of the role of limits on knowledge of others but also how unbearable what we already know about others can be:

> How could I have failed to be suspicious, no matter how many years later, when I found philosophers asking such questions as, "Do I know your pain the way you do?" My principal problem was not that of doubting my knowledge of the feelings of others but rather of standing apart from them, or failing to. Not to know them would require exorcism.
>
> (*Little Did I Know*, pp. 19–20)

Whereas analytic philosophy conventionally sets out to avoid the spectre of doubt and find a way to certainty through correct procedure, Cavell learnt that some certainties could have their own appalling spectre, for which doubt would be a relief. Some examples of certainty that Cavell offers in an ostensibly non-autobiographical text, *Disowning Knowledge*, are nonetheless revealing: Cavell proposes that I am as certain that I am unable to change the outcome of a performance of *King Lear* except by interrupting it as I am that "I cannot choose the contents of my dreams or suffer my daughter's pain or alter my father's childhood" (*Disowning Knowledge*, p. 90). Theatre, dreams, parenting and being a child can have a similar kind of certainty, despite their variedness as domains of experience, since in each the terms of what we mean to others are foregrounded. Cavell was intensely aware of the social conditions of being recognisable and acknowledged by others, and felt that in any case of genuine moral or existential significance there could be no single protocol to find the single right answer – as most analytic philosophy would wish. He argues that learning how others decide whether we are worth understanding is something every child must face:

> My meaning anything, my making sense, depends upon others finding me worth understanding, as if they might just decide that I am without sense. Childhood is lived under this threat. It is no wonder Melanie Klein describes the child's world as hedged with madness, negotiating melancholy for paranoia, reparation for destructiveness.
>
> (*Philosophy the Day after Tomorrow*, p. 264)

Across his autobiography, Cavell examines the influence of both his parents, but above all his father, on his experience and choices, his drive and his errors, his wish for and fears of recognition. In this relationship with the figure and then memory of his father, Cavell documents ongoing moments of difficulty, but also some moments of repair. For instance, the day after the defence of his doctoral dissertation at Harvard, he returned briefly to see his parents in Atlanta. His father surprised him by offering to pay to outfit Cavell in a PhD robe in Harvard colours. Cavell surprised himself by accepting:

> It was a private ceremony in a process of forgiving each other, to whatever extent coloured by insincerity, yet clear and not without immediate effectiveness. Ceremony in human existence is no more measurable by its utility, though philosophers sometimes seem to argue otherwise, than the possession of language is.

This is demonstrated, both in literature and in life, by "the role of ceremony in the lives of creatures vulnerable to tragedy and madness (shown in King Lear as the consequences of the perversion or negation of ceremony)" (*Little Did I Know*, pp. 15–16). In offering Cavell this ceremony of acknowledgement, some connection and repair was achieved both *despite* and *because* of the fact that father and son knew that the distance between them ultimately remained. The mutual understanding of this fact, combined with the gesture of the father's offering and the son's acceptance of the fitting, permitted an interaction that gained its generosity through the doubts felt by each for their relationship with the other.

Do I know your pain the way you do?

In philosophy, the problem of sceptical doubt has two dimensions. A first is object scepticism: how do I know that anything in the external world is real? A second dimension is scepticism regarding other minds: how do I know that you have experience like mine? In the *Philosophical Investigations* (§253), Wittgenstein asks whether these two problems are like or unlike one another:

> "Another person can't have my pains." – Which are my pains? What counts as a criterion of identity here? Consider what makes it possible in the case of physical objects to speak of "two exactly the same", for example, to say "This chair is not the one you saw here yesterday, but is exactly the same as it".

In his magnum opus *The Claim of Reason*, Cavell's great concern is this comparison in Wittgenstein between object scepticism and scepticism regarding other minds. In the course of his reflections, Cavell comes to the conclusion that though the two may have a similar formulation, they are actually radically different in how we actually go about living our lives. Their social meaning is largely different, in large part because knowing about facts is only a small part of what we spend our time doing. When someone tells us 'I am in pain', except in particular specialist medical contexts it is rare that they are making a statement pointing to a specific inner object. More often they are making a claim on us that may be acknowledged or not acknowledged and in doing so puts our relationship with the speaker into question – and this includes in the medical context as well. The more general point, for Cavell, is that the contexts of the two forms of scepticism differ substantially. Object scepticism is something that appears on particular occasions, within a sea of everyday certainty. For instance we may meaningfully ask "Is this really a biscuit?" in the specific context of a legal case about tax payable on chocolate-covered biscuits but not on chocolate-covered cakes (e.g. United Biscuits (UK) Ltd (No 2) (LON/91/160) VAT Decision 634 on the classification of Jaffa Cakes). This question then has some purpose, and criteria can be drawn up and debated, and then used to support or contest a decision. However, to ask the question "Is this really a biscuit?" without such context is to end up freewheeling, to lose contact with the ground and friction of meanings provided by everyday life and its ordinary demands.

However, this situation stands in stark contrast to scepticism regarding other minds. Rather than the exception as with objects, it is the *rule* that we find ourselves considering and weighing and worrying about our perceptions of what others are experiencing. Most of our days are taken up with this activity. One example is considering, weighing and worrying about the suffering of others – or the variety of activities we use to avoid engaging or being open to the pain of others. "For me to know your pain", Cavell writes,

> I cannot locate it as I locate mine, but I must let it happen to me. My knowledge of you marks me . . . My knowledge of myself is something I find, as on a successful quest; my knowledge of others, of their separateness from me, is something that finds me. I might say that I must let it make an impression upon me.
>
> (*Remarks on 'Language and Body'*, pp. 97–98)

To take another example besides pain as a point of comparison – a different, familiar example in our lives of concern we have regarding other minds – relates to what to accept under the name of *love* within our lives, with its promises and compromises, with its capacity to absorb and tame intensities. As the cases of the pain or love experienced by others reveal,

> with respect to the external world, an initial sanity requires recognising that I cannot live my scepticism, whereas with respect to others a final sanity requires recognising that I can. I do.
>
> (*The Claim of Reason*, p. 451)

Cavell does not think that we can therefore escape scepticism regarding other minds: we simply cannot remove from our lives the issues that make us wonder about the minds of others, "problems of trust and betrayal, of false isolation and false company, of the desire and the fear of both privacy and union" (*Claim of Reason*, pp. 453–454). Cavell argues that our knowledge of others is always subject to comparison, consciously or in phantasy, with an unreachable harmony, transparency, union. We wish for and fear the kind of acute and stable knowledge of others that we *do* have, to a large degree, about external objects. Against this idealised image, our actual successes at knowing or being known by others are broken, inadequate things.

As described in the previous section, in his autobiography Cavell gives an account of his early impression – or rationalisation perhaps – that it was his sense of distance from or ignorance of his father that was the cause of his father's rage at him. In his philosophy, in the shadow of this early experience, Cavell emphasised that

> in everyday life the lives of others are neither here nor there; they drift between their inexpressiveness and my inaccuracy in responding to them.
>
> (*The Claim of Reason*, p. 84)

He expresses frustration, then, at the analytic philosophy of his day for making knowing others a procedural or methodological problem divorced from life. Analytic philosophy misrecognises as a problem of epistemological method the existential predicament that there are both painful and protective limits in what humans can show one another and what we can conceal about ourselves. The problem is not that we are distant knowers of the minds of others, but that in everyday life we worry about others as distant and/or overclose. In this way,

> philosophers deny how real the practical difficulty is of coming to know another person, and how little we can reveal of ourselves to another's gaze, or bear of it.
>
> (*The Claim of Reason*, p. 91)

Cavell aligns himself with the argument, proposed by object relations theory, that our minds and our lives are fully social from the beginning, though certainly spaces of isolation are subsequently made when others shut the door on us or we on them. To get the other fully out of us would require an exorcism. Even a coded, private diary or an internal conversation – as Wittgenstein (1953, §258) and Milner (1987) show – is prompted by the social and emotional terrain we share with others, with concepts invested by these encounters, and with effects on the self that we can sustain in future social interactions:

> The extent to which we understand one another or ourselves is the same as the extent to which we share or understand forms of life, share and know, for example, what it is to take turns, to take chances, or know that some things we have lost we cannot look for but can nevertheless sometimes find or recover; share the sense of what is fun and what loss feels like, and take comfort from the same things and take confidence or offence in similar ways.
> (*Themes out of School*, p. 223)

Given this, the problem of knowing others does not come from the need to bridge some great original separateness between human beings. It arises, Cavell argues, when we face others' doubts and denials of us, in the regular situations that reveal that "my relations with others are restricted, that I cannot trust them blindly" (*Claim of Reason*, p. 432).

It is *then* that questions about the minds of others are ignited within us. Where our encounters with others are either (1) superficial or (2) adequately trusting, the sceptical question simply does not arise with any traction. In *Themes out of School*, Cavell recalls how effective his father was at putting strangers at ease, with superficiality and trust supporting one another in achieving mutuality and convivial pleasure. In his interactions with strangers, Cavell's father was able

> to act on what nobody could fail to know, and to provide what nobody could fail to appreciate, even if in a given moment they could not return it. Call it sociability. At such a time I felt I would be happy to have my father as an acquaintance, to be treated by him to a serious regard, if somewhat external, for my comfort and opinion; to count not as an intimate but as an equal.
> (*Themes out of School*, p. 105)

Cavell observes that scepticism is sometimes framed as a kind of scrupulousness or precision, an attempt to ensure that we do not make mistakes when attempting to penetrate the minds of others. However, he suggests that this is a front, overgeneralised from some very specific occasions like law courts where it might be pertinent. In truth, scepticism is generally motivated, he thinks, by experiences or worries about being disappointed and depleted by others in the context of our *continual exposure* to them. Influenced by Freud's *Psychopathology of Everyday Life*, Cavell urges recognition that with every hesitation, with every gesture, we risk revealing things about our experience to others, and that this potential for revelation is beyond our capacity to fully control. While it is true that a great deal of our experience is generally only acknowledged by others when we speak of it, Cavell emphasises that there is nothing within us for which this is entirely true.

Any aspect of our inner lives or past can threaten to be potentially available for exposure without our volition, depending on how our encounters with others go. Others may catch the direction of our gaze, discerning lines of desire or identification we had otherwise kept hidden. They may note the lines around our eyes that speak of waking early with anxiety and memories heavy upon us. They may see actually how much reassurance, even pleasure, we take from grumbling about the familiar things:

> With each word we utter we emit stipulations, agreements we do not know and do not want to know we have entered, agreements we were always in, that were in effect before our participation in them. Our relation to our language – to the fact that we are subject to expression and comprehension, victims of meaning – is accordingly a key to our sense of our distance from our lives.
>
> (Cavell, *In Quest of the Ordinary*, p. 40)

Most of the time, if we are in a state of comparative mental health, our inner lives are kept unavailable from one another, whether or not by conscious choice. We roll through life within the placeholders made available by convention, knowing one another well enough generally to muddle through, without demanding too much openness from ourselves or others except at circumscribed and ritualised moments (e.g. medical examination, religious confession, heart-to-heart conversation with a friend, pillow talk with a lover). Cavell recalls learning about the role of these placeholders in puzzling about the behaviour of his parents, trying to understand:

> how these two human beings that I called my parents, who were capable of these intensities, had nevertheless come to their accustomed economy of life.
>
> (*A Pitch of Philosophy*, p. 48)

We may be fearful that if we know others too well we will either be damaged by this or feel infinitely, unbearably responsible for making things right for them. It is hard not to be distrustful of the patience and inventiveness of others in their capacity to know us, and so hold back from letting them see those aspects of ourselves that we worry might create a bad impression. We may also doubt our ability to engage others, with anxiety about our inexpressiveness, or our capacity to deserve or sustain the other's interest. These fears about being known by and knowing other people are not simply irrational: there may be very good, protective reasons for them. This point is well illustrated by findings by attachment researchers that an avoidant response to loved ones in the context of distress is especially common among those individuals who have learnt from experience to expect painful rebuff or excessive interference (Ainsworth et al., *Patterns of Attachment*; Mikulincer & Shaver, *Attachment in Adulthood*).

However, even in the context of avoidant strategies or the platitudes of everyday convention that keep others at bay, Cavell emphasises that there is always the potential for knowing others and for being known, beyond our intentions. In this, the present acts as the poorly sutured wound of the past, continually threatening to bleed through:

> I cannot at will give my past expression, though every gesture expresses it, and each elation and headache; my character is its epitome, as if the present were a pantomime of ghostly selections.
>
> (*Must We Mean*, p. 295)

It is for this reason that we cannot know ourselves alone. In Cavell's view active conversation, with sufficient trust, is needed for us to truly *learn from* what we

Table 11.1 Hoping and fearing knowing and being known

	We can know or learn about others	*We will not know or learn about others*
Hope that . . .	e.g. we might learn spontaneously when to be tender with a child or parent.	e.g. the child's or parent's love in which we find happiness and vitality is perceived by them as nothing special.
Fear that . . .	e.g. in knowing about the child/parent we will end up infinitely responsible for their needs and pain.	e.g. we will be exiled and cut off from any meaningful sense of community or belonging, left in isolation and abandonment by our child/parent.
	Others will know or learn about us	*Others will not know or learn about us*
Hope that . . .	e.g. that we might be recognised and acknowledged when we try to convey to others something about our life, so that their response is to *us* in some true sense, not just what we do in our role as a child/parent.	e.g. that our child/parent will not learn some of the private things we still despair at ourselves for having done in the past.
Fear that . . .	e.g. that our tone and gestures will betray us to the child's/parent's interest and insightfulness, revealing our contradictory or embarrassing commitments and wishes – even ones we don't ourselves fully know.	e.g. that our words will be met with scorn or bafflement, due to the child's/parent's lack of understanding, patience, inventiveness, or interest.

Note: Hopes and fears about how a child or parent may know us can be about the same thing, for instance how much effort it can take for us to cope with and get through a day.

say and do, as we live our inheritance in ways that exceed our intentions or ready ways of knowing ourselves. Without others engaging our actions with seriousness and patience, Cavell worries that we stand little chance of understanding our partly willed orientation within the world, and to sense our own lives as morally intelligible. In his autobiographical account, Cavell's experience of psychotherapy, of teaching, of (his second) marriage, of friendship and of being a parent to young children are each described as important sources of personal strength in his adult life, and provide him with the exemplary cases of this process of coming to know oneself in serious, patient dialogue.

The problem of love

For Cavell, the problem that philosophy calls scepticism regarding other minds is, in fact, the substantive concern of our everyday lives, motivated by desires and fears about what our lives may hold. This is formulated by the philosophical tradition through questions such as "Is my pain the same as your pain?" However, one of Cavell's most important insights is that the same issue of the intelligibility of others faced by philosophy is also one of the great animating topics of literature and film, as crystals in turn refracting the concerns of everyday life. Literature provides a space where we come to know ourselves and others, precisely though the way that literature traces the varied ways that knowledge of others is achieved or not achieved. Cavell's son, Benjamin, in an interview about his collection of short stories *Rumble, Young Man, Rumble*, reports literature (and boxing, in fact) as a space of non-identification but of love and knowing in his relationship with his father:

> I felt as though I couldn't be a philosopher. What would be my dream? My dream would be to be my father in some way. And that didn't appeal to me. Certainly, he influenced the way I thought about the world. I have always had this feeling for writing that I am sure is due in part to his influence and his love for writing and writers.
>
> ('Benjamin Cavell, Interview')

Unlike Stanley Cavell, who changed his name as one index of his disidentification with his father, Benjamin Cavell's account seems to speak of a more negotiated position of dependence and independence. *Rumble, Young Man, Rumble* is a beautiful collection of stories about young masculinity and detachment as an achievement, training attention on the banter, boasting and anger used both to express and to mask desire for affection and to feel a little less lost in the world.

In his own scholarship, Cavell finds in Shakespeare, like in no other writer, the most acute attention to a version of the sceptic's doubt regarding the mind of the other: "How do I know that she loves me?", perhaps alternately formulated as "Is she satisfied and is the satisfaction directed at me?" Each tragedy holds this concern in a different way. Indeed, "a map of the territory of scepticism provides, or is, a map of Shakespearean regions" (*Disowning Knowledge*, p. 19). Beginning perhaps with the simple wish to test a truth, the tragic hero pursues a line of doubt to the point of violence in response to a fear about his or her relationship with and vulnerability to others. Othello murders Desdemona in despair at finding evidence in the world that can prove conclusively that she loves him; the doubt is motivated ultimately by the fear that she might not, given that he has no idea why she actually came to love him in the first place. The same logic can be seen in *The Winter's Tale*: in his doubt whether he is the father of Hermione's child, Leontes ruins his family and harms his kingdom to the point that the miraculous happy ending to the play comes out of the blue and rings uncomfortably hollow. The insistent truth of the ghost of Hamlet's father deprives the son of the chance to mourn, with the consequence that Hamlet is unable to enter into and trust life with others, and their interactions take on a skeletal or theatrical quality for him.

In each case, tragedy arises from an individual unwilling to the point of violence to give up on doubts about others around him. Othello, Leontes and Hamlet hold a bar for acknowledgement so high that their real, everyday life cannot reach it, and for this reason they indict and destroy this life as *sickening* or *worthless*. This is the mythological quality of tragedy. It dramatises the consequences of a temptation common to all humans – but especially likely under conditions of disappointment or restlessness – to distrust the terms of our poor, ordinary mutual attunement and vulnerability to one another. In contrast to most humans, who have other options, a tragic hero is, for whatever reason, constituted in some indelible way that makes them unable to make sense of their relationships in terms other than doubt:

> In normal periods, tragic acts are skirted by one's cares remaining superficial enough or mutually compatible enough for them not to suffer naked exposure. In the typical situation of tragic heroes, time and space converge to a point at which an ultimate care is exposed and action must be taken which impales one's life upon the founding care of that life – that in the loss of which chaos is come. . . . That the love becomes incompatible with that life is tragic, but that it is maintained until the end is heroic.
>
> (*Must We Mean*, pp. 349–350)

Our lives are generally superficial enough or mutually compatible enough that we do not come to exposure. And when we do, it often turns out that what is exposed is not something that cannot be altered, and tragedy averted. In drawing this conclusion, Cavell has a great sense of the malleability of human nature, and, following Freud, for him it is based ultimately in how they engage what history has made of their present (Cavell's debt to Freud in this regard is pervasive in his writings, but especially documented in his article 'Freud and Philosophy'). For Cavell, sceptical doubt and failures to acknowledge others are not inevitable. They are formed by particular circumstances from childhood:

> Men do not just naturally not love, they learn not to. And our lives begin by having to accept under the name of love whatever closeness is offered, and by then having to forgo its object.
>
> (*Must We Mean*, p. 300)

Despite his analysis of the theme of scepticism across Shakespeare's tragedies in general, the central play for Cavell's study of scepticism is Shakespeare's *King Lear*. Fisher (2000: 977), writing in the *International Journal of Psychoanalysis*, has called Cavell's work "one of the most penetrating essays on this play" across the long history of Shakespeare scholarship. In Cavell's essay on *Lear*, the angry father, full of rage and incomprehension, is taken as the paradigm of the sceptical predicament. There is a limited sadness in the fact that this analysis, so laden with themes from Cavell's childhood, would precisely have the greatest role to play of all his writings in catapulting him to international renown as a scholar, to the acknowledgement and respect from others his father yearned for and never received. But there is also a limited happiness in this as well, that through Cavell's impassioned analysis of a father's avoidance of acknowledgement a son would find a way beyond his father, never escaping the incinerating inheritance of his father's rage entirely, but making headway.

On Cavell's interpretation, the opening scene of *King Lear* reveals the stakes of the play. Lear stages a ceremony, announcing that he will divide his realm among his three daughters, and that the largest share will go to the one who loves him the most. Goneril and Regan flatter their father, and receive a share of the inheritance. Cordelia, however, refuses to flatter Lear through public declaration of platitudes. Lear is enraged by this, and he disinherits Cordelia. But what *was* Lear attempting to achieve with this ceremony? Why ask his daughters whether they love him, and why do so in public? Cavell suggests that, as king, Lear was unable to feel sure whether his daughters loved him for his power or out of attachment. Lear worried that without power, he would be unworthy of their love, and that increasing powerlessness was inevitable as he approached old age. The ceremony, on Cavell's interpretation, was a strategy designed to avoid learning whether this fear was true. In "exchanging his fortune for his love at one swap" (*Must We Mean*, p. 289), Lear avoids the question of whether he was worthy of love by asking only for its public profession, nothing more genuine. In exchange, he offers his kingdom, but no true feeling of his own. However, Cordelia's response threatens this defence:

> Cordelia is alarming precisely because he *knows* she is offering the real thing, offering something a more opulent third of his kingdom cannot, must not, repay; putting a claim upon him he cannot face. She threatens to expose both his plan for returning false love with no love, and expose the necessity for that plan – his terror of being loved, of needing love.
>
> (*Must We Mean*, p. 290)

In hiding from our fears and wishes, Cavell argues, we hold on to doubts about ourselves and others, rather than allowing uncertainties to be worked out with others in the ordinary ways humans can go adventuring and getting matters done with one another.

The raging incomprehension of Lear, like Cavell's father, make him a hard act to follow, casting a great shadow across his children. Rage does so in part by taking those that feel it away from the ordinary space of mutual attunement and change, where things can remain either superficial enough or mutually compatible enough that we can be together without the need to doubt one another beyond what the relationship can sustain. In considering the role of rage in this regard, it is uncomfortable but helpful to imagine what it would have been like for Cavell's father, forced to acknowledge or not acknowledge his son's thinking and accomplishments. One clue to what it was like for Cavell's father is given in the book on Shakespeare where Cavell reports that his father joked that, rather than a student of philosophy, his son must be a researcher in chemistry. Otherwise how could it be that he was able to turn tuition money into shit? (*Disowning Knowledge*, p. 172). Yet another clue lies in the father's offer to pay to have Cavell fitted in the Harvard PhD robes. The fitting allowed father and son to symbolise the way that each had overshadowed the other, and nonetheless claim kinship and attachment and a certain need for one another. Such demonstrations of believing in one another and of returning the other's love are complex and indirect, but achievable and real. The autobiographical scene of the robe fitting stands in contrast to the ceremony that begins *King Lear*, which Cavell interprets precisely as a way of avoiding acknowledgement of the wish to be loved. In his angry doubts about his own value and that of his loved ones, together with his occasional attempts to do better, Cavell's father is less a tragic hero of the consistent and brutal Shakespearean type than one aspect of the ordinary family member each of us remains.

References

Ainsworth, M. D., Blehar, M., Waters, E., & Wall, S. (1978). *Patterns of Attachment: A Psychological Study of the Strange Situation*. Hillsdale, NJ: Erlbaum.

Cavell, B. (2003). 'Cavell, Interview' www.identitytheory.com/benjamin-cavell/

Cavell, S. (1969). *Must We Mean What We Say?*, Cambridge: Cambridge University Press.

Cavell, S. (1979). *The Claim of Reason*, Oxford: Oxford University Press.

Cavell, S. (1984). *Themes Out of School*, Chicago: University of Chicago Press.

Cavell, S. (1987). 'Freud and Philosophy' *Critical Inquiry*, 13: 386–393.

Cavell, S. (1987). *Disowning Knowledge in Seven Plays of Shakespeare*, Cambridge: Cambridge University Press.

Cavell, S. (1994). *In Quest of the Ordinary: Lines of Skepticism and Romanticism*, Chicago: University of Chicago Press.

Cavell, S. (1996). 'Comments on Veena Das's Essay "Language and Body: Transactions in the Construction of Pain"' *Daedalus*, 125(1): 93–98.

Cavell, S. (2002). *A Pitch of Philosophy*, Cambridge, MA: Harvard University Press.

Cavell, S. (2006). *Philosophy the Day after Tomorrow*, Cambridge, MA: Harvard University Press.

Cavell, S. (2010a). *Little Did I Know: Excerpts from Memory*, Stanford: Stanford University Press.
Fisher, J. (2000). 'A Father's Abdication: Lear's Retreat from "Aesthetic Conflict"' *International Journal of Psycho-Analysis*, 81(5): 963–982.
Mikulincer, M. & Shaver, P. (2016). *Attachment in Adulthood: Structure, Dynamics and Change*, New York: Guilford.
Milner, M. (1987). *Eternity's Surprise*, New York: Virago.
Wittgenstein, L. (1953). *Philosophical Investigations*, Oxford: Blackwell.

In religion and family life

Chapter 12

The eye begins to see

Personal reflections on a fragmented father–son relationship, and other related matters

Howard Cooper

The essay that follows reflects in a deeply personal way on the contrast between a man open and caring to the outside world, yet experienced as largely emotionally closed to those 'on the inside', with whom he appeared able to put his feeling life into words, yet only in writing. This dynamic is seen, en passant, in the context of Jewish immigrant parents whose sons felt pressured into following certain professional careers, often against the next generation's best interests.

Evidence is brought of the way in which living in the shadow of a parent in the public eye has often affected a particular group of contemporary Jews in England: the sons and daughters of rabbis. And – to widen the perspective – a case study is also presented of a patient who was the son of a Church of England minister, whose life felt very much lived 'in the shadow of his father'.

My father died when I was 24 years old. From 1977 onwards I lived in the shadow of the age he was when he died – 59 – an age which gradually took on a dark, almost mythic dimension. Somewhat to my amazement I have now outlived him by a number of years, but I remember how impossible it seemed during all that time that I could ever become as old as, let alone older than, my own father.

His death was sudden: a coronary thrombosis. It was the fourth evening of Passover and, back home for a few days, I had gone to the cinema with friends. We parked the car and, as I moved forward to get out of the back seat, someone swung back into my face the metal clasp of the front seat belt and it broke the left lens of my glasses.

The sentiments in the film – Sidney Lumet's Oscar-winning *Network* – about a television company's manipulation of news anchorman Howard Beale (Peter Finch), who announces mid-show that due to falling ratings he will kill himself live on air the following Tuesday – "I'm mad as hell and I'm not going to take this anymore" – have remained fused inside me with the events of that April evening. When we arrived home, stirred by the film's themes and Finch's barnstorming performance – which turned out to be his last (Finch had died a couple of months before, suddenly, of a heart attack, a young 60-year-old.) I was puzzled to see the Rabbi's car parked outside our house. My father had died – it turned out – at the same time as the lens in my glasses had shattered. I attended my father's funeral and the subsequent nights of *shiva* (Jewish mourning) with one eye seeing clearly out of the remaining lens, and the rest a blur.

'Synchronicity' is a handy label, though not an explanation, for events such as these. Just as 'counter-transference' is a convenient reach-me-down term, but not an 'explanation' for what transpires in the consulting room. It seems to me that in the space-time continuum we call life things are linked in ways that as yet defy our understanding. As if the world operates more like a poem than a science textbook. And this leaves us to ascribe – or withhold – meaning as we see fit. Theodore Roethke's reflection comes to mind, and underpins this essay: "*In a dark time, the eye begins to see / I meet my shadow in the deepening shade*" (from his poem *In a Dark Time*, 1961).

I'm a rationalist, like my father. Yet I think – or maybe I like to think – that he believed, as do I, that the world is far larger and more mysterious than our rationality-dominated mental apparatus can readily accommodate; that we are more than our means to know gives us to know.

Today one of the only things I recall from the meagre conversations we had over the years was his belief that probably 75% of the patients he saw were suffering from psychosomatic symptoms – that the physical complaints they brought to him were rooted in emotional distress. (This was a conversation many years before I had any thoughts of training as a psychotherapist; and many years before general practitioners [GPs] might have begun to think, as part of their training, about the complex relationship between psyche and soma.)

My father was a GP who trained as a doctor in the early years of the National Health Service. He was the traditional family doctor who now exists only in an older generation's fading memories: he would go out to patients who phoned in the middle of the night; he knew his patients by their first names and would stop (or, more often, be stopped) on the street for a chat or a mini-consultation; he remained in one GP practice all his working life, so he eventually attended to (and would remember to enquire after) several generations within a single family; he would come home late after an evening surgery, ashen-faced with tiredness after seeing anyone who turned up with or without an appointment; and he apparently had a caring and dedicated bedside manner that knew what to say, how to elicit information, how to handle young and old, how to impart difficult news with compassion. After his death, my mother received several hundred letters and cards from grateful patients shocked and upset by his untimely death.

But at home he was silent. The conversations he was (apparently) so skilled at having in his professional life did not exist at home. For complicated reasons that I came to understand more about only after his death, he had drawn a veil over his deeper emotional life, and so was never able to relate to or attend to my mother's feeling life or the deeper, non-practical, needs of my sister and me. (Material needs were another matter: he would go miles out of his way to buy a book that might be useful for my homework, or a new set of stamps for my philately collection, or to pick up a spare football ticket offered to him by a grateful patient.) At home his silence, his inwardness, his unwillingness (no, his inability) to relate in a more personal, emotionally open way, left me – although I did not know it at the time – as 'mad as hell'; though his premature death meant that I was never able to say that "I'm not going to take this anymore".

> Everything around me is evaporating. My whole life, my memories, my imagination and its contents, my personality – it's all evaporating. I continuously feel that I was someone else, that I felt something else, that I thought something else. What I am attending here is a show. . . . And the show I'm attending is myself.
>
> (Fernando Pessoa, *The Book of Disquiet*)

As I sit and write about this enigma of a man, I have in front of me one of the only artefacts I possess that once belonged to him. It is a small ivory-handled penknife. Closed up, it is less than a couple of inches long. Opened up, the blade is dull: it has lost its cutting edge, though the tip of the blade is still sharp. As I handle it, rub my thumb along the smooth but mottled ivory, I recall holding my father's hand. He had soft hands. And immaculate nails, which he pared regularly. I bite my nails.

Yes, I can remember his liver-spotted hands, the way his greying hair curled up on his collar when it grew time for a cut, the sound of the key in the front door when he arrived home at night and something in me instinctively relaxed. But I hardly remember a single conversation we ever had. No words of advice, or warning, or wisdom. Of course he talked – he would spend hours with me as I struggled with my Latin homework and tried to keep at bay the secret shame that accompanied my inability to get the better of a language he was more adept at than I was – even though it'd been more than 30 years since he'd studied it at school. He did talk – but it was focused-on-the-situation pragmatic talk, the-only-way-he-knew-how-to-speak-in-an-intimate-setting talk. And the rest was silence. The complex legacy of that silence resides in me to this day.

Many years after my father's death, a rabbinic colleague of mine who'd been a student rabbi at the synagogue that our family attended – and that my father had helped establish and to which he became the honorary secretary – told me that at regular council meetings they both attended my father rarely spoke, but that when he did speak the room went quiet and people listened: that he had a natural authority that people recognised and respected. He didn't argue, he just spoke clearly and quietly and to the point. And that this would, more often than not, sway the meeting.

I am told that the same is true of me (though I am perhaps not best placed to judge): this is not a case of people who knew the father projecting certain qualities onto the son – people who remember my father are few and far between. But as I grow older I am intrigued by the ways I am my father's son. In spite of years consciously charting my own way through life, forging a professional and personal life very different from my father's, and recognising the multiple ways in which I am quite unlike my father – particularly in my capacity for, playfulness and the joys of human connectedness – I can trace (sometimes contentedly, often disconcertingly) hidden lines of continuity that others never see, and which I may only rarely catch glimpses of myself.

'Forging' a life is of course a usefully ambiguous term. I think there were aspects of his work that my father gradually, over the 30 years he practiced, grew to hate – like the unceasing and repetitious demands on his time and patience – sentiments that nobody knew about, that he swallowed in silence, and that merged into his silence. He just forged ahead regardless, making it up as he went along. Though I recognise myself in this characterisation of my father, I don't think this is merely a projection. Whatever he privately felt about his work, and some of the impossible expectations he faced from colleagues and patients alike (and probably from himself as well), I think he acted the part of a caring and dedicated general practitioner until he became one. But I also think, I speculate, that this performance of a persona eventually killed him.

Although I grew up with a father in the public eye – as both a local GP and a synagogue official – I never consciously felt daunted by this, nor have I discovered, in spite of many years of analysis over the decades, ways in which I felt unconsciously daunted by his public roles or personae. Although many people knew him – and knew me to be his son – I don't feel I have ever lived my adult life 'in his shadow'. From my twenties onwards – though did he have to die for this to happen? – I consider that I became my own man in ways that are both idiosyncratically satisfying for myself and stimulating, nurturing and productive for others.

And yet.

What does it mean that I have developed a pair of careers that so closely mirror his own enthusiasms? Whatever else it might be, psychoanalytic psychotherapy is a 'caring' profession. Like my father, I too have my patients. Like my father too, I approach my work with devotion, diligence and what I take to be – on a good day – an intelligent sensitivity. And like my father – not coincidentally, of course – I see how many of my patients suffer from psychosomatic symptoms. My advantage over my father is that I have a framework within which to think about this, and a feeling language with which to communicate my understanding of their suffering and (sometimes, if things go well) help alleviate it.

And what is my rabbinic career but a continuation of, and maybe a transformation of, his love of Judaism? He had grown up with a traditional Orthodox Jewish background – there was no other way in pre-war Glasgow – but he was no slavish adherent to rituals, traditions or beliefs. Indeed he was moved in 1963 to leave the Orthodox community to which we had belonged in Manchester and help set up a new Reform community in the wake of what became known in Anglo-Jewry as the 'Louis Jacobs affair'.[1]

My father's approach to religion was much influenced by his reading of his fellow Scot Sir James Frazer's anthropological dissection of religious myth and ritual in *The Golden Bough*. This comparative study of religion and mythology – published in 12 volumes between 1906 and 1915 and hugely influential at the time – argued that humanity progresses from 'magical' thinking to 'religious' belief to 'scientific' rationality. Although such a schema is now seen as hopelessly passé, my father was an enthusiast of Frazer's views – and kept his abridged version of *The Golden Bough* on our family bookcase next to his personally annotated and heavily underlined volume of the *Complete Works of Shakespeare*.

This is almost too neat a symbol of the ways in which the rational pragmatist and the poetic soul nestled side by side within my father. One of my father's problems was the way in which he never found a way of truly integrating that latter side of his nature into himself: it was as if the romantic within him was a secret feeling-based self that had to be split off and kept away from public view, and maybe from himself. He had written love sonnets as a young man but I only discovered them in an old wallet after he died. He was a good classical pianist but only ever played on his own, in the lounge, and would stop if anyone would enter the room.

Unlike my father, I have found the tension and interplay between my rational and poetic selves – if I can revert for a moment to such simplifications – creative and life enhancing. I have been known to characterise myself, somewhat whimsically, as a mystically inclined rationalist. That is to say, I have a need for intellectual coherence, and the cool discipline and rigour of a logical approach to life situations – we have *reason* to believe – that can challenge irrationality and call out illusionary and wishful thinking. And I have a need for a life lived attendant to the mystery encoded within being, the awareness that there is always more going on than meets the eye, the perception that the unconscious is the great *subverter* of our knowingness and wish for intelligibility; a life lived attuned to what John Keats famously described as 'Negative Capability': when a person "is capable of being in uncertainties, mysteries, doubts, without any irritable reaching after fact and reason". One of the lessons I learnt – indirectly, unwittingly – from my father is that one may pay an unforeseen price in failing to honour the multiple selves that exist within us.

Apparently – so my mother told me in more recent times – my father had harboured a growing wish over the years to retrain as a lawyer. It seemed that he'd inquired about both correspondence courses and night school. But how seriously he'd contemplated this, or why he hadn't proceeded (though, as satirist Peter Cook would say – *he had the Latin*) I have no idea: something else he never spoke to me about. Yet, unbeknownst to me, his desire to study Law had a significant influence on my own early academic choices.

Aged 16, I was an intellectually precocious but emotionally choked adolescent who, when it came to applying to university, had no idea what I wanted to study. History and English were my strongest subjects; physics, chemistry and biology my weakest. So I couldn't have applied for medicine even if I'd had the slightest interest in doing so, which I didn't. (My sister lived in the shadow of a father she idealised, followed in his footsteps, and ended up an unhappy doctor who struggled for years to get out of general practice.)

But what was I to do? The application forms for university entrance arrived and they needed to be filled in. It was suggested to me – by my mother – that I should apply to read law. My father's inhibition in having a feeling-based conversation with me meant that he'd told my mother that I'd be suited for such a career; she duly conveyed this to me; and I passively went along with it. As I write this, I still find it hard to credit that this describes accurately the family dynamic that existed. But it pains me to have to say that this is how it was. I applied to Sussex University to read law.

Many of my current (male) contemporaries tell me how they went into professions determined by a parent's spoken or unspoken wishes: they became dentists, doctors, accountants and lawyers – and successful ones – but often struggled during their careers with the feelings generated by a growing awareness that they had never felt as if they themselves had freely chosen what to study and what profession to follow. These are not men whose parents had been in the public eye; but they were men with aspirational parents – Jewish immigrant parents who believed that the route to social and financial betterment (and, not unimportantly, the route to the *fantasised* security of assimilation) lay in educational success followed by entry into one of the 'professions'.

I remain unsure to what extent my father suffered from those external parental pressures – his own father, a gentle and rather unworldly soul, had arrived in Glasgow from Poland as a teenager at the turn of the century and worked as a tailor all his life; his emotionally possessive mother came from a Viennese background, was orphaned young and forced to marry 'beneath' her, subsequently bearing a large chip on her shoulder. One of my father's brothers became a baker; another was in America when war broke out, stayed there afterwards, and entered the world of business consultancy.

Although my father went to a leading Glasgow grammar school and was a diligent student, he didn't go from there to university: money was short in the family and he became a sanitary inspector; and then, during the war, served in the army Medical Corps. By the time he entered medical school after the war, he was already nearly 30. Why medicine and not law – if that was what he really wanted to do? Or do the fantasies about being happier in another profession only emerge once one feels oneself drowning in a tide of dissatisfactions about one's chosen career? I won't ever know – perhaps a small example of how children never really know what goes on in their parents' inner worlds. However, what is clear is that my father's frustrated desire to study law was displaced onto his son. Without my knowing it, with my mother the secret bearer of my father's wishes, my application for law was over-determined.

Fortunately the system at Sussex in those days was to require students in the humanities to take two terms of 'contextual' subjects before starting their 'major' degree subject. Because I had taken a gap year, it was more than two years between my initial application and the beginning of the law courses. That's a long time in an impressionable teenager's life. In that time something in me had changed – I hesitate to say 'matured', but I suppose that's what I mean; although when I think back to how I spent that year off, travelling across America in thrall to *Easy Rider* and the anti–Vietnam War protests, I can see that the anti-authority trope is writ large. So maybe 'matured' is not quite right. My gap year was both a protest against parental constraints and expectations, as well as an unconscious quest for a different kind of fathering. At any rate, by the time I started at Sussex University I had become clear in my own mind that the career I wanted to pursue was not law but the rabbinate. Becoming a rabbi meant going to the Leo Baeck College rabbinical school for a further five years of study after my undergraduate degree. What better preparation for these later studies than to major at Sussex in religious studies?

Perhaps surprisingly, the rabbinate was attracting a new generation of young Jewish men. During my teenage years I had met several charismatic trainee rabbis, students from the Leo Baeck College who came to work with, teach and preach at the new Reform congregation my parents had helped set up. Often these men in their twenties and thirties came to stay in our home, for the weekend or longer. They were knowledgeable, engaging, fascinating to listen to and – fatefully as it turned out – interested in my thoughts and views in ways that my own father couldn't find it in himself to express. This was very seductive for a teenager who was developing a growing fascination for the universal phenomenon of religion and religious belief, for the questions of meaning and human purpose they purport to address, and for Judaism and its post-Holocaust dilemmas and possibilities.

These trainee rabbis were involved in a religious project that combined personal spiritual adventurousness with the rebuilding of European Jewish life after the *Shoah*. Meanwhile, old verities and truths were up for grabs, strands of revolution and societal change were in the air – it was the 'Age of Aquarius', and youthfulness was synchronous with hopefulness – and these dynamic, iconoclastic father figures seemed to me to be forging a new Jewish mythology out of the fragments of a faith that had been shattered by history. This was all a heady mix. My own father didn't stand a chance against these expressive and passionate figures. I became set on a rabbinical career where (in my mind) I could make a difference to people's lives. And although I did not think about it like this at the time, I can now see that – just as my father with his own work – I was intent on a so-called caring profession through pastoral work that was a daily part of a rabbi's life.

This decision to change courses, with a view to an eventual rabbinical career, wasn't discussed with my parents. I (thought I) knew my own mind – though I didn't yet have a language to speak personally to either of them about what I really wanted to do. But during a visit home during that first year at university I must have alluded to my plans to change direction, because I have in front of me one of the only letters I ever received from my father.

It is handwritten on several smallish pieces of his surgery notepaper – Dr A. S. Cooper, M.B., CH.B. – and dated Sunday, 20 February 1972. The envelope is written in my mother's handwriting – a neat piece of symbolism: he did the thinking for both of them, she acted as container of his rare emotional outbursts. I had never re-read the letter until thinking about the themes of this essay (though, self-evidently, I had kept it), but having dug it out and looked at it for the first time in almost 45 years, I hesitatingly realised that it contained something close to the heart of what I wanted to write about today.

It opens with a rebuke:

> *Dear Howard,*
>
> *I am writing primarily because of your failure to phone here last night as promised and the fact that we have been unable to contact you this morning.*

My father would never say he was disappointed, or hurt, or upset. Or angry. Though I was frightened of his anger.

What follows is an uninterrupted transcription of the rest of the letter from my father. I have retained his exact flow of words, although there are places where one could say that the structure of the sentences seems to breakdown under the urgency and pressure of what is being said.

> *My second reason for writing is to urge you while there is still time to be absolutely positive of what you want to do before you commit yourself to theology. It would be facile to say that it requires a lot of thought and it would be impossible, even if it were desirable, to show you the kind of thing in which you are involving yourself. You are by now aware of the manifold duties imposed on what I would call, for want of a better word, the conventional type of Rabbi and even if these were not daunting enough, your future may be in the hands of people like myself, who, when faced with the choice of the appointment of one or other rabbi must be guided to some extent, or rather influenced is the word, not by the obvious sincerity, maturity of outlook, spirituality of one candidate but* assume *that most ministers have these in varying degrees, but cast your die in favour of one who by his social graces, charm and apparent ability not only to be all things to all men but have a special gift to attract a large membership in double quick time.*
>
> *A man's future may well depend on these qualities in varying degrees. To the type of Rabbi who sees something different in religion and hopes to have some message for mankind, I would say that such ideas have been in the forefront of many a man's mind in every religion before and after Christ, without much success. To think that influence can be brought to bear on man's inhumanity to man is like denying the existence of the rich and the poor. And at all times to have to live in the public eye, a pillar of rectitude whose every word and gesture and action one must not only justify but appear to be beyond reproach to an unintelligent public.*
>
> *From the above you may assume that I am advising against the course of study you now appear to have set your heart on. But truthfully I am not. My only desire in the past and in the future has been that your life should be led in the way you yourself want it to be, and most of all that you should be*

happy and confident in that choice. *So once again I am saying be very sure, for once committed to theology only two things can happen either you will go forward to Leo Baeck or end up with a degree able to cope with social studies of some kind.*

I should have thought that by maintaining your previous choice of law and staying with it for at least three years you could if you were still unhappy about it and intent on Rabbinics, then enter Leo Baeck. It may take longer that way but it has the great virtue of being safer – and anyway what is time in an undertaking which has as its ultimate aim an understanding of religion.

I will close now by assuring you most vigorously on two counts. First, that I have only your interest at heart, and that I will be equally pleased with whatever decision you make – after thought.

All my love,
Dad

His brilliant disguise: passionate, eloquent, opinionated-but-thoughtful, emotionally self-expressive, caring – my father was able to put into words on the page what he could never speak out loud. From what "you . . . have set your heart on" to "I have only your interest at heart", this text is the kind of heart-to-heart conversation we never had, and that I sorely missed – though I was not conscious of that sadness until years after he was gone: *my* brilliant disguise.

> *It was hard for Satan alone to mislead the whole world, so he appointed rabbis in different localities.*
>
> (Rabbi Nachman of Bratslav, 1772–1810)

> *Between the idea / And the reality / Between the motion / And the act / Falls the Shadow.*
>
> (T. S. Eliot, 'The Hollow Men')

The aim of this book is to explore the psychological challenges that parents, many of whom live in the public eye, can present to their offspring. As I have suggested, in my eyes my father was a semi-public figure, which is why I have thus far focused on our relationship, but there is one cluster of people within the Anglo-Jewish community who most definitely have had the experience of growing up in the shadow of such a parent: *faute de mieux*, this is the children of rabbis.

When I raised it casually with one young man in his thirties, the son of a prominent Progressive rabbi, he immediately told me that his overwhelming experience as a teenager was that he found himself reacting to the oft-expressed expectation (by those outside his family): "Oh, you'll do well because you are X's son". This pressure led him to under-achieve at school, sabotage important exams, and induced, he felt, an 'intellectual laziness' that it took him some time to shake off. He said he'd struggled during his twenties to find his feet, but now sees himself as having a successful professional career as well as being a devoted father. Yet he's still aware that his father has indeed been a hard act to follow.

This is not an unfamiliar story – though with cases I know where children of rabbis have experienced personal failures or problems (whether they be drug or alcohol abuse, dysfunctional relationships or gambling addiction) each, of course, has complex roots and specific dynamics that make any generalisation otiose. Maybe we are best to adapt Tolstoy's famous fictional dictum and suggest: "Happy rabbinic families are all alike; every unhappy rabbinic family is unhappy in its own way".

One daughter of a congregational rabbi shared with me her own experience and insights:

> *Being shy and unconfident* [*sic*] *I had to wear a series of Laura Ashley dresses and white tights. Being pointed out to other people's kids, by their parents, as looking so neat is not the way to make yourself popular with peers. No-one would be your friend because you must be a goody-goody, being the Rabbi's daughter. But no-one would be horrible to you, because you were the Rabbi's daughter. Everyone treated you as if you knew the answer to everything and had great knowledge – but in fact I got away with never being put on the spot and asked to answer questions in cheder [religion school] – so I felt a fraud and not very knowledgeable.*
>
> *I was pretty good at talking to adults – having handed round the nuts and olives at endless dinner parties and presented many a bouquet to various mayoresses – but I struggled to feel comfortable with my peers. . . . I dealt with it all by hiding behind music, pursuing pretty wild behaviour with my music school friends, whilst maintaining my Laura Ashley facade for my parents, as I could never disappoint them.*

Now married and, with her two teenage children, active in synagogue life, she is able to look back on these difficulties with a degree of detachment – an example of how it is possible in time to work through these issues and find a satisfying way of re-integrating into a community that had caused her such upset.

One rabbi's son, however, told me how fortunate he felt growing up with a rabbi as a father. He had had a very positive role model and could think of nothing that was detrimental about the experience. That it meant that his father was only able to come and see him play for his school football team once a year made that one-off visit really special, he said, rather than engendering a feeling that he was missing out. Growing up, he once heard his father talk to his mother about 'the children' only to realise his father was not talking about him and his siblings but the children of the congregation. He took this in his stride, emphasising to me that it was an honour to follow his father into the rabbinate – his career choice was a source of great pride to both his parents. How much of this narrative involves denial of the difficulties involved is perhaps a moot point.

No doubt disappointing a parent is an experience many children have or fear as they grow up: It doesn't require one's parent to be in the public eye for children to feel the shame or anger or sense of inadequacy engendered by the experience of (or fantasy of) letting them down. There may even be a sense for any child whose parent is out of the house, *in the working world*, that their parent is in 'the public eye'.

Some decades ago a teacher in his thirties, the son of a Church of England vicar, came to me for therapy following a series of failed relationships with women. He described his father as aloof and cold, a man who shut himself away each Friday to write his uplifting sermons full of exhortations to Christian piety, love and neighbourliness. The son felt he was closer to his depressed and anxious mother, who lived in awe of her husband, as did – according to the son – his father's parishioners, particularly some of the women who fawned over this upright man (much to my patient's chagrin). The son was overweight, and bullied at school. But his father refused to intervene. The message was that one had to learn to 'turn the other cheek', put up with the taunts and kicks, and consider oneself 'better than them'. A feeling of moral superiority became my patient's primary defence against his sadness and anger – along with a secret identification with 'Jesus, meek and mild' which gave his own suffering a 'higher' purpose.

As a teenager he had a print of St. Veronica's handkerchief on his wall, a picture that he found both comforting and disturbing. The woman moved with pity at Jesus's plight on the road to Golgotha, who used her veil to wipe the sweat and tears from Jesus's face, became a key image in the therapy. The fantasy of finding a woman with the degree of selflessness that this image of St. Veronica evoked proved hard to relinquish. It took a number of years for him to begin to unravel ways in which his identification with his father had led him to have a secret disdain for women, whom he ended up treating as his father had his mother; and how his frustrations with his mother – who saw food as the only resource she had available – had led him to feel that women would be unable to meet his sexual and emotional needs.

Although he had resented how much time his father had devoted to others, we gradually saw how his own career as a teacher – with his own 'flock' of youngsters following him – had been influenced by an unconscious belief that this is how you get women to 'look up to' you: at his all-girls' school he was surrounded by young (and not so young) women teachers, as well as his cohorts of students. In some ways this was a dangerous place for my patient to be working but, although he had rejected his father's Christian beliefs, there was a residual moral framework within him (and plenty of repression) so that he didn't end up acting out in a destructive way his need for emotional (and sexual) intimacy. Over time he recognised enough of these dynamics to leave the teaching profession and pursue other paths (in the arts) – and eventually find a woman with whom he could settle down and start his own family. This might sound like a therapeutic 'success story' but what remained unresolved was his relationship with his father, who became a senior figure in the church hierarchy, and from whom, when he moved abroad and ended therapy, my patient had become estranged. Clearly, it is not just rabbis' children who may find their clerical parent a 'hard act to follow'.

***

> April 2015: "*The most we can do is to write – intelligently, creatively, critically, evocatively – about what it is like living in the world at this time*".
> (Oliver Sacks, 1933–2015, neurologist and author)

My father was right of course. In many ways the congregational rabbinate wasn't for me – apart from anything else, I lacked, in his canny formulation, the "*social graces, charm and apparent ability . . . to be all things to all men*". Already by my fourth year at Leo Baeck, having 'served time', so to speak, as a student rabbi working in various congregations, I was having doubts about a rabbinic career, a career filled with "*the manifold duties imposed on what I would call, for want of a better word, the conventional type of Rabbi*". I was beginning to be drawn to counselling/psychotherapy training and I nearly left the college. I was persuaded by a rabbinic mentor that I should stick it out for a final year and get my rabbinic diploma (it could do no harm to have one) and then see what I wanted to do.

I realise now that this crisis occurred within a year of my father's premature death. Was there a link? Is there a link? Even if he had lived, I doubt I would have turned to him to talk about my doubts and misgivings – what would have been the point? Yet my father had an inkling that I would not be able to sustain a career as a '*conventional type of Rabbi*' – I heard from my mother some years after his death that he'd told her that if I did pursue this career successfully it would be by becoming a rabbi in the mould of Rabbi Lionel Blue (whom my father greatly admired): someone who was not a congregational rabbi but was a Jewish teacher speaking to a wider audience; a rabbi working at an idiosyncratic tangent to the day-to-day need to be '*all things to all men*' and not fitting into the conventional "*pillar of rectitude whose every word and gesture and action . . . must . . . appear to be beyond reproach*".

Although this comparison somewhat embarrasses me as I set it down in print, I have always held close to my heart this small window into my father's thoughts about me. That my own professional career has been quite unlike that of Lionel Blue is not the point. But that my father viewed me as having the potential to forge a rabbinic career in any way similar to such a prestigious rabbinic figure in the Reform community seems to me extraordinary. And that my father never let me have any clue about this was, of course, par for the course. It makes me sad, and angry, and opens up the chasm of regret in me about what failed to happen between us.

No doubt I am still looking at our father–son relationship through my broken glasses, as it were: part of what I see, I am imagining I see clearly; part is blurred and fragmented. That I have gone on to craft a professional career combining psychoanalytic psychotherapy, the rabbinate albeit without a congregation, and authorship is something in which I imagine he would have taken a lot of (quiet) pride.

I am glad I ignored the well-meaning advice he offered in that long, emotionally laden letter. I am sure I never acknowledged to him that I had even received it. Maybe this essay is my belated act of acknowledgement. As well as a belated act of gratitude. In spite of his silence, it was clear that he cared. That he cared more than words could say. Our mutual loss.

Note

1 Rabbi Louis Jacobs was a dedicated and scholarly Orthodox rabbi of immense learning who had published a book which acknowledged that the Torah – the Five Books of Moses – was a document written not by God but by human hands. For this alleged 'heresy' – historical-critical Biblical scholarship was unacceptable to the Orthodox powers-that-be – he was not allowed to take over as head of the UK's leading Orthodox rabbinical seminary, Jews' College; and the subsequent furore tore the Jewish community apart.

(My father was an admirer of Rabbi Jacobs (he'd also happened to be his GP) and supported his views about the need for Judaism to balance tradition with modernity. I grew up with this debate raging around me before I had any real understanding of what it was all about. But I recall that as I approached my teenage years Louis Jacobs's book *We Have Reason to Believe* was in our house, and although I don't remember being actively *encouraged* to read it, I was intrigued enough by the passion generated by this 'affair' to work my way slowly though its somewhat dry pages – which I had gathered were a kind of Jewish dynamite.)

Reflections in fine art

Other than in music and, of course, the theatre – which for our purposes I have 'subsumed' under opera (Chapter 2) – it is surely in the visual arena where we are most literally 'on display' – where we open ourselves up for comparison with others, be family, friends, colleagues, characters in our present or figures from the past. For the London artist Gayna Pelham,[1] it was the original title of our book, *A Hard Act to Follow*, that brought to mind a range of artist parents who surpassed in fame their artist offspring, and conversely, artists more famous than their parents. With permission, I am offering Gayna's comments as a postscript below.[2]

It is of course far beyond the scope of this book to consider, for example, the lives of the great artists of the Renaissance and post-Renaissance (Mannerist, Baroque or Rococo) periods, for example, though one might well ponder the father–son relationships – and, in at least one case, the father–daughter relationship – of the artistic greats of those times.

For our purposes, however, our book concludes with two chapters focusing on the creative lives of two very different contemporary artists and their respective experiences of their artist parents. In both cases, the question "Isn't your father the well-known . . ." or "Aren't you the daughter or son of . . ." is sensitively discussed. I am grateful to our two authors who are clearly *not just* the 'sum of their parts' but, drawing on *internal* resources, continue to pursue their respective journeys far beyond *the shadow;* and indeed, with emotional development borne of maturing experience, have allowed themselves to shine in their own light.

Notes

1 In London, Gayna Pelham lectures mainly at the National Gallery, the Portrait Gallery, the Courtauld Institute and the Wallace Collection.

2 Gayna's selection of artists more famous than their offspring included:

- Jorge Manuel Theotocópuli – son of El Greco (Doménikos Theotokópoulos) – spent much of his time producing copies of his father's paintings.
- Pieter Brueghel the Younger and Jan Brueghel – sons of Pieter Brueghel – arguably never as successful as their father, and certainly Pieter spent most of his career producing copies of his father's paintings.

- Domenico Tintoretto – son of Jacopo Tintoretto – with his brother Marco and sister Marietta became artists in their father's workshop and assisted him in his paintings. Their careers, however, declined after their father's death.

Artists who became more famous than their parents included:

- Jacopo Bellini and his sons Giovanni and Gentile, both of whom were very successful in their own rights.
- Artemesia Gentileschi – daughter of Orazio Gentileschi.
- Hans Holbein the Younger, son of Hans Holbein the Elder.
- Canaletto – son of Bernardo Canal.

Chapter 13

Shadow, colour, glass

The family I knew and the family I never knew

*Ardyn Halter**

Our penultimate chapter presents us with yet a further disturbance in a father–son relationship and this despite the overarching love that existed between the two. It was a relationship that, for all its expression, could not be anything but deeply influenced by the tragic events of the Holocaust.

In the chapter that follows, the artist Ardyn Halter reflects on his relationship with his father, the artist and architect Roman Halter – a man who devoted much of his life to expressing his experiences in the Holocaust, in word and image. Ardyn's father was a charismatic man who led a creative life, yet who, surprisingly, blurred the line between his own achievements and those of his son. The interview below with Jonathan Burke reveals the tension between this and the deep filial love felt by Ardyn towards his father. The chapter continues to open up for our consideration the subject of inherited memory – very much the leitmotiv of our book, emphasising The Shadow of the Parent.

As the title of our book clearly implies, we are concerned here with living in the shadow of a parent – whether consciously experienced or not. Your father was an artist and you are an artist.

AH: My father was many things. He was an architect. He was designer and maker of the Royal Coat of Arms for the Queen. He was also a designer and maker of stained glass. He was a natural raconteur and author of a book. He was a survivor of the *Shoah* (the Holocaust). And when after he died, David Glasser, director of the Ben Uri Gallery in London, thought long and hard under what title, what category to celebrate his life in the visual arts, before deciding upon *Roman Halter, Life and Art through Stained Glass*. The choice of title was not obvious. I thought then and I think now that his greatest creation was his own persona. I do not mean this condescendingly. You could not forget him. The force of his personality.

Strangely, professionally, I was an artist before my father made his name as an artist. This was thanks to the encouragement he gave me when I was a child. He himself painted at different periods of his life, but his chosen career was architecture.

The wording of your subject of living in the shadow of a *parent* is very relevant in my case. Because for me, his shadow was more the shadow of his *persona*, than of his work. The shadow, if shadow it was and is, is what he had lived through, and his desire to pass on the baton of memory of genocide, that it be known and not forgotten.

But in order to answer your questions relating to the subject of the degree or nature of the influence or 'shadow' of my father on me, or on my work as an artist, I suppose the reader should know something more of his background.

Yes, could you tell me more about him?

AH: My father, Roman Halter, came from Chodecz, a small town in central Poland. Before 1939 the population was roughly evenly divided, half Jewish and half Christian, though the Christian population was divided between the Lutheran *Volksdeutsch* and the Polish Catholics. In total there were 1,500 people in the town.

Apart from my father, in all six Jews from Chodecz survived.

At the start of the Second World War he was 12 years old, the youngest child in his family. By the winter of 1942 his parents, five brothers and sisters, their children – his first cousins – had all been killed. They died of starvation in Lodz, were gassed to death in the Chelmno extermination camp, killed in the Warsaw Ghetto, in Treblinka, and his brother Izaak, the communist, was killed in Russia. With some of his family my father was transferred to the Lodz Ghetto where his father died of starvation.

He was with his mother on a transport to Chelmno, escaping as they left Lodz and, returning alone, found work as a slave labourer in a metal factory whose workers were sent to Auschwitz when the ghetto was liquidated. From Auschwitz the group of metal workers were moved to the Stutthof concentration camp by the Baltic and then to Dresden, still as slave labourers, working in munitions up to and during the Allied bombings.

At the end of the war he joined the Jewish orphans gathered in Theresienstadt, from where they were flown to England. In England he was taken on as an assistant draftsman in an engineering office. He went on to study and teach architecture at the Architectural Association, London and eventually formed his own practice.

In parallel with his architectural work, my father always sketched and painted. In the 1970s, mid-career, when he was in his fifties, he quit architecture, and took six months off to work on a series of paintings, in Israel, setting down his Holocaust memories. He ran out of money, saw that he would never make a living in art in Israel and returned to the UK, using his skills in engineering and design to begin a different career designing and making the Royal Coat of Arms for the Queen, while at the same time designing and making stained glass windows. Then towards the end of his life he resumed painting, mostly small format watercolours.

As an artist his oeuvre was not large, but part of his main series of paintings was exhibited in Tate Britain, the only *Shoah* survivor artist to be exhibited there. The paintings were later acquired by the National Art Fund for the collection of the Imperial War Museum, London.

This is the thumbnail biography. Missing from it is his love of sport, swimming in particular, and skiing: his capacity to enjoy life. Also missing is his compulsive occupation with the *Shoah* that dominated the final two decades of his life. During that period he also organised, voluntarily, claims for slave labourers who had laboured under the Nazis. He came to be one of the best known voices of the *Shoah* survivors living in Britain. His autobiography, *Roman's Journey* was published in the UK by Portobello Books and was serialised on BBC radio. He was often interviewed on TV and radio, and when he died there were full-page obituaries in the major British newspapers. He was a loving, domineering, creative and attractive man.

How would you say that he influenced your working career as an artist?

AH: He regarded creativity as the apogee of human endeavour. As a child, if I wanted to take a part-time job at the weekend he would do his utmost to discourage me. My father encouraged me and my sisters' abilities in art and writing, almost bribing us to do this. When Aloma, my older sister was 11 years old and I was nine, he encouraged her to stop reading Agatha Christie and me to leave Tintin and get our teeth into Dostoyevsky and Tolstoy, Chekhov and Turgenev. And so we did. Why the Russians? Well he hadn't read the classics of English literature.

It was your father who encouraged you to paint. Can you tell me more?

AH: Yes. It was marvellous. From the age of six, he gave me watercolours, crayons and industrial paints manufactured by Bromell. Large tins, big brushes and a large tarpaulin to spread on the floor of my room so I could paint there. He bought me $6' \times 4'$ hardboard sheets and coloured tissue paper and brushes for house painting. I would paint during the weekends. He arranged for my first exhibition when I was nine years old at the Haringey Library Exhibition space, used at the time for shows by the Hornsey College of Art. I'm not sure how many great artists they produced but they were a hotbed of student demonstrations in the 1960s, with sit-ins and fervent politicking until the school was closed down. My own solo show was covered in the British and European Press, and on Pathé News (cinema). My subjects were happy. Clowns, fish, birds. A second show followed when I was 12.

Just as an aside, I've been meaning to ask you about your unusual first name.

AH: My father felt beholden to no one and, in a sense, felt he was creating his own life and could do what he wanted, so inventing a name for his son was part of that.

How old were you when you first became conscious of your father's and your mother's past?

AH: Perhaps I was first conscious of this when I went to a school friend's birthday party. I was nine or ten years old. The living room of my friend Gore (grandson, I think, of the artist Frederick Gore), near Hampstead Heath. It was jam-packed with his family . . . grandparents, uncles, aunts, cousins. I was aware how different the atmosphere in the Gore house was from ours. I had just one aunt, my mother's sister, living in North London and that was it. And I had a grandmother in Budapest, who came to England a few years later, for the last years of her life. I suddenly realised that all my uncles, aunts, grandparents and cousins on my father's side were dead. I think that I knew this, but there, at that party, the reality of it registered. It was the end of the party, we were lying down, playing 'dead lions' and I thought about all the family I did not have.

On my mother's side I had one aunt and some great-aunts, but my second cousins were from ultra-Orthodox Jewish families and they had been told by their parents that my mother was killed during the *Shoah*, for they preferred the fiction of her death to the shame of their children knowing that she did not follow in the path of Orthodox Judaism. This I only discovered many years later.

Not long after this I came upon three books in my father's workroom. They showed photos of the concentration camps. Black-and-white stark photos of gas chambers, photos of piles of emaciated bodies. I leafed through the books until I could stand it no longer, then closed them, replacing them carefully positioned as they had been on the shelf. I felt guilty looking at those books. This was not something my father had spoken about, but I *knew* that this was part of his past, part of his experience. I wondered why my father needed these books if he had been there and experienced this. Did he need to be reminded of this? Was it a form of proof? And had he left the books there in order that my sister Aloma and I would find them? Were these things to know about and not to speak of?

Round about that time he began dictating his wartime experiences to my mother and we came to hear more. Snippets of events. And then there were his friends from the *'45 Society*, orphans brought over with him to England, from Theresienstadt after the war, who stayed in touch, many of them living in London. They shared knowledge and a black humour. They seemed to *know* more than the other adults I saw around us, or those who were friends of my parents from the world of architecture or swimming.

And can you recall a day when your father sat you down to talk to you about his past?

AH: No. There was no such unlocking of a door or formal narrative – the kind one sees in filmed documentaries of survivors telling their children about their past, as though for the first time.

By the time I entered my teens, my father spoke more frequently about the *Shoah*. This increased as he penned draft after draft of his autobiography. Remember that this was the pre-computer era. And when personal computers did enter the public domain he never used one, preferring pen and ink. Both

Aloma and I read literature at Cambridge. Assuming our support, he would send us his versions to read and edit. And when I moved to Israel, and Aloma followed a year later, he continued posting us his writing and revisions, often sending the same text to both of us. It seemed that the writing of his book would never end. The subject obsessed him and he demanded our response and work on his text both as a form of filial piety and because he felt a sense of duty to those murdered. To record their names was to save them from oblivion. For him it was a responsibility. Back then there was no Holocaust Memorial Day. There was no museum dedicated to the memory of the 1.5 million Jewish children murdered during the *Shoah*. My father and I created that: *Yad LaYeled (The Children's Memorial Museum)* at the Ghetto Fighters Museum in the Western Galilee in the 1980s–1990s. The message, back then in the early 1970s, now repeated to the point of sounding hackneyed, made hollow by history and subsequent genocides, was *Never Again*. And *Remembering for the Future*. There was the belief and hope that to know would be to prevent. Following the *Shoah*, the Western world did not know about or report on further genocides. The statistics on Mao Zedong's and Stalin's vast programmes of killing were either not known or not 'credited', in part due to Western socialist and communist sympathies. And this was before the Cambodian genocide which took place between 1975 and 1979, the Rwandan genocide of 1994, Kosovo in 1998, and Darfur since 2003.

And I shared my father's belief that it would be possible to teach and to prevent. If a student's mind were taught, made aware of the poison of racist incitement then, we thought, both my father and I, that this would plant a seed, help the person to recognise racism for what it is. The individual might act differently when the time came. I believed and still believe in education: it is surely what can help us to make the right decision when confronting a fork on the path of our lives. This was something my father and I discussed at length. I wrote a charter for *Yad LaYeled* distilling my ideas succinctly, defining the educational function and purpose of a centre commemorating genocide.

My father also wanted us to share his memories and take on the responsibility of memory of the *Shoah*. And when it came to the subject of the *Shoah*, it could not wait. Nothing was more important to him. He demanded immediate attention to his manuscript. Sensing the great pain deep within him, his ever-present trauma, my sisters and I, in some strange measure, as so many children of survivors, assumed the role of our parents' parents, or guardians. We, as the next generation, were replacements for the murdered generations.

Paradoxically, while speaking with increasing regularity about the *Shoah*, my father would always vocalise how wonderful life was. The 1960s and 1970s in England, the time of my childhood and adolescence, the secure post-war society was characterised by the pleasures of peace. My father wanted me to recognise (constantly) how marvellous our adolescence was, compared to his, and to savour it. He would say that a lovely morning, a calm and beautiful sea, an enjoyable event were a *Mechaya* (literally 'a reviving' or 'life-giving' event – certainly a replenishing and enhancing one). The word was spoken from the soul, with enormous, disproportionate joy, whose proportion by inference bore with it consciousness of the torment of the years he had faced between the ages of 12 and 18 in the Lodz Ghetto, Auschwitz, Stutthof and Dresden. Any difficulties of the growing child were seen as non-existent when compared with the horrors experienced by my father, and so growing up I truly thought that I could have none, because everything was compared to life and death, suffering and murder, starvation and genocide.

The enduring effect this has had on me is that I find that I measure the happiest moments of life against the nadirs of human experience. In the same way, at the end of a Jewish wedding ceremony, under the *Huppa* (the wedding canopy) the glass is stamped on by the bridegroom, in memory of the destruction of the Temple.

So I grew up with, perhaps, an exaggerated version of the adolescent's dilemma: respect your parents, care for them, and at the same time, leave home, break away. Only here I felt that I needed also to support my father and accept a baton he wanted to pass to me. In addition to this, while pursuing my career as an artist I tried to ignore the fact that this was what my father originally willed me to do. During my childhood his over-encouragement could be intrusive. I remember him sometimes wanting to do my homework. This might seem a blessing to most schoolchildren. But he wanted to do this because he had not been to a good school, and his own schooling at that age was in concentration and slave-labour camps. He craved what he had missed out on.

For all this, you should not get an impression that he was emotionally clinging. He encouraged me to travel, on my own. It was safe to travel in the 1960s and early 1970s. And I did – in Europe, Israel, Canada, the USA, Mexico and later in Iran and Afghanistan. There was no Internet and my parents did not expect phone calls. When away for three months between school and university, once every fortnight I might reverse the charges through the operator who would ask my parents if they would accept the charges of a call from, say, Vancouver, Flagstaff, Knoxville. They would reply: *No*. And before the operator cut off the call I might hear my mother or father say *He's in Flagstaff*. They never accepted the call. I really do not think that they worried about me. (No GPS or email/Skype or a WhatsApp umbilical cord that characterises the connection between children travelling today and their parents.)

Yet after university I left home and England. But not to get away from my parents. I moved to Israel to establish my home and work there. Despite this, or perhaps in order to remain in contact, I worked with my father on a few projects, whilst pursuing my own career in painting and printmaking. The only constant invasion on my space came in the form of his manuscript, penned and revised, endlessly revised over a number of years that demanded filial attention, not just for my father's sake but, implicitly, for that of our murdered family.

Eventually, thankfully, my sister, Aloma took his manuscript in hand and edited the unwieldy thousand pages into the published book. This sealed the process. We would receive no more scripted versions of the manuscript. And both she and I made clear that we would edit no more of his writing. But that was in 2006.

Having moved away from home I painted a large series of oil paintings titled *The Family I Never Knew*. It is about the limits to the sympathetic imagination, about what I feel someone born to a survivor, after the *Shoah*, can truly say. Visually I make the point that my father's experience is not my own, that while relating to the subject I am not claiming that experience as my own. The paintings are about distance and about the context of incitement, and also about tolerance.

Tell me a bit about your mother

AH: My father never really considered my mother to be a survivor because she escaped from the march out of Budapest to the trains in 1944, the trains that led her friends to their deaths in Auschwitz. She sensed that she and her school friends would never return from wherever they were being taken. And with pluck and timing, she managed to escape and returned to the city, surviving the period until the Soviet invasion. Because she had never been in the concentration camps and because almost all her aunts, uncles and cousins survived, my father dismissed her wartime experiences, belittling her experience, certainly giving it no space for expression. And she did not like to dwell on the war or talk to me about it, though she had lived through danger and witnessed death and humiliations. She preferred to accentuate the positive and loved to live in the present.

Physicality and sport were central to both my parents and to my childhood. Susan (née Nador) my mother was an Olympic swimmer, representing Hungary in the 1948 London games, and representing Great Britain thereafter. My father achieved minor success in swimming, mainly in lock-to-lock distance races in the Thames, and he also played water polo. Both my parents celebrated my successes in swimming, taking me training before school in the morning. When I won first place in the British national age-group competitions, my success served as a vicarious reflection of my parents' self-image.

My mother trained me till I was 12 years old. Her methods, 20 years out of date, were the same as those of Saroszi, the legendary Hungarian coach, who had been her coach in 1946–1947. I did not realise my full potential, though I enjoyed the fellowship of her company.

And when did your father begin to talk to you about his past? And your mother about hers?

AH: There was no continuous narrative, just the occasional vignette. Somehow these must have influenced me because when I was 12 years old I participated in a painting competition organised, by the *Jewish Chronicle*, the only Jewish newspaper at the time in the UK, titled 'Our Ghetto Heritage' – I could not relate to the ghetto in the sense of the Jewish *shtetl*, but to concentration camps. Besides which I knew very little of Eastern European Jewish history and what I had seen of it in the work of Marc Chagall struck me as sentimental and self-indulgent.

I painted two *katzetniks*[1] behind barbed wire. I won first prize. And when my parents took friends upstairs to the loft studio in the house to view my painting, I felt deceitful, for I had painted something I had not actually witnessed myself. It was as though I imagined I could imagine that. I knew, deep down, that this feeling and my painting were false. I had adopted an experience as though it was my own. The key point being a lack of self-scrutiny and humility.

What would you say is the nature of the shadow of your father on your life?

AH: Shadow or illumination, or perhaps both. We do not live our parents' lives. We live our own. We carry our parents' and grandparents' genes. They influence our make-up, but they don't determine our actions, our achievements, our goals and our thoughts. Or only insofar as we allow them to. The present is grounded in the past. Some events in history and some individuals affect the course of the future well beyond their own lifetime, creatively or negatively.

My father was a larger-than-life person. I don't feel his life shadowed or shadows mine nor, when I work, do I think of his style of work or of his life. But the past is with us. Our parents, when they have died, live in our minds and memories. Picasso liked to spread the story that when he was 12 his father gave him, the precocious genius, his brushes and paints, as though resigning, emasculating himself. For Picasso to enjoy creative *Lebensraum* he had to destroy his father as an artist.

I have made a life in art, which is what my father truly wanted to do for himself, but only did for certain periods of his own life. I do feel a strong sense of gratitude to my parents for their support and for the wonderful childhood I enjoyed. They are now dead. I think of them both. Perhaps now I think more about my mother who even more than my father had a great capacity, a talent, for living in the present, savouring each day as a gift. Swimming, sketching, visiting museums, enjoying the company of friends, she was extraordinarily positive. During their lives, when I would be with them, my father dominated. But my mother's life was remarkable, and perhaps most remarkable of all was the way she crafted her end. For when she knew that her death was close, when she knew that her illness was terminal, she welcomed her death, opened her hands, palm upwards, refused any morphine, let go of life. Her soul departed her body a full day and half before she died. I was there. I witnessed this. It was like when you park your car, walk away and still hear the engine ticking over, the fan belt cooling the motor. She was not there, but the mechanical sound of her breath still went on. Yet she was gone. I felt that she had gone. The body was there but the room was empty. For the first time I came to actually understand the meaning of the word 'soul'. She accepted death. It was an extraordinarily graceful ending: a lesson, an illumination.

My father, by contrast, struggled to the last, gripping on to life, saying *there is nothing but life*. He was a very creative man, but I do not think it unfair to say that his greatest creation was his own persona. Anyone who met him felt that – his blue eyes boring into you like gimlets.

He was hounded by the trauma of his past. The older he grew, the more his past dominated him. Day and night, nightmares and visions of the past were there with him. In his final decade, the terrible things he had witnessed were there before him, they seemed to him more real than the present. And because he spent much of his final two decades painting, writing about and talking about his past, it came to dominate his life. Almost everything he read related to the Second World War. It was as though he was trying to find a rational explanation for the trauma he experienced.

The narrative of our family's past is compelling, but for me it is part of an even broader message. One-third of the Jewish people were murdered during the Second World War. It is true that had Hitler and Nazi Germany had their way then every Jew on the planet would have been exterminated. As a Jew this is something sobering to remember, commemorate and teach. Yet the broader message and lesson I have taken from this is that in all human society, and perhaps it is in our DNA, there is the capacity for prejudice, incitement, discrimination, violence and, yes, even genocide. Learn, teach, remember, all in order to prevent.

This is why in 2003, when my father and I were commissioned to create stained glass windows for the National Genocide Memorial in Rwanda I said *Yes. I want to be associated with this project*. The organisers had seen *Yad LaYeled*, the memorial centre my father and I had planned in the north of Israel. They loved our concept of commemorating the creativity of the children's lives, rather than dwelling on the murderous ways in which those lives were taken. This was expressed in the stained glass windows we had made there, based on the children's drawings from Theresienstadt.

I was, however, surprised by my father's response. He told me he was not interested. Why? Perhaps because he had suffered his quantum of pain during the *Shoah*, could not feel beyond his own trauma, and did not have space in his mind or emotions to commemorate another people's genocide. I tried to reason with him: *If* ***we*** *do not care, you a survivor and me the next generation, then who will care? If we Jews do not show understanding of the genocide of 1994 in Rwanda, then who should?* But he was not interested. He told me: *I am having nothing whatsoever to do with this project*. My repeated attempts at persuasion met with the same stony reply – *I am having nothing to do with this project*.

I went on to design and make the two large stained glass windows alone. One was called *Descent to Genocide*, full of downward motion, dark blues and greys and deep scarlet all thrashing down, like machetes towards skulls heaped to one side at the base of steps whose passage is barred by instruments of slaughter. The second window is called *The Way Forward* and shows the same staircase but with the skulls at the centre base and two swirling forms motioning the eye up the steps, whose passage is open, towards a sky that is lighter and bears promise. The simple message in this window is that perpetrator and victim need to recognise the reality of the incitement and the genocide if there is to be any chance of future coexistence. I worked intensively on these two windows for the better part of five months. Completed, I installed them in Rwanda and attended the opening of the Genocide Memorial Centre in April 2004.

After my father died in 2012. I organised a retrospective exhibition of his paintings with the Ben Uri Gallery in London, and a book accompanying it, focusing on his career. Almost immediately after that, my sister Aviva and I chanced to discover a number of effusive letters, one from the head of an Oxford College, another from the Emeritus Chief Rabbi, the Lord Sacks,[2] thanking my father for his letter in which he had informed them of the windows *he* had made in Rwanda and congratulating him on his work. How laudable, they wrote, for a survivor that he should embrace the pain of another people and empathise with them. And how good that he engaged his son to help him on this project! I was dumbfounded. Amazed. Struck between the eyes. Having told me that he'd have nothing to do with the project, here he was taking full credit for something he had opposed and in which he had done nothing.

Now *this* is indeed a shadow, or perhaps a barb, one that has remained. Let's assume that you have written a book, laboured long at it. It is published and you discover that your father's name has usurped yours on the cover. How do you deal with such knowledge? Now consider also that my father was dead and that whatever I would now say would make me appear like some ungrateful revisionist, seeking to take advantage of the fact that my father was not around to respond. The bizarre truth was that while I was working on the windows, my father was writing to everyone he knew, telling them that he was doing this, with a bit of assistance from me.

All I can say is that somewhere he mixed jealousy with pride and emerged with his own proprietary solution.

How would you characterise the two of you as artists – the similarities and the differences?

AH: He was an extrovert and also very charming. I have always been suspicious of artists who dress and look like artists, conforming to the stereotypical image of artists, but I do not think this is because of him. I dislike the Bohemian show. Eliot wrote that poetry is a desk job, and he was a banker. Henry James looked like a banker. Georges Rouault looked like a cross between a baker and priest. Matisse looked like a lawyer, Braque like a blue-collar worker.

My father liked to be thought of as an artist. He wore a Basque beret, but perhaps this was simply to keep his head warm.

My father liked to work with other craftsmen. Perhaps this was why he chose architecture as his first profession and why there were relatively few periods in his life when he painted, in his studio, alone. He liked the interaction with clients and craftsmen when making stained glass windows or the Royal Coat of Arms.

I, on the other hand, am used to working alone. And when I need company I sketch from life. I am fascinated by the presence of a person sitting to be drawn. My father did not draw from life. He actually liked to sit for me to draw him and I did so on several occasions, also painting his portrait twice, once after I had painted Henry Moore; liking the work, he said he was willing to sit for a portrait on a similar scale. And when he was dying and did not wish to talk, he was happy for me to draw him. In hospital I sketched him once each week during the final six weeks of his life.

Is the theme of parents and children present – overtly or in more representative forms – in any of your respective pieces of art? If so, could I ask you to describe and comment on these pieces of art?

AH: My father drew his own parents, from memory twice, as though conjuring them from oblivion. The works are expressionistic and express pain. He was closer to his maternal grandfather than he was to his own father and so his grandfather appears more in his work.

My own paintings do not focus on my parents, apart from the actual drawings/paintings I made of them when they sat for me. My subjects are water, people, the passage of time, existential threat, environmental change and the complexity of human experience, expressed recently in a series of paintings titled *Concordance*.

Are there pieces that you or your father have made, separately or together, that you feel in some ways represent your relationship with one another? By the way, how did the two of you experience working together?

AH: It is possible to enter the mind-set of another artist, rather in the way a translator enters the mind of a writer. It is also possible for artists to share the same atelier, as least for a period, either when one is learning from the other, for example, technique. Or two artists may share the same studio when their explorations converge, as did Braque and Picasso for a year or so. But in my experience, it is almost impossible for two artists to design a single work.

I recall one commission, for a stained glass window for the *Beit Midrash* (Study Hall) of the St John's Wood Synagogue in London. My father and I were commissioned to present designs. *Which of us should design the window?* I asked. My father said that we should both submit designs and whoever did not win would support the other, working as assistant to him. I sensed that this sounded more egalitarian than realistic. I felt uneasy as to the practicality, but agreed.

The client selected my design. I enlarged it (the window measured over 3 × 2 metres in size) and consulted with the head of the foundry to check my design was technically feasible, that the filigree was not too thin in places for the metal to flow during casting – as my father and I worked in cast metal, bronze or aluminium rather than with traditional lead cames. Seeing my enlarged design, my father derided it, adding that technically it would not work because the metal would not be able to flow, some of the divisions being too thin. So I worked on the project alone, but because we had both been commissioned, I put his initials besides my own at the base of the window.

I regretted that he would not work with me, in the way he himself had suggested from the start. I resolved to try and avoid such situations in the future. We did not work together again and I think it was for the best. If you have a vision for a piece of art, it is hard to compromise on colour or allow another's sensibility to direct the work, you have to be faithful to your inner voice and trust your own judgement.

Stylistically, did your father influence you as an artist?

AH: Not really. The light of the great artists of the past illuminates artists working in the present. Nothing is born of a vacuum. The influences of art or literature are not genetic. Growing up in London I was exposed, as would any artist growing up in the metropolis, to the riches of the great museums and galleries.

Philip Roth spoke a harsh truism when he said: "a writer should write as though his parents are dead". Creativity should be free of considerations of kin, embarrassment or filial responsibility, unless, that is, the artist or writer chooses these as his subject. And perhaps then the artist should strive all the more to ignore the trammels of those considerations.

Ardyn, I wonder if you might comment on how it has felt for you to answer these questions that have largely centred around your father and your relationship with him.

AH: Since my father died in 2012 I have sought to perpetuate his memory, for example, in an exhibition, and by collaborating with the BBC's Fergal Keane and Fred Scott in a film they have made about him. So I am comfortable talking or writing about him. I do not feel that your questions have picked raw scars. These are things I have thought about. The dead live with us.

Notes

* Ardyn Halter is the artist of the book's front cover, *Vault* (oil on canvas).

1 KZ (pronounced 'Ka-Tzet') is the German acronym for Konzentrationslager (concentration camp). In camp slang, a Ka-Tzetnik is a prisoner.

2 Rabbi Dr Jonathan Sacks served as the Chief Rabbi of the United Hebrew Congregations of the Commonwealth from 1991 to 2013.

Chapter 14

Paddle your own canoe

Negotiating the shadows

Jane McAdam Freud

Our final chapter begins with an overview of an unusual sort. Indeed we wrap up our book with a paper that in some ways flies in the face of our earlier papers – one that is without doubt as unique as its author and her art.

"'If it ain't broke, don't fix it!' and other hackneyed phrases come to mind when I think of myself in the shadow of my father, Lucian Freud, and also perhaps of my great-grandfather, Sigmund Freud," writes our author. "One precious phrase though, and one that greatly influenced me came via my mother: 'Paddle your own canoe, Jane'".

Please note*: All images presented in this chapter show sculpture and artworks conceived and made by the contemporary artist Jane McAdam Freud.*

As all children do, I would ask my mother many questions but for one type of question her strange metaphoric answers ring clear – like a bell that never stops chiming.

Within my mother's responses: 'mind your own business' and 'paddle your own canoe', there was an instructional element: to do *my own thing* and *go on* even against the odds – but certainly to do it on my own terms. In my interpretation the meaning was approximately "Do something you might throw yourself into and everyone else will mind *their* own business".

Unlike so many others I knew, I always associated art with something that might save one from the judgement of another and from society's projections. It was my mother who directed me to make my own way, without recourse or reference to my father. This excellent advice allowed me to strive for recognition in my own right.

In point of fact, seeing myself in the shadows was a later consideration for me as, up until my thirties I always worked under my mother's name, McAdam, with no recourse to my father and great-grandfather. So thankfully, having my work acquired by the British Museum at aged 21 in the name Jane McAdam, I experienced personal success without the connotation. To 'come out' as a relative of Freud, in public, in my thirties, was quite bizarre for me yet, looking back it seems no surprise that then and still now I work with the subject of identity. Though

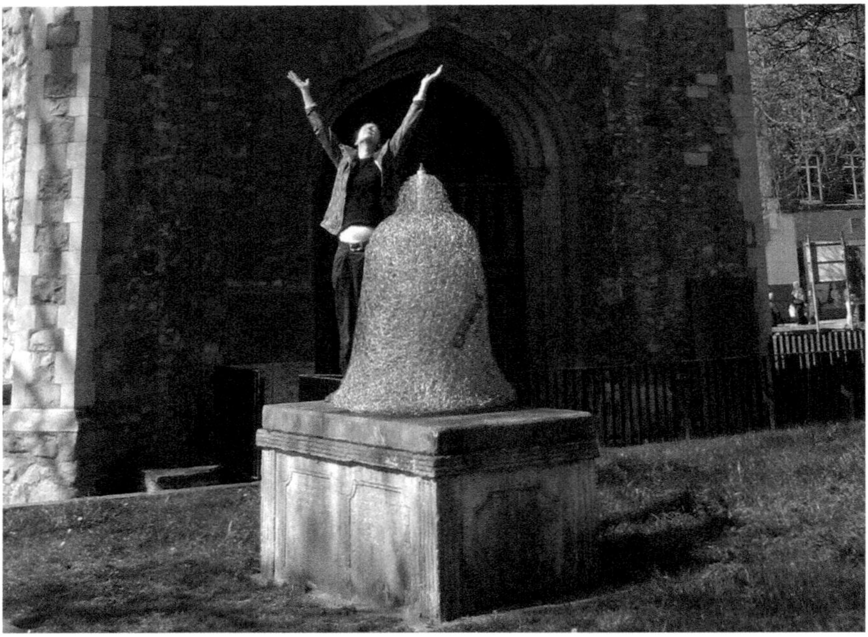

Figure 14.1 *Ding Dong*, 2015, Galvanised steel netting and found objects, 132 cm H × 97 cm D

life seems to speed up as I get older, still the very thought of working *under the shadow* feels relatively new to me. After all, even now at the age of 59, I have lived for more than half my life without the Freud 'label'.

To clarify: in 1990, aged 32, as Jane McAdam, I was invited to receive the 'Freedom of the City of London' on merit for my contribution to the public collections of works housed at institutions in the city, including the British Museum and the Worshipful Company of Goldsmiths. It was only in the preparations for this ceremony that my relationship to Freud(s) was discovered. Along with swearing allegiance to the Queen, I was compelled to provide my full birth certificate as part of the ritual of accepting this ancient honorary decree.

What might we mean by 'succeeding the shadow'? I would use this term to imply 'knowing' success in one's own right. Success is difficult to define. If feedback is *always* in relation to the 'shadower', one can understand this as negating or invalidating for the 'shadowed'. By this, I echo Martin Freud's point (shared by Jonathan Burke in his preface) that if all the attention on the subject is only by way of referencing his or her predecessor then it might well have a negating effect on any personal triumphs that the subject may achieve.

In contrast to this, however, I would consider my own situation to be a curious case of a *reversal* of events. I experienced coveted museum acquisitions of my works early in my career before taking on the Freud mantle. In fact while I longed to be 'seen' publicly, for who I really was, that is my father's daughter (almost seeking the shadow), this only happened (as far as the projected view is concerned) *after* I had already celebrated success in my own right. So I wasn't adversely affected in the way I may have been. One might put this down to my expectation through the examples I had experienced. I brought my perceived information of events to my expectation of 'what I believed to be a predictive truth' as in Helmholtz cognitive illusions. So it could be that I applied 'unconscious inference' not in terms of visual perception but as related to experiential stimuli. I witnessed (by association) several examples of success in the face of shadow figures. It could be said that I unconsciously expected to succeed in the face of the oppressive Fathers (including the cultural fathers).

Both precedents and names, of course, affect us all on some level and I think I was primed to look out for them and their consequences while growing up. What I noticed became my instruction, furthermore my norm. I find it fascinating that my father's great friend (at one time) was Francis Bacon. Interestingly when I was very young and one referred to Frances Bacon it was not the artist they intended but the great philosopher, statesman and scientist. Now we immediately think of the painter Frances Bacon rather than the father of empiricism and the scientific method. What must it have been like for the painter following in this namesake? Could this predecessor namesake have operated as both shadow and instructor to the young Frances? And what were his parents thinking?

Beyond succeeding the parental figures, the concept of *succeeding the shadow* is embedded in Western culture. An example from nineteenth-century art relates to the French sculptor Auguste Rodin (1840–1917) who asked the protégé sculptor Constantin Brancusi to work in his studio. After one month Brancusi declared with implicit knowledge: "young shoots cannot flourish under the shadow of great trees". I will come back to this point later in reference to my father succeeding my great-grandfather. After all, in hearing the name without context, one might *also* wonder to which *Freud* reference is being made, both being equally distinguished in their respective fields.

'Shadow' as a general concept relating to the object's cast also serves to describe the unconscious aspect of the personality in Jungian terms. Sculpturally speaking, an object in a certain light, throws a shadow. In a physical sense, the larger the object the greater the shadow cast. For the psychological characterisation of the shadow we might look to Jung who understood the merit of the 'shadow side' and its important role in balancing the psyche in the interest of promoting personal growth. "Everyone carries a shadow and the less it is embodied in the individual's conscious life, the blacker and denser it is". We might read this sentence by Jung (1940) to indicate that awareness is freedom.

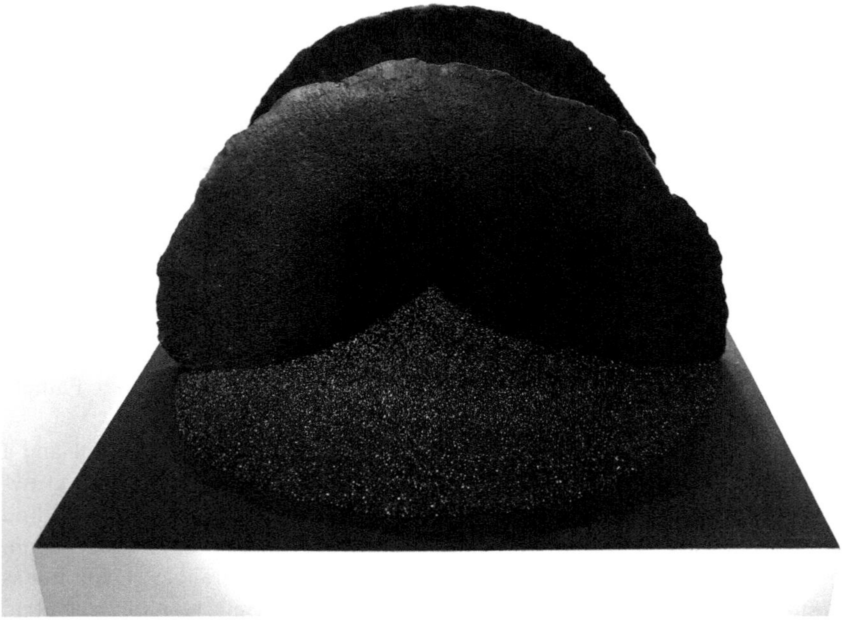

Figure 14.2 Hidden Light, 2010, painted stoneware and grit, 23 cm H × 76 cm W × 46 cm D

Recalling my works from the early 1990s when my productive period really started, I note that this productivity coincided with me embracing my shadow side – the Freud side. I found freedom and focus within my practice and I began to trust my instincts, allowing them to *drive* me. I look at how I chose somehow *to embody* these shadows in what was, and still is, an absorbing and creative experience. I will look at the factors that had an impact on my situation and the relevant aspects that helped me to operate, against the odds. The factors for deliberation include early experience and predilection, individuation, sublimation, relationship with immediate family and female experience. Finally I will look at the important relationship I had with my paternal grandmother.

Early experience

At a very early age I had a sort of epiphany and it was in the sandpit. So my first sculptural experiences came at nursery school, with the feel of water, sand and chocolate powder. These are my strongest memories of early childhood, and I see them as the forerunner experiences to making sculpture. I would have been around three or four years old. I still recall that powerful sensory impression that transported me, creating its own sense of meaning.

The reason I make sculpture is because it is my nature, my nurture, my oxygen. It started on the breast and then in the sandpit and the sensory appreciation developed through feeling my mother's materials – the silk, the satin and taffeta she worked with.

Making sculpture completely absorbs me. It is as though the process neutralises all conflicts. But more than this, the creative act (sculpture) is *my religion*. It gives me that quiet spiritual feeling that others might get in a church, synagogue, temple or mosque. In this sense I am a great *believer* in art. It gives me that feeling I desire – of being at one with the world and doing exactly what I am meant to be doing.

Creating meaning through making sculpture was, and still is, a sort of saviour – a saviour from boredom, from the mundane and, in the end, from the fear of obscurity in death. My desire, *an ancestral instruction* perhaps, is for my works to SPEAK. I say this in regard to Sigmund Freud and his exclamation about his beloved antiquities – 'Stone Speak'.

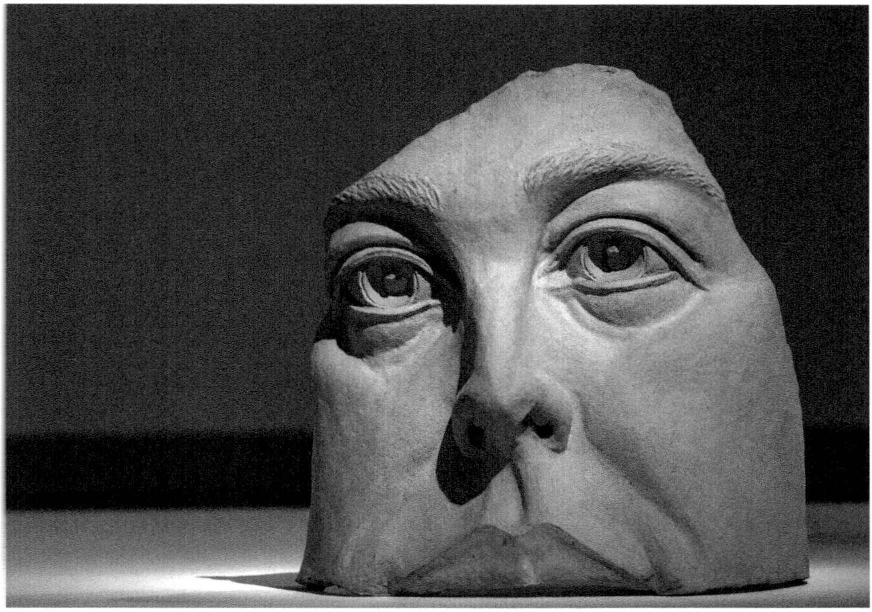

Figure 14.3 Stone Speak, 2010, stoneware, 76 cm H × 69.5 cm W × 50 cm D

Sublimation

In hindsight, I realise I have channelled my feelings through my works. In the early 1990s, my works were concerned with "the flattening of objects via random acts of crushing".

Perhaps the significance for me was that I was symbolically dealing with these potentially 'crushing' shadows by channelling formerly repressed feelings which contained the sensation of not being whole, that is missing the presence and authority of my father. The metaphors became my medium and I created conundrums, convergences and new meaning through art.

I first began exploring the relief form in 1980 with my Picasso medal, a decade later developing the series *Sculpture – On the Edge* based on crushed found objects.

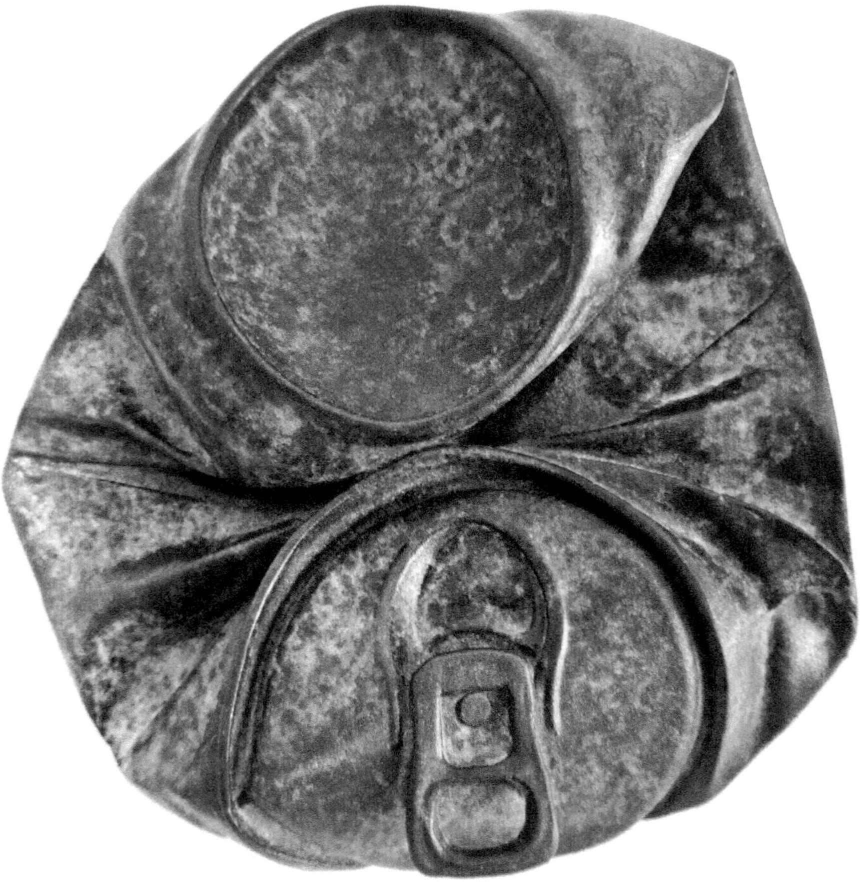

Figure 14.4 Decoration of the Rim, 1995, patinated bronze, 10 cm Di × 2 cm D

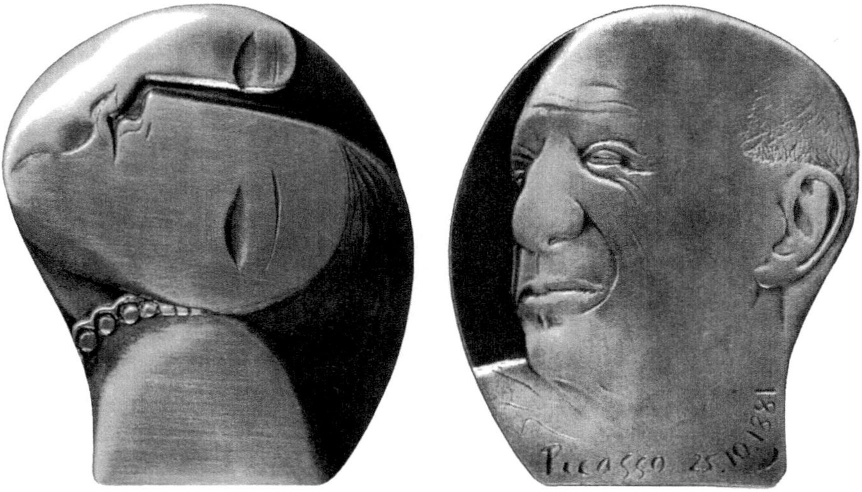

Figure 14.5 Picasso (obverse and reverse), 1980, bronze, 9 cm H × 7 cm W × 0.5 cm D

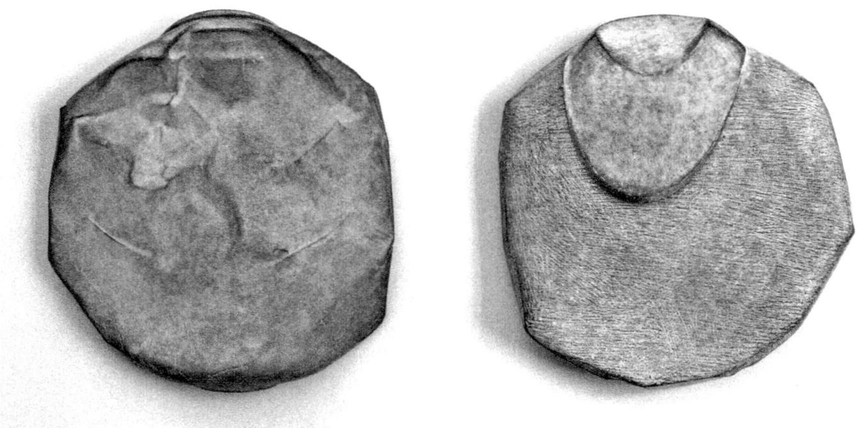

Figure 14.6 Rim as Motif (obverse and reverse), 1995, patinated bronze, 10 cm H × 9 cm W × 1 cm D

These developed into modelled works involving compression of the human figure with the series *After Bacon*.

I think that my past and its unpicking have shaped my creativity. These works and their processes all seem very symbolic – in hindsight; but at the time of the sculpture's inception I worked with unknown instincts and only a drive to look for form and poetry via objects and subjects.

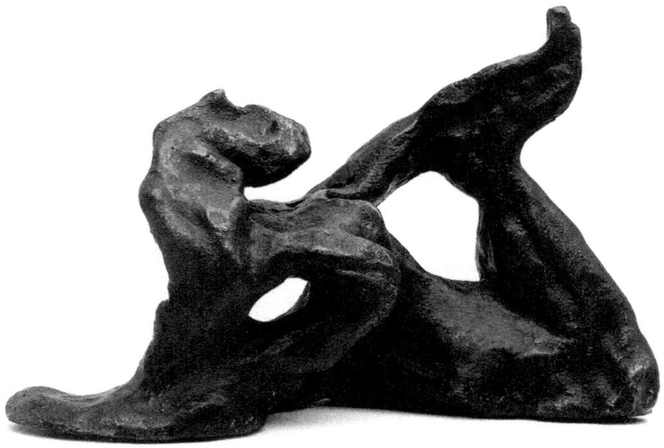

Figure 14.7 After Bacon, 1992, bronze, 17 cm H × 16 cm W × 10 cm D

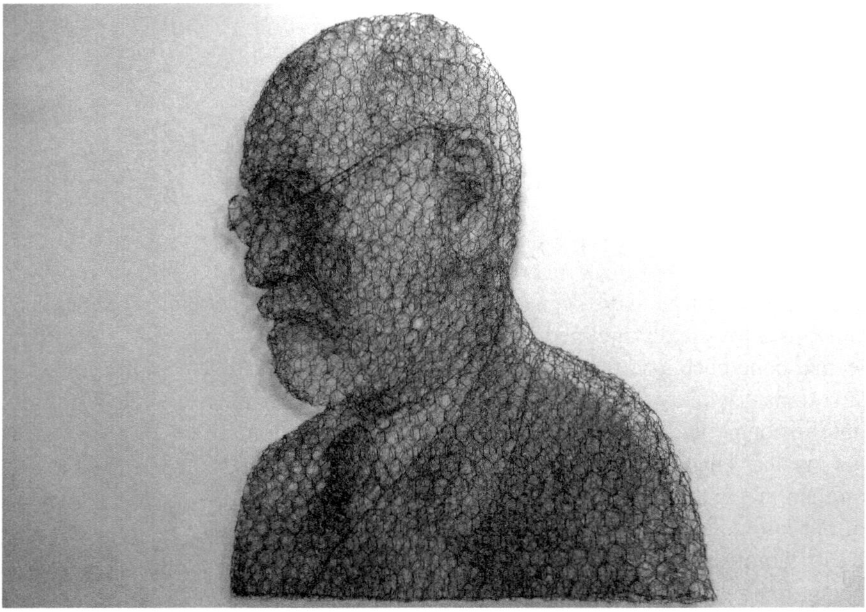

Figure 14.8 Are you ready for me now?, 2014, galvanised steel netting, 107 cm H × 92 cm W × 2 cm D

I note that often I prefer a dimmer light to both produce and display my wire-mesh relief portraits and they work best when viewed in this low light.

I function well in the shadow and several works function well in the dark. I note also that they function very well too, when seen obliquely. By this I mean that the

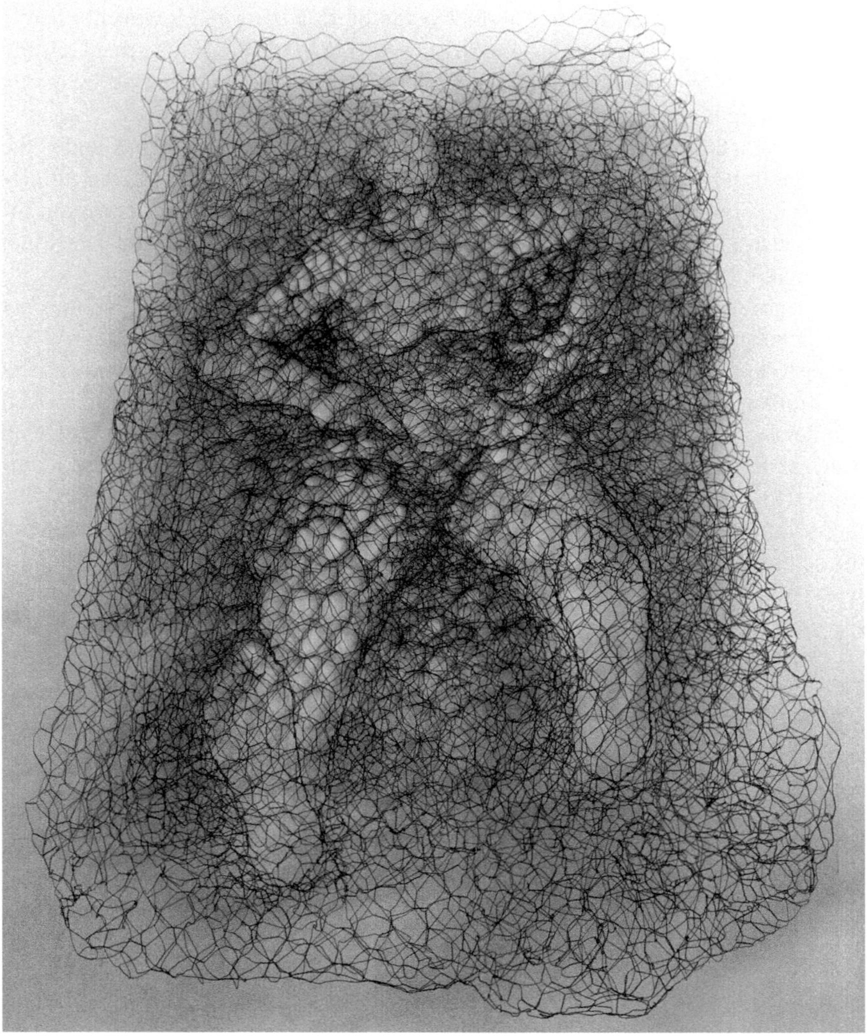

Figure 14.9 Foreshortened, 2017, rusted steel netting, 170 cm H × 136 cm W × 2 cm D

images contained in the works are seen most clearly in a dim light when one is standing at an angle to the work, that is not directly in front of it. The dimmer the light the more three-dimensional these large relief works become, with the figures emerging in the foreground. The works take on their correct perspective with the foreshortened limbs projecting and the dark background disappearing.

It seems I have channelled my 'shadow affects' into 'creative process' by turning what could be a hindrance into a helper by working with it to re-appropriate the disavowed shadow, treating it as a virtue by indulging it. However, where I can see clearly that I did 'suffer' the shadow was in the 1980s. I note that I simply took my early successes for granted rather than seeing being collected by museums as something to celebrate.

I make sculpture and my father made paintings. They both come under the same umbrella of fine art. However, I think I chose sculpture as I had an affinity for the tactile from the very beginning. But I believe there is a further reason for my choice. I think it was their choice. By 'their' I intend the forebears. I feel that I am making sculpture on behalf of *them*.

My mother, father *and* also my great-grandfather loved sculpture. My mother and father each told me that "sculpture was their first choice of medium". My father told me it would have been too difficult to succeed in his *first* choice, and my mother said she had to think of the practicalities of making a living. And I understand Sigmund Freud as a sort of 'shadow' sculptor, one who collected rather than made sculpture but who placed his collected works in the way a conceptual sculptor might do today. He symbolically placed his antiquities on his mantel and on his desk, with the bear in the west and the monkey in the east, with the central part reserved for Athena symbolising the classical world and the cyclic wars (of which he was so nearly a victim).[1] Sigmund Freud collected sculpture (in the form of his antiquities) and I make sculpture.

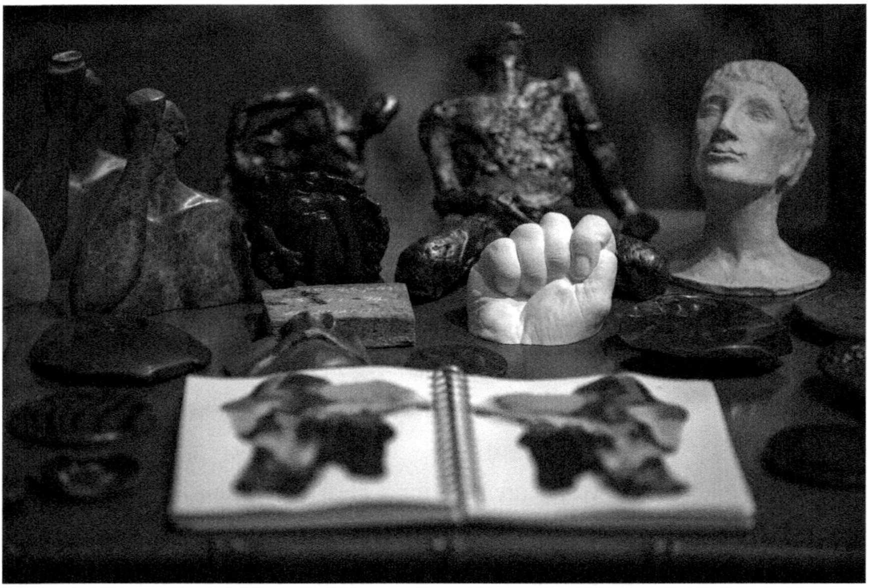

Figure 14.10 Freud Study Merge-Desk, 2015, materials: various, size: variable

During my residency at the Freud Museum in 2005–2006 I learnt to appreciate that we had a parallel sensibility and a mutual receptivity to sculpture. However, despite the near misses with sculpture in the lives of Sigmund and my parents, my immersion in the concerns of sculpture seems so separate from them, something so totally mine – and timeless in terms of when my relationship with materials began. It was always there: from the sandpit to the silk and satin of my mother's creations and the sensory beyond.

Mother

My mother, being the dominant parent, was my main influence. I think my story gets mixed up with hers in the way all our stories are mixed up with their stories because we are so much the product of our parents.

According to the retorts of my siblings, it seems that I was my mother's favourite or at least the one she watched most closely and for whom she seemed to have more time when I was a child. Added to this I became the surrogate daughter of my aunt, my mother's sister. She lived with us for quite some time. I think in my mother's case this favouritism was perhaps because she was a very practical person and I was the first, so it was prescient for me to lead the way. I was her instructor, in terms of what was to come. I was also quite merged with her emotionally. This of course was not always easy for my mother or my siblings but at least the turbulence resulted in individuation. I broke the ties and fought for my independence. Perhaps it was this inner battle (with myself as much as anything else) for that independence that left me feeling liberated.

Regarding his *sure* status as the favoured one, Sigmund Freud notes: "When you were incontestably the favorite child of your mother, you keep during your lifetime this victor feeling, you keep feeling sure of success, which in reality seldom doesn't fulfill".[2] However, I do think it interesting that Freud's sentence contains this pairing of negatives. So instead of 'often fulfills' he says 'seldom doesn't fulfill'! It leaves me feeling curious. Is this pairing of negatives (a positive?) intentional, unconscious or a glitch in the translation? Ideas to explore for another paper perhaps – although I think it relevant here that there is a sort of negative–positive conundrum going on in the battle to save yourself from yourself in terms of being merged with the mother who is both your nurturer and your nemesis! It is a battle against oneself of sorts. We are part of the mother after all. We were *her* once.

I am the eldest of my mother and father's four children. Interestingly, my three siblings, although working happily for many years in other careers, have latterly turned towards painting. I used to wonder if I was making art on their behalf, so that they were in a way freed from the need. However, perhaps my father's death allowed them the space to pursue it or maybe gave them a reason.

Another difference between my siblings and me is that they didn't rebel as teenagers. I always think that my own teenage rebellion was against my mother or at least against turning into her. On the other hand I strove to succeed on her behalf

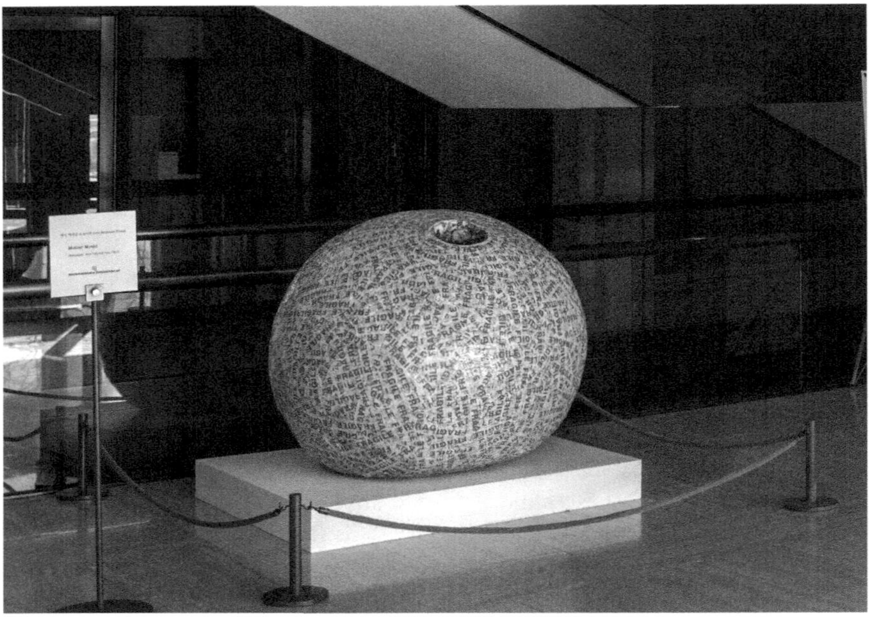

Figure 14.11 *Mother Mould*, 2015, newspaper, tape, 107.7 cm D

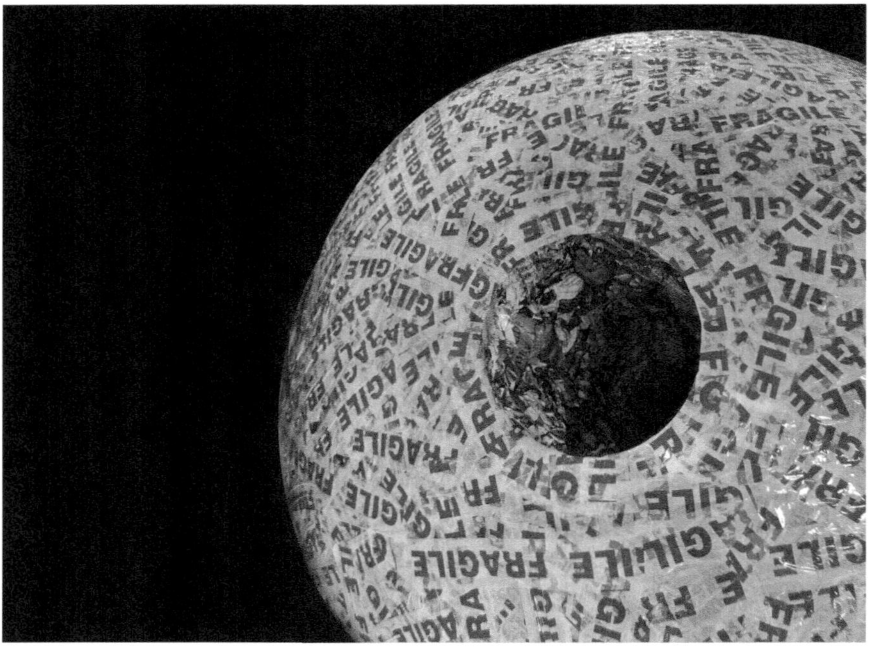

Figure 14.12 *Mother Mould detail,* 2015, newspaper, tape, 107.7 cm D

because she didn't get to indulge her own great talent and as a child I greatly admired her work. Instead she had children.

My mother studied fine art for two years at St Martin's School of Art, followed by fashion for a further two years. To go to art school was a rare thing at that time for a 'convent' boarding school girl. While we were young she worked as an art teacher and in fashion houses, although these were just jobs to assist in her main, all-consuming job as a mother.

Just as likely, my determination was *despite* her, as in reality there were rarely any clear instructions to rebel against (although these instructions are often so subtle as to be imperceptible to 'reasoned thought'). These feelings are of course ambivalent. Might my early drive and ambition be just as easily interpreted as acts of defiance, perhaps against her seemingly laissez-faire attitude?

My mother didn't have strict rules, and her answers to my many questions were always cryptic and abstract, leaving me with the sense that some things are unknowable. Even *this* though was subsumed into art. Asking unanswerable questions, not coming down on either side is the artist's way. Not to judge but to observe; avoidance of the didactic and embracing the philosophical. These were early introductions by my mother who related to me in this way; and her way, *by default*, became my way.

At the time, of course I found my mother's 'way' infuriating and so I was often defiant. But everything has its counter-balance, and it was perhaps helpful on another level, as in the arts one needs to be driven by having something to say. It doesn't matter if it is a thought-out thing or simply propulsion in defiance? This is quite evident in Sigmund Freud's 'victory dream'. As a boy of eight, Freud intentionally urinated in his parents' bedroom and was dismissed by his father who said, "Nothing will come of this boy!" Freud said that this comment should have deeply afflicted him. He wrote, "in my dreams the scene often repeated, always accompanied by an enumeration of my works and successes, as if I intended to say: 'You see, nevertheless I became somebody!'"[3]

Gender

One's expectations and even drives may differ in relation to one's gender. For example, being a daughter with male shadows will not bring the same things to bear as being a *son* with male shadows or, indeed, a daughter with female shadows. The identification *shifts* may be enough to save one.

Of course for my mother and perhaps, more generally, for women in the West today, the expectation and research indicates that we are not as dependent as men on work-related successes to satisfy our ego needs. There are, of course, gender differences in regard to 'ego needs'. Might it be said that the male superego drives the competition between men, between father and son and that this has continued symbolically, metaphorically or otherwise, from biblical times through to today.

Whether I identify more readily with my mother than my father (though I cannot say that this is the case), succeeding my mother might well be empowering enough for me. Or at the very least a satisfying substitute. So as a female with a mother who also trained as an artist but who didn't pursue her art career in the way she wanted, I have perhaps succeeded *her* in at least doing that. In fact, I do have a powerful memory of opening the acceptance letter and celebrating my entry into art school, by jumping on her back! – a symbolic act indicating that first step perhaps?

Within the *gender* context there is, of course, also the social context, that is the societal expectation of the *female* within society. In my mother's time women were made to feel outside the cut and thrust of life. Even linguistically, in English, and dare I say in other languages, being female suggests something 'applied': FeMALE, WoMAN, LADy, mADAM, MATErnal, MENoPAUSE. The use of language, as we know, influences our concepts and vice versa. This 'applied' status starts with the Bible and goes on; and I have approached the subject in some of my works, including, of course, those that evoke biblical figures.

Perhaps standing, in general, outside 'the cut and thrust' may explain why women's achievements do not so readily get recognised. It is as though they aren't important in HIStory – as though history was itself a sort of phallocentric shadow figure. Outside the family saga, I think a part of my determination to succeed is an act of solidarity on behalf of my fellow females.

My mother certainly felt oppressed by the expectations of society – I remember her saying to me: 'It's not about us, Jane'. By 'us' she clearly meant women in

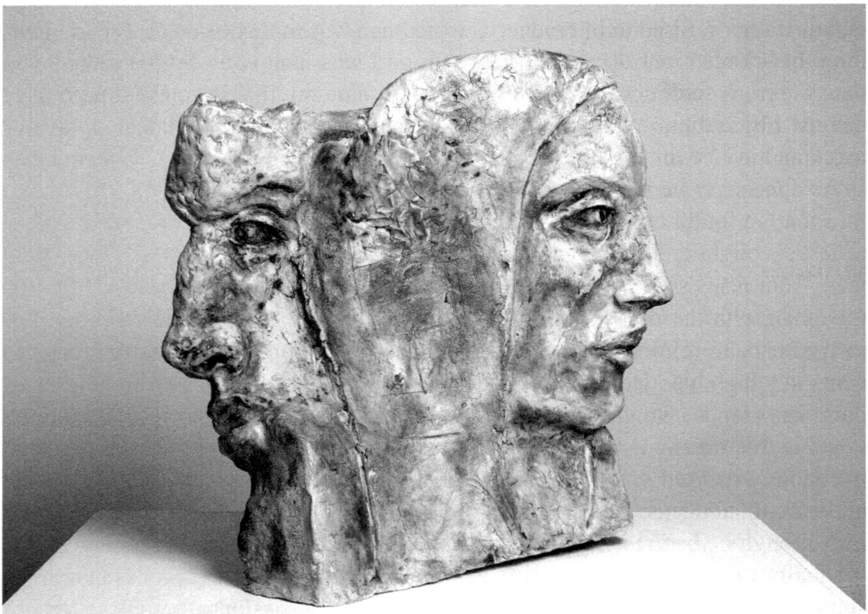

Figure 14.13 mm & mm, 2009, painted stoneware, 54 cm H × 55 cm W × 12 cm D

general – women in the world of men's things. When I think about it, of course, she was quite right and very aware for her time. She talked of medicine as a body of knowledge based on men and then applied to woman's bodies and so forth. Her statement 'It's not about us' I found infuriating, but I think that, on some level, it freed me from thinking that, as a woman, I had to compete. If 'it's not about us' means that we are not taken notice of, then on the positive side, this statement is completely liberating because you cannot fail if you are noticed. Put another way: if female success does not seem to be valued in society, the path to success is made clearer. A greater freedom (despite this or because of it) is afforded to woman. It matters less to society whether you succeed or fail so the pressure is off! Does the pressure cause men to suffer more from being in the shadow of their fathers?

Father

Moving on to *my* father, I must declare that – SHADOWS are multifold in my paternal family – Sigmund, Lucian, Clement and the list goes on. My favourite story, as mentioned earlier, is about Rodin and Brancusi, two important and inspired sculptors of the past. As for Brancusi's response to Rodin, I think about how this was not true for Lucian. He certainly flourished under the shadow of the great tree of Sigmund. Lucian succeeded his legendary grandfather *and* with so much of Sigmund in the mix! They certainly both analysed people on a couch without saying how long it might take. I see my father's success while under the shadow of Sigmund not only as an example but more – as an instruction.

My father was absent for much of my early childhood, but his exhibition catalogues and his powerful, silent presence lingered. I felt his absence as a type of *absent presence*. Not that he was *never* there – he was in fact present, but in an *in-and-out* sort of a way. With his studio virtually opposite our home, he was certainly often 'indoors with us'.

Still, exceedingly driven, my father's focus was on his work and he had time for little else. In fact, he fits Danielle Knafo's model of the genius about whom Knafo writes "the working demands of the 'genius' may be so all-consuming, or at least be experienced as such that often little time whatsoever is left for their children and their emotional growth".[4]

While regretting his absences, I was all the more delighted to have re-connected with him privately (through my sister Bella) on my return from completing my sculpture scholarship in Rome in 1989. Indeed there was an eight-month period in 1990 when we sat for one another making sculptures. I found it exciting, challenging and revealing. He would often ask me about my art – inviting me to bring images of my works from Rome in to show him; and when I did he was totally engaged with it – facially animated when he liked something and annoyed if I interrupted his 'looking'. I remember a work I gave him at the time, a medal I made in Rome that featured a zebra. I called it *Moments and Memories*. Interestingly this work, was titled in an almost prescient way quite some time before our reunion.

Since my father's death in 2011, I recognise that both the image of my father and the theme of *Shadows* has become more clearly a part of my making process and also my conceptual process. Sculpture involves objects and materials, which invariably throw shadows. Sculpture can be differentiated from painting in this way, as a painting is in fact a flat surface, an illusory device. Painting doesn't employ the physical use of objects, which throw actual shadows. Instead painting involves the illusion of those objects (via rendering them on a flat surface). There is something similar about painting and sculpture and at the same time something very different.

Around the time of my father's illness I made the work *Us*.

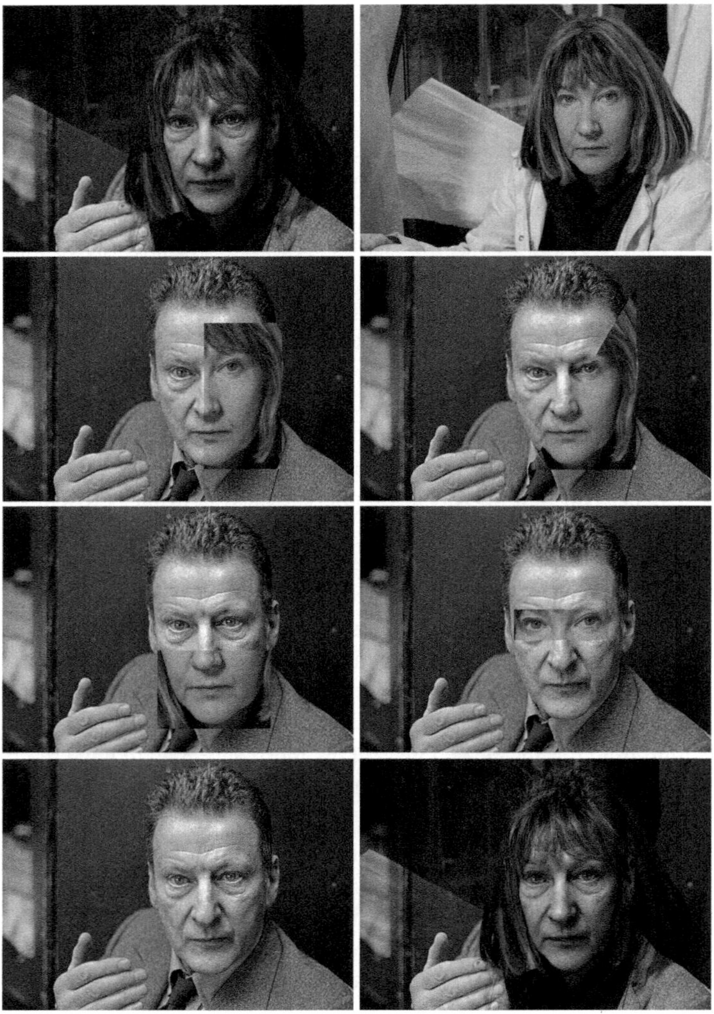

Figure 14.14 *Us*, 2011, photo, 86 cm H × 63 cm W

I suppose this was a way of uniting us, at least in an image form. Conversely, it could of course, be seen as me appropriating my father's persona – as in the work by Marcel Duchamp called *L.H.O.O.Q*, where Duchamp appropriates Leonardo Da Vinci's *Mona Lisa* for himself. After all, I share both my father and my great-grandfather, and my work is a way of coveting them, having them for myself. Their public and private faces have the same features, yet the face has public ownership. There was a point in my childhood when I realised I shared my father Lucian Freud, as Lucian did with his grandfather Sigmund Freud. Fathers, dead or alive, are your finest motivator and best oppressor and so, making works in that context, I am clearly driven by my internal environment as much as external stimuli.

Interestingly, while my father was alive I worked a lot with object-based sculptures that physically create shadows, and when he died I immediately made a large two-part installation, one half of which represented the broken parts of a shadow, and I lay it down on the floor. I put it down. The thing I had symbolically picked up in the work *Us* (his image), I metaphorically put down in the work *Shadow*. Or did I throw it down (it was in pieces) as a reference to my inner world exhibiting that *I* was in pieces?

Lucian himself spent his early adult life under a dual shadow. My father was not only in the shadow of his grandfather Sigmund, but also of his younger brother Clement, which must have infuriated him, as they never did get on well. Clement

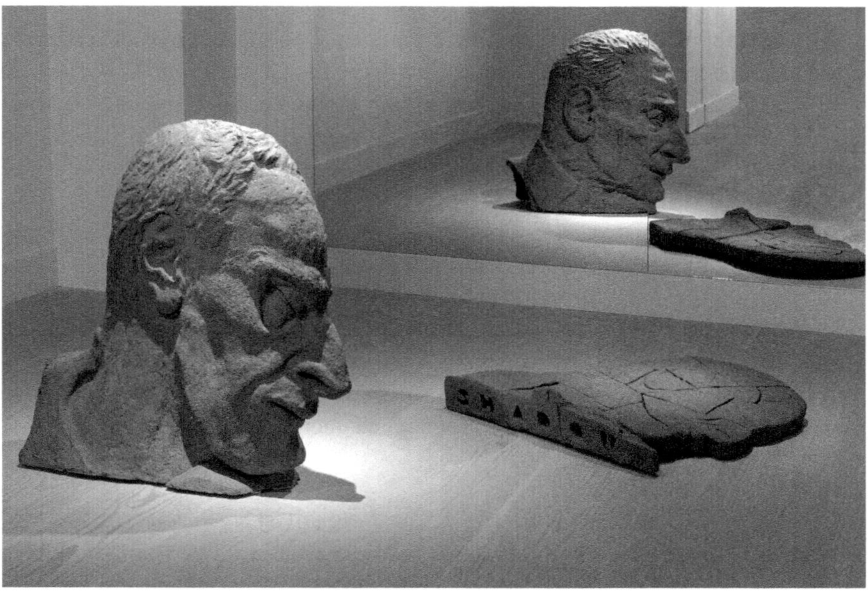

Figure 14.15 *Earthstone Triptych* and *Shadow*, terracotta, 2011, 88 cm H × 88 cm W × 38 cm D, 88 cm H × 88 cm W × 20 cm D

overshadowed Lucian during his early adulthood and during my childhood. He was a member of Parliament, an author and television chef, who featured regularly on television and radio. He was a household name, in fact something of a celebrity.

As for my father, I watched his rise through the media, seeing him supersede Clement by becoming better known and respected. This was another instruction that entered my psyche from afar. Things change. People evolve in their own time.

Grandmother

This account would not be complete without the mention of my grandparents, particularly my paternal grandmother, Lucie, who played such an important role in my early life. She was the discipline, the rational figure who gave me strong reigns through her clear instructions. This led me to do what I always wanted to do: to be making sculpture *freely*; and in turn to be unexpectedly freed by the self-same process. In considering this close early relationship to my paternal grandmother, Lucie Freud, I muse on the fact that this was the same mothering experienced that my father had. (After all, my father, Lucian Freud, was quite clear about what he wanted to do from the outset, his own shadowing by Sigmund notwithstanding.)

My paternal grandparents were quite formal and conservative – with their Viennese whirls and their Austrian ways. I loved this sense of belonging and in the only place where my taught knowledge about the world fitted with my actual experience of it. Sometimes I think in marrying my adored husband, who is also quite formal and very rational, I need to thank Ernst and Lucie for showing me what a good relationship is like.

My paternal grandparents had quite an influence on me and introduced me to Sigmund's theories indirectly though their work in translating *Freud's Diaries – In Words and Pictures*. They edited this work during the period of my early schooling. My father may have resented his mother's intrusiveness, but I relished the attention! Having both sets of grandparents ever-present gave me the sense of identity I needed early on.

Although we spent much time with my mother's sister and some with my maternal grandparents these relationship became more distant as the years went by. Following the death of my maternal grandfather, my residing memory of my grandmother, by then, more reclusive, was her retort 'NO VISITORS TODAY JANE' from the little doorway opening onto her London flat. She was quite distant in her way. Interesting for me that in choosing my father, my mother also chose a distant partner, echoing her mother's character. A familiar trait.

Conclusion

The above, I hope, goes some way towards an explanation as to why I feel I have escaped, to a certain extent, the suffering that may generally go hand-in-hand with having famous antecedents, which have so commonly overshadowed the creative flow of their progeny, particularly when working in the same field.

Ars longa, vita brevis is the motto inscribed on entry to the art department at the famous public school *Harrow*, where I recently (July 2017) completed a two-year artist residency. In art, the judgements as to whether one's work has contributed or not – come after one's demise, so in that way – are none of our business. One can live *and* die in hope! – the hope of measuring up against the father(s) in death at least, if not in life.

On one occasion, while speaking to my father about art, he described the art object as something that people liked and valued so it didn't get thrown away. In that way it lasts and outlives us. This seems to be a strange equalling of the inanimate and the animate, the object and the offspring. After all, our children outlive us and are a creation too.

There is something totemic about the hugely successful. My father, with his primal performance was more 'totem' figure than father figure. However in hindsight I think he served me well, if not as a role model, definitely as a totem. Perhaps, just as it was in the distant past, "the totem – can be not only the progenitor of the family, but also the genius to protect".[5]

I have looked at how potential blocks have been rendered impotent, leaving me feeling that I can *go on* in Beckett's simple yet wonderful words: "You must go on. I can't go on. I'll go on" This, given all those factors that could conspire against the probability of feeling that my efforts are fruitful. I conclude by again echoing Jonathan Burke – "succeeding *a hard act to follow* is all about the manner in which the transmission itself is experienced".

Notes

1 Artist in Residence, Freud Museum January 2005–September 2006. Working with Freud's antiquities.
2 Freud, S. (1900) *Die Traumdeutung*. Leipzig & Vienna (translated by James Strachey: The Interpretation of Dreams, Macmillan, 1913). www.freudfile.org/childhood.html.
3 Freud, S. (1900) *Die Traumdeutung*. Leipzig & Vienna (translated by James Strachey: The Interpretation of Dreams, Macmillan, 1913). www.freudfile.org/childhood.html.
4 Danielle Knafo in Danielle Knafo: *Dancing with the Unconscious: The Art of Psychoanalysis and the Psychoanalysis of Art*.
5 Author quotes the words by Claudio Costa from Costa's artists book called *Totem and Taboo* created in 1988. This book was made as Costa's artist's interpretation of Freud's work Totem and Taboo. Costa illustrated and wrote accompanying notes in his book of the same name. Costa (1942–1995) was an important Italian contemporary artist.

References

Beckett, S. (2010). *The Unnameable*, Series: The Trilogy #3. London: Faber and Faber (final 3 lines) You must go on. I can't go on. I'll go on

Freud, S. (1900) *Die Traumdeutung*, Leipzig & Vienna (translated by James Strachey: The Interpretation of Dreams, Macmillan, 1913)

Jung, C. G. (1940) *Collected Works, Vol. 11: Psychology and Religion: West and East* (translated by Adler, G. and Hull, R.F.C.). Princeton: Princeton University Press, 1969.

Knafo, D. (2012). *Dancing with the Unconscious: The Art of Psychoanalysis and the Psychoanalysis of Art*, Psychoanalysis in a New Key Book Series, Vol. 14. New York: Routledge.

Index

Note: Page numbers in italics indicate figures on the corresponding pages.

Abraham, Karl 95–96, 99
Abraham (from Genesis) 11–12, 18
Acropolis 79–81
Adler, Alfred 159
Admetus 37
Aegisthus 27, 28–29
affect 64
After Bacon 230
Agamemnon 23, 27, 33
Agamemnon (play by Aeschylus) 29–30
Akedah 11, 12–17
Albany, Duke of (from *King Lear)* 50
Alkestis 37
Amphion 39n32
anomie 121
Apollo 27, 39n30, 39n32
Are you ready for me now? 230
art 62; and genocides 219–220; *see also* sculptures; theatre
Artemis 27, 33, 38n11, 39n32
artists 209
Ataturk, Mustafa Kemal 146
Athena 30
Athens 77, 78–79
Atreus 27, 33, 40n43
attributions 165–166
Auschwitz 118–119
authoritarianism 171–172
avoidant strategies 186–187

Bacon, Francis 225
Bastiaans, Jan 137
blindness 12–15
Blue, Lionel 206
Book of Deuteronomy 2
Brancusi, Constantin 225
Brazil 65–66
British Secret Service 116
Bronstein, Lev Davidovich *see* Trotsky, Leon
Büyükada 147–148

Cassandra (prophetess) 27, 33
castration anxiety 85
Cavell, Benjamin 188
Cavell, Stanley 179–180; and knowing others 183–188; and love 188–191; relationship with father 180–182; and scepticism 183–185
child analysis 96–97
children of perpetrators 109–114; and acceptance 116–118; and evil 123–124; and guilt 118–123; and idealisation 114–115; and repudiation 115–116; types of 114
Children's Memorial Museum, The see Yad LaYeled
Chrysothemis 34, 36
Churchill, Winston 150
Clytemnestra 27–30, 34, 38n14
colonialism 65–66
compassion 16–18
concentration camps 112, 118–119, 214, 222n1
Cordelia (from *King Lear*): death of 45, 55–56; maturity of 54; and nothing 50–51, 54; and prayers 51–52; silence of 43–44, 45–50
Costa, Claudio 241n5
critical hermeneutics 44

Davies, Oliver Ford 1, 3n1
Day-Lewis, Daniel 1, 3n1
Decoration of the Rim 228
déjà vu 81
depersonalisation 81
derealisation 86
derealization 76, 78, 81
Der Vater 115
dharma 174n5
diasporic communities 10
Ding Dong 224
Dionysus 32, 39n30
disillusionment 47
'disturbance of memory' 76, 81
doctors 196; as fathers 61–62
Dolan, Xavier 168
doubt 181–183
drugs 58, 61, 67
Duchamp, Marcel 239
duty 110, 112

Earthstone Triptych 239
Eastman, Max 159n2
Edgar (from *King Lear*) 50
Eitingon, Max 97
Elektra 23; and Agamemnon 33; characterization of 28–29; death of 36–37; and grief 30–32
Elektra complex 29, 38n19
Elektra (opera) 23, 25
Elektra (play by Euripides) 28–29
Elektra (play by Hofmannsthal) 30–37; staging of 39n26
Elektra (play by Sophocles) 28
empathy 16–17
envy 99, 166
Esau (from Genesis) 13
evil 106–107, 123–124, 125n9

fascism 172
Federn, Paul 85
Feigenbaum, Dorian 85
femininity 60
Ferenczi, Sandor 94, 95
Foreshortened 231
Frank, Hans 114, 115, 119
Frank, Niklas 114, 118, 119; and evil 123–124
Frazer, James 198–199
Freiberg 90n1
Freud, Amalia 88–90
Freud, Anna 84, 97, 101
Freud, Clement 239–240
Freud, Jacob 88–90
Freud, Jane McAdam: and art 223–226, 240–241; childhood of 226–227; father of 237–240; and gender 235–236; grandmother of 240; mother of 233–235, 236–237; and sculptures 227–233
Freud, Lucian 239
Freud, Lucie 240
Freud, Sigmund 2; and the Acropolis 79–81; and Anna Freud 84; and the Bible 10; and death 47–49; and favorite children 233; and his parents 88–90; and Jane McAdam Freud 223–224, 232; and Lucian Freud 239; and mediums 25; and Nazis 101; and necessity 46; and Oedipal experiences 81–84, 87; and Romain Rolland 76, 78–79; and writers 38n21
Freud Study Merge-Desk 232

gender 235–237
Genesis 11
genocides 215, 219
Glasser, David 211
Gloucester, Earl of (from *King Lear*) 55
Glover, Edward 98–99, 103
gods 32–33
Goering, Bettina 116
Goering, Hermann 116
Golden Bough, The 198–199
gratitude 165
Greek drama 25–29
guilt 118–123

Haddad, Amir 59
Hagar (from Genesis) 12
Halter, Aloma 214–215
Halter, Ardyn 211; as an artist 218, 220–222; childhood of 213, 215–216; and the Holocaust 217–218
Halter, Roman: as an artist 211, 212–213, 220–222; and the arts 213, 219; and the Holocaust 212, 213–216
Halter, Susan (Nador) 217
Hamlet 1, 29
Hamlet 26, 65, 189
headaches 110–111
Hess, Rudolf 116
Hess, Wolf-Rudiger 116
Hidden Light 226
Himmler, Gudrun 116

Himmler, Heinrich 116, 117–118
Himmler, Katrin 117–118
Hippocrates 60, 61–62
Hoess, Ingebirgitt 112, 116, 117
Hoess, Rainer 115
Hoess, Rudolf 112, 115
Hoffman, Eva 105–106
Hofmannsthal, Hugo von 23; and *Elektra* 30–37; and Greek drama 25–30
Holocaust 105–106, 113–114, 125n6, 127; and Alice Miller 130–131; and the arts 217–218; lessons from 219; and Roman Halter 212, 213–214
homosexuality 169–170
Horney, Karen 95
Hotel and Spa of Madness 59

Iago 52
idealisation 115
identities 9–11
illiteracy 119–120
immunology 64
improvisation 64
Inquisition 66
Iphianassa 33, 39n29
Iphigenia 27, 38n11
Isaac (from Genesis): binding of 11; blindness of 12–15; and love 14–16; and masculinity 16–19; sacrifice of 11–12
Ishmael (from Genesis) 12
It's Only the End of the World 168

Jacob (from Genesis) 13
Jacobs, Louis 207n1
Jewish identity 9–10, 132; and the Bible 16
Jews: and Louis Jacobs affair 198, 207n1; and uncleanness 169–170; *see also* Holocaust; rabbis
Joffe, Adolf 159
Joseph (from Genesis) 10
joy 67
Jung, Carl 63, 225

Kafka, Franz 161–162; and homosexuality 170; relationship with father 162–165, 167, 174; work of 171
Kafka, Hermann: and homosexuality 170; relationship with son 162–165, 167, 174; and 'withoutness' 167
Keats, John 199
Kent, Earl of (from *King Lear*) 50
Kertesz, Imre 121
King Lear 3n1; and death 56; ending of 55–56; Freud's interpretation of 46–49; interpretations of 43–45; and love 53–54; and prayers 51–53, 56; and scepticism 190–191; and silence 45–46, 49–51
Klein, Arthur 94, 95
Klein, Erich 94
Klein, Hans 94, 99–100
Klein, Melanie 2, 84, 93–104
Knafo, Danielle 237
knowing 183–188
Kronfeld, Arthur 153, 159

Levi, Primo 118–119, 172
love 53–54, 188–190; and Isaac (from Genesis) 14–16; redemptive 44–45
Lumet, Sidney 195
Lvovna, Alexandra 149–150, 155
Lvovna, Nina *see* Nevelson, Nina (Lvovna)
Lvovna, Zinaida *see* Volkova, Zinaida (Zina) (Lvovna)

manic depression 100
masculinity: and destruction 61; and homosexuality 170–171; and Isaac (from Genesis) 16–19; unheroic 14
masks 59, 68
matriarchy 65
mediums 25
mental illnesses 60; *see also* psychiatric patients
Midrash 19n2
Miller, Alice: career of 135–136, 138–141; celebrity of 136–138; and Holocaust 129–131; as a mother 131–134
Miller, Andreas: career of 135; as father 131–135; and Holocaust 130–131
Miller, Martin 127; childhood of 131–134; as psychotherapist 137–141; schooling of 134–136
mm & mm 236
Molinier, Jeanne *147,* 153, 154
Molinier, Raymond 153
moral order 121
mother figures 48
Mother Mould 234
mothers 82
My Nazi Legacy 114
myths, ancestral 9–10

Nador, Susan *see* Halter, Susan (Nador)
narcissistic injury 116–117
National Genocide Memorial 219–220
Nazis 125n5; children of 112–117; and the Holocaust 129–131; and Jewish persecution 132–133; precursors to 172
necessity 46–47
'Negative Capability' 199
Nervi, Mauro 162, 174n2
Network 195
Nevelson, Nina (Lvovna) 149–150
nightmares 108, 111
Niobe 39n32
Nise da Silveira Institute 60
nothing 50–51

object loss 85–86
'oceanic feelings' 78–79
Oedipal experiences 81–84, 90; and rivalry 167; and Zinaida Volkova 158
Oedipus Rex 26
Olivier, Laurence 3n1
Oresteia 27–28
Orestes 27–29; characterization of 40n43; and Elektra 35
Othello 189

parthenogenesis 83, 84
Pasha, Izzet 148
patriarchy 29–30; and mental illness 60
Payne, Sylvia 102–103
Pelham, Gayna 209
'Permanent Revolution' 146
perpetrators 105–107; children of 109–114; families of 125n4, 125n7; Nazi 108–109, 112, 125n5
personal narrative 128
Pfemfert, Franz 153, 154
phallic awe 91n5
Picasso 229
Picasso, Pablo 218
possibility 50–51
poverty 65
prayers 51–52
professions 200
projections 138; parental 171; of uncleanness 169–170
prototypes 9
psychiatric patients 62–63; *see also* mental illnesses
psychosomatic symptoms 196, 198

rabbis 201–207
racism 215
rams 12
rationality 62
Reader, The 119–120, 121–122, 125n8
reassurance 101
Rebecca (from Genesis) 13–15
religious mythology 198–199, 202–203
restorative hermeneutics 44
resurrections 19
Richard III 3n1, 25
Rim as Motif 229
Rio de Janeiro 59
Riviere, Joan 96, 99
Rodin, Auguste 225
Roethke, Theodore 196
Rolland, Romain 76, 78–79
Rome 76–78
Rumble, Young Man, Rumble 188
Russell, Bertand 180
Russia 145–146, 159
Rwanda 219

Salome 37
Sands, Phillipe 114–115
Sarah (from Genesis) 11–12, 14–15, 17
scepticism 183–185, 188–191
Schlink, Bernhard 113, 119–120, 125n7
Schmideberg, Melitta 93–94, 104
Schmideberg, Walter 97–98, 101
screen memory 82
sculptures 227–233, 238
Second Coming, The 173
Sedov, Lyova 145, 153–154, 155; and studies 160n7; and teaching 160n4
Sedova, Natalia *see* Trotsky, Natalia (Sedova)
Senin, Adolf *147*
separation 90, 91n4
sexual relationships 205–206
Shadow 239
shadow sides 225–226
shame 118–119, 121–122
Sharpe, Ella 98, 103
Shoah see Holocaust
silence 47–50; and love 49–50; and perpetrators 112–113; and relating 196–197
Silveira, Nise da 59, 63, 64
Sobolevicius, Abraham *see* Senin, Adolf
Sobolevicius, Ruvin *see* Well, Roman
social organizations 171–172

Solar Gods 61
speechlessness *see* silence
Spinoza, Baruch 64, 67
Stalin, Joseph 146–147, 148, 159n1
sterilisation 116
Stettbacher, Konrad 139–141, 142n2
St John's Wood Synagogue 221–222
Stockholm syndrome 131
Stone Speak 227
Strachey, Alix 96
Strachey, James 96
Strauss, Richard 23
sublimation 228
sublime 87
success 224–225
swimming 217

teaching 205–206
Terra, Reginaldo 67–68
theatre 58–60; and change 65; as cure 63–64; and improvisation 64; and mental health 66, 68; *see also* art
Thyestes 27
tragedies 49, 106
traumas 106
Trial, The 161
Trotsky, Leon 2; exile of 145–149; relationship with daughter 149–153, 155–159
Trotsky, Natalia (Sedova) 145, 152
Trump, Donald 61, 162
Turkey 146

uncanny 86–87
Us 238

vampires 61
vaudeville 23–24
Vaz, Nelson 64
violence 11–12
Volkov, Platon 150
Volkov, Seva 154
Volkova, Zinaida (Zina) (Lvovna) *147,* 149–151, 160n5; death of 153–155; relationship with father 151–153, 157–159

Wächter, Horst von 114–115
Wächter, Otto von 114–115
Weber, Sara 151
Well, Roman *147*
Welles, Orson 161
Wilde, Oscar 37
Winter's Tale, The 189
witches 60
'withoutness' 166–167
World War II 129; *see also* Holocaust

Yad LaYeled 215
Yeats, William Butler 172–173

For Product Safety Concerns and Information please contact our EU representative GPSR@taylorandfrancis.com Taylor & Francis Verlag GmbH, Kaufingerstraße 24, 80331 München, Germany

Batch number: 10726493

Printed by Printforce, the Netherlands